Anesthesia for The High

Risk

Anesthesia for The High Risk Patient

Second Edition

Edited by

Ian McConachie MB FRCA FRCPC
Associate Professor of Anesthesia and Perioperative Medicine
University of Western Ontario

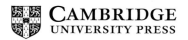

CAMBRIDGE UNIVERSITY PRESS
Cambridge, New York, Melbourne, Madrid, Cape Town, Singapore, São Paulo,
Delhi, Dubai, Tokyo

Cambridge University Press
The Edinburgh Building, Cambridge CB2 8RU, UK

Published in the United States of America by Cambridge University Press, New York

www.cambridge.org
Information on this title: www.cambridge.org/9780521710183

First published 2002
Second edition 2009
Reprinted 2010

Printed in the United Kingdom at the University Press, Cambridge

A catalog record for this publication is available from the British Library

Library of Congress Cataloging in Publication data
Anesthesia for the high risk patient : anesthesia and perioperative care / edited by Ian McConachie. – 2nd ed.
    p. ; cm.
Rev. ed. of: Anaesthesia for the high risk patient / edited by Ian McConachie. 2002.
Includes bibliographical references and index.
ISBN 978-0-521-71018-3 (hardback)
1. Anesthesia – Handbooks, manuals, etc. 2. Anesthesia – Complications – Handbooks, manuals, etc.
3. Geriatric anesthesia – Handbooks, manuals, etc. I. McConachie, Ian. II. Anaesthesia for the high risk
patient. III. Title.
[DNLM: 1. Anesthesia – adverse effects – Handbooks. 2. Perioperative Care – Handbooks. 3. Risk
Factors – Handbooks. WO 231 A5325 2009]
RD82.2.A535 2009
617.9′6–dc22
                                                                                              2008045116

ISBN 978-0-521-71018-3 paperback

Cambridge University Press has no responsibility for
the persistence or accuracy of URLs for external or
third-party internet websites referred to in this publication,
and does not guarantee that any content on such
websites is, or will remain, accurate or appropriate.

Contents

Foreword

The current practice of anesthesia is characterized by advanced age and increased co-morbidity in high-risk patients for an ever-growing spectrum of surgical interventions. Thus, clinical anesthesia practice has become much broader and more complex than just the provision of intraoperative anesthesia, now encompassing perioperative medicine. Anesthesia techniques have developed with preoperative admission screening, modern anesthetic agents and regional anesthesia procedures, postoperative pain and fast-track recovery management. These, and advances in perioperative monitoring, all contribute towards improving care of the high-risk patient.

This concise and practical book edited by Dr. Ian McConachie is updated from the first edition and provides a useful guide to the anesthesia management of high-risk adult patients undergoing elective and emergency surgery. This book provides a succinct, problem-oriented source of practical information based on current literature and the experience of senior clinicians. The outstanding contributors selected by Dr. McConachie from both sides of the Atlantic have presented a full spectrum of preoperative, intraoperative and postoperative management of high-risk surgical patients undergoing anesthesia care.

All practitioners are likely to benefit from refreshing their knowledge of the principles and approaches presented in these chapters with the goal of improving the care of high-risk surgical patients.

Davy Cheng, MD, MSc, FRCPC, FCAHS
Professor & Chair/Chief
Department of Anesthesia & Perioperative Medicine
London Health Sciences Centre and St. Joseph's Health Care London
University of Western Ontario
London, Ontario
Canada

Preface to the second edition

This text:

- Is aimed primarily at trainees in Anesthesia, although more experienced practitioners may find it useful as a refresher in recent concepts and advances. A basic knowledge of physiology, pharmacology and anesthesia is assumed.
- May be a useful "aide memoire" for postgraduate examinations in anesthesia.
- Exclusively discusses adult anesthesia. Pediatric and neonatal anesthesia is outside the scope of this text.
- Aims to provide practical information on the management of high-risk patients presenting for surgery, as well as sufficient background information to enable understanding of the principles and rationale behind their anesthetic and perioperative management. We hope it will prove useful, but we would emphasize that this, or any other book, is no substitute for experienced supervision, support and training.
- Is not a substitute for the major anesthetic texts, but concentrates on principles of management of the most challenging anesthetic cases.
- Aims to provide guidance to help manage these patients in the perioperative period in line with modern concepts of critical care, and the potential role of the anesthetist as perioperative physician.
- Emphasizes cardiovascular risk, cardiac disease and cardiac management, as these are undoubtedly the most important aspects of perioperative anesthetic risk.
- The choice of topics is selective, but should appeal and be useful to the majority of practitioners. Important information not readily available in similar texts is also included.
- The format is designed to provide easy access to information presented in a concise manner. We have tried to eliminate all superfluous material. Selected important or controversial references are presented as well as suggestions for further reading. The style of the chapters varies. This is deliberate. Some relate more to basic principles, physiology, pharmacology, etc. – bookwork. Others are more practical in nature, discussing the principles of anesthetic techniques for certain high-risk situations.
- The authors are all experienced practitioners working with a high proportion of sick, elderly patients presenting for both elective and emergency surgery. The authors are committed to providing a high level of perioperative care of patients undergoing anesthesia. We make no apologies for repetition of important principles and facts – a second perspective on a subject is often useful.
- The editor has enlisted contributors active in both practice and training from institutions on both sides of the Atlantic. The aim has therefore been to produce a text of international relevance.

- One aim has been to discuss high-risk situations and patients presenting to the generalist. Therefore specialist neurosurgical and cardiothoracic anesthetic chapters have not been included.

- The second edition builds on the success of the first and contains several new chapters as well as revisions of older chapters – all have been completely rewritten.

- By way of disclosure, many drugs discussed in this text and many trials reported and discussed involve use of drugs in "off-label" situations. Use of drugs in such situations is at the discretion of individual physicians after full evaluation of the circumstances at that time. Similarly, dosages presented in this text represent dosages commonly found in the literature, but physicians should always seek guidance from appropriate pharmaceutical literature.

Ian McConachie MB FRCA FRCPC
Associate Professor
Department of Anesthesia & Perioperative Medicine
University of Western Ontario
St. Joseph's Health Care London
London
Ontario, Canada

Contributors

A. Adams MBChB BSc FRCS FRCA
Department of Anaesthesia, Lancashire
Teaching Hospitals NHS Foundation
Trust, Preston, UK

S. Balasubramanian MB FRCA
Department of Anaesthesia and Intensive
Care, University Hospitals, Coventry and
Warwickshire, UK

D. Cheng MD MSc FRCPC FCAHS
Department of Anesthesia and
Perioperative Medicine, University of
Western Ontario, London Health Sciences
Centre & St Joseph's Health Care, London,
Ontario, Canada

C. Clarke MD
Department of Anesthesia and
Perioperative Medicine, University of
Western Ontario, London Health Sciences
Centre & St Joseph's Health Care, London,
Ontario, Canada

J. Cupitt MB FRCA
Department of Anaesthesia and Intensive
Care, Blackpool Victoria Hospital,
Blackpool, UK

**M. Cutts MB ChB BSc (Hons) Physiology
MRCP FRCA**
Department of Anaesthesia and Intensive
Care, Stockport NHS Foundation Trust,
Stockport, UK

P. Dean MB FRCA
Department of Anaesthesia and Intensive
Care, Blackpool Victoria Hospital,
Blackpool, UK

S. Dhir MD
Department of Anesthesia and
Perioperative Medicine, University of
Western Ontario, London Health Sciences
Centre & St Joseph's Health Care, London,
Ontario, Canada

C. Dunkley MB FRCA
Department of Anaesthesia and Intensive
Care, Blackpool Victoria Hospital,
Blackpool, UK

G. Evans MD
Department of Anesthesia and
Perioperative Medicine, University of
Western Ontario, London Health Sciences
Centre & St Joseph's Health Care, London,
Ontario, Canada

J. Granton MD FRCPC
Department of Anesthesia and
Perioperative Medicine, University of
Western Ontario, London Health Sciences
Centre & St Joseph's Health Care, London,
Ontario, Canada

C. Harle MBChB FRCA
Department of Anesthesia and
Perioperative Medicine, University of
Western Ontario, London Health Sciences
Centre & St Joseph's Health Care, London,
Ontario, Canada

P. S. Hegde MB MD FRCA
Department of Anaesthesia, University
Hospital of Wales, Cardiff, Wales

N. Imasogie MB FRCA
Department of Anesthesia and
Perioperative Medicine, University of
Western Ontario, London Health Sciences
Centre & St Joseph's Health Care, London,
Ontario, Canada

P. Jones MD FRCPC
Department of Anesthesia and
Perioperative Medicine, University of
Western Ontario, London Health Sciences
Centre & St Joseph's Health Care, London,
Ontario, Canada

R. Kishen MB FRCA
Department of Anaesthesia and Intensive
Care, Hope Hospital, Salford, UK

I. McConachie MB FRCPC FRCA
Department of Anesthesia and
Perioperative Medicine, University of
Western Ontario, London Health Sciences
Centre & St Joseph's Health Care, London,
Ontario, Canada

N. Moreland MB BS MRCS FRCA
Department of Anaesthesia and Intensive
Care, Royal Preston Hospital, Preston, UK

P. Morley-Forster MD FRCPC
Department of Anesthesia and
Perioperative Medicine, University of
Western Ontario, London Health Sciences
Centre & St Joseph's Health Care, London,
Ontario, Canada

C. Railton BSc MD PhD FRCPC
Department of Anesthesia and
Perioperative Medicine, University of
Western Ontario, London Health Sciences
Centre & St Joseph's Health Care, London,
Ontario, Canada

Dominic Sebastian MB, FFARCSI
Department of Anaesthesia and Intensive
Care, Royal Blackburn Hospital, Blackburn,
UK

R. Sharma MBBS MD FRCA
Department of Anaesthesia and Intensive
Care, Royal Albert Edward Infirmary,
Wigan, UK

T. Turkstra MD M Eng P Eng FRCPC
Department of Anesthesia and
Perioperative Medicine, University of
Western Ontario, London Health Sciences
Centre & St Joseph's Health Care, London,
Ontario, Canada

S. Vaughan MB MRCP FRCA
Department of Anaesthesia and Intensive
Care, Blackpool Victoria Hospital,
Blackpool, UK

Abbreviations

AAA	abdominal aortic aneurysm
AAGBI	Association of Anaesthetists of Great Britain and Ireland
ABW	actual body weight
ACC	American College of Cardiologists
ACE	angiotensin-converting enzyme
ACS	acute coronary syndrome
ADH	anti-diuretic hormone
ADQI	acute dialysis quality initiative
AHA	American Heart Association
AIMS	Anaesthetic Incident Monitoring Study
AKI	acute kidney injury
AMPA	α-amino-3-hydroxy-5-methyl-4-isoxazolepropionic acid
ANF	atrial naturetic factor
APACHE	acute physiology and chronic health evaluation
APS	acute pain service
ARA	angiotensin receptor antagonist
ARB	angiotensin receptor blocking
ARF	acute renal failure
ASA	American Society of Anesthesiologists
ATN	acute tubular necrosis
AV	arteriovenous
AWS	alcohol withdrawal syndrome
BIPAP	bilevel positive airway pressure
BMS	bare metal stents
BNP	brain natriuretic peptide
BPI	bactericidal permeability increasing (protein)
BRAN	(Benefits, Risks, Alternatives, Nothing)
BUN	blood urea nitrogen
CABG	coronary artery bypass grafting
CaCB	calcium channel blockers
CAD	coronary artery disease
CBF	cerebral blood flow
CCF	Congestive Cardiac Failure
CEPOD	Confidential Enquiry into Peri Operative Deaths
CHF	congestive heart failure
CIN	contrast-induced nephropathy
CNA	central neuraxial analgesia
CNST	Clinical Negligence Scheme for Trusts
CO	cardiac ouput
COPD	chronic obstructive pulmonary disease
CPAP	continuous positive airway pressure
CPB	cardiopulmonary bypass
CPK	creatine phosphokinase

CPX	cardiopulmonary exercise
CRRT	continuous renal replacement therapy
CV	closing volume
CVP	central venous pressure
DCLB	diasprin cross-linked hemoglobin
DDAVP	1-deamino-8-D-arginine vasopressin
DES	drug-eluting stents
DIC	disseminated intravascular coagulation
DM	diabetes mellitus
DNAR	do not attempt resuscitation
EA	epidural analgesia
eGFR	estimated glomerular filtration rate
EPO	erythropoietin
ERV	expiratory reserve volume
EWS	early warning score
FDP	fibrin degradation products
FEV	forced expiratory volume
FFP	fresh, frozen plasma
FRC	functional residual capacity
FVC	forced vital capacity
GA	general anesthesia
GFR	glomerular filtration rate
Hb	hemoglobin
Hct	hematocrit
HDU	high-dependency unit
IABP	intra-aortic balloon pump
IBW	ideal body weight
ICD	implantable cardioverter-defibrillators
ICP	intracranial pressure
ICU	intensive care unit
IHD	Ischemic Heart Disease
ISB	interscalene block
ITP	intrathoracic pressure
IVRA	intravenous regional analgesia
IYDT	if you don't treat
KIM1	kidney injury molecule 1
LA	local anesthetic
LV	left ventricular
LVEDP	left ventricular end diastolic pressure
MAC	mid-arm circumference
MAC	minimum alveolar concentration
MAMC	mid-arm muscle circumference
MAP	mean arterial pressure
MBT	massive blood transfusion
MDRD	modified diet in renal disease
MET	medical emergency team

MET	metabolic equivalent
MEWS	modified early warning system
MI	myocardial infarction
MMA	multi-modal analgesia
MODS	multi-organ dysfunction syndrome
mTAL	medullary thick ascending part of the loop of Henlé
MUST	malnutrition screening tool
NCCG	Non Consultant Career Grade
NCEPOD	National Confidential Enquiry into Perioperative Deaths
NDMR	nondepolarizing muscle relaxants
NG	nasogastric
NGAL	neutrophil gelatinase-associated lipocalin
NIBP	noninvasive blood pressure
NMDA	N-methyl-D-aspartate
NNH	number needed to harm
NNM	number needed to monitor
NNT	number needed to treat
NRI	nutritional risk index
NRS	numerical rating scale
NRT	nicotine replacement therapy
NYHA	New York Heart Association
OCP	oral contraceptive pill
ODC	oxyhemoglobin dissociation curve
OR	operating room
OSA	obstructive sleep apnea
PACU	postanesthetic care unit
PAFC	pulmonary artery flotation catheter
PART	patient at risk team
PCA	patient-controlled analgesia
PCEA	patient-controlled epidural analgesia
PCI	percutaneous coronary intervention
PCT	proximal convoluted tubule
PCWP	pulmonary capillary wedge pressure
PE	pulmonary embolism
PEEP	positive end expiratory pressure
PEM	protein energy malnutrition
PFT	pulmonary function test
PNS	peripheral nerve stimulator
POCD	postoperative cognitive dysfunction
POISE	Perioperative Ischemic Events Trial
PORIF	perioperative renal insufficiency and failure
POSSUM	physiological and operative severity score for the enumeration of mortality and morbidity
PPC	perioperative pulmonary complications
PPV	pulse pressure variation
PSS	physiological scoring system

PVD   Peripheral Vascular Disease
PVR   pulmonary vascular resistance
QAL   quality of life
RA   regional anesthesia
RCRI   revised cardiac risk index
RCT   randomized controlled trials
RIFLE   Risk, Injury, Failure, and outcome of Loss and End-stage
          kidney disease
ROC   Receiver Operating Characteristic
RPP   renal perfusion pressure
RRT   renal replacement therapy
RVR   renal vascular resistance
SGA   subjective global assessment
SIRS   systemic inflammatory response syndrome
SVR   systemic vascular resistance
TEA   thoracic epidural analgesia
TGF   tubulo-glomerular feedback
TRALI   transfusion-related acute lung injury
TRBF   total renal blood flow
TRICC   Transfusion Requirements in Critical Care
TSF   triple skin-fold thickness
TXA   tranexamic acid
UO   urine output
US   ultrasound
VC   vital capacity
VILI   ventilator-induced lung injury
VIP   ventilation, infusion and perfusion
VTE   venous thromboembolism
AS   aortic stenosis
AI   aortic incompetence
MS   mitral stenosis
MR   mitral regurgitation
IE   infective endocarditis
LA   left atrium
PAOP   pulmonary artery occlusion pressure
PA   pulmonary arteries
CEA   carotid artery endarterectomy
NIRS   near infrared spectroscopy
SP   stump pressure
SEP   somatosensory-evoked potential
TCD   transcranial Doppler
RBF   renal blood flow

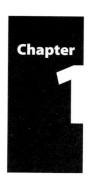

Chapter

1

Risk and risk assessment

N. Moreland and A. Adams

Risk

- Risk is a concept that denotes a potential negative impact to an asset or some characteristic of value that may arise from some present process or future event.

- Implicitly negative, risk is suggestive of potential danger or hazard and is therefore associated with discomfort and loss, and not gain or well-being.

- *Risk* is often used synonymously with the *probability* of a known loss.

- Paradoxically, a probable, or possible, loss may be uncertain and relative in an individual event, but may be much more certain over an aggregate of multiple events.

- Risk is the probability of an event occurring that will have an impact on the achievement of objectives. Risk is measured in terms of impact and likelihood.

- In 1983, the Royal Society in the UK defined *risk* as "the probability that a particular event occurs during a stated period of time or results from a particular challenge." They defined a *hazard* as a situation that could lead to harm. The chance or likelihood of this occurring is its associated *risk* [1].

- Risk is part of life whether we like it or not [2]. All medical interventions carry risks, but anesthesia is often perceived to be especially risky, although in general the risks of anesthesia are small. Risk communication, understanding and perception are fundamental to all decision-making including consent for surgical operation.

- Risk evaluation by individuals is not a purely statistical phenomenon. It is widely accepted that individuals tend to evaluate risk not solely on statistical data but on many other subjective qualitative aspects of risk. This means that the assessment and perception of risk may incorporate subconscious, subjective, personality-dependent factors and may not follow any rational or methodical pattern [3].

Identifying risk

There are numerous potential hazards and we have many ways of predicting and quantifying the risks associated with these hazards. Experience of each procedure undertaken gives us an idea of the hazards associated with it. Pooled experience within a department gives us the experience of our colleagues too, but this requires openness and a platform from which this information can be shared. Peer-reviewed journals and specialist literature, freely available now on the Internet, allow us to evaluate not only our own practice, but that of others throughout the world.

Frequently occurring adverse events are fairly straightforward to identify simply because they are common. The rarer an event occurs, the less likely it is that an individual practitioner will encounter such an event during his/her practice. Without accurate reporting these events

Anesthesia for the High Risk Patient, ed. I. McConachie. Published by Cambridge University Press.
© Cambridge University Press 2009.

may go undocumented and lead to inaccuracies in the pooled data. For a very rare event, this will cause large discrepancies in the estimated risk level for that event.

For very rare adverse events, or for procedures that are not performed regularly, it may be difficult to recruit enough patients for a study to be adequately powered to show anything meaningful. For this reason, one must be cautious in interpreting the results of many smaller studies. Multi-center co-operation is increasingly being organized to produce data from large numbers of patients that could not possibly be recruited from a single center.

An alternative method of producing some relevant conclusion from a number of smaller studies, which themselves do not show anything statistically significant, is to conduct a meta-analysis. This pools the patient numbers from smaller studies so as to give a number large enough to reach significance. One must be wary in interpreting these results, as it is often difficult to find studies that are similar enough to be comparable.

The timing of an adverse outcome will affect both our ability to identify and report it, and the way in which patients will perceive it. Immediate events are identifiable by staff caring for patients in the postoperative period, either in OR, the post-anesthesia care unit (PACU), or on the wards. Immediate adverse outcomes will also be reported by the patient themselves. Later complications may be reported less frequently by the patient especially if deemed not to be too serious. If there is a long lead-time between treatment and complication the association may go unnoticed.

Perceiving risk [4]

The timing of the event can have an effect on the way risk is perceived. Early complications, for example, often have a greater impact than those that are delayed. These tend to have a diminished perceived risk value.

The duration of an adverse event can also affect risk perception. Similarly, the ease with which something can be treated will reduce the severity of risk perceived. The possibility of postoperative pain or nausea is usually transient and easily treated, and is therefore perceived as having lower risk severity than a possible longer-term or irreversible disability.

Many studies have been done to evaluate the particular aspects thought to be relevant to the way risk is perceived, and many mental biases exist to prejudice our view [5]. These characteristics include both conscious and subconscious elements:

- magnitude,
- severity,
- vulnerability,
- controllability,
- familiarity,
- acceptability, and
- framing effect.

Risk probability or magnitude

This is usually expressed as a mathematical probability. As already mentioned, these numbers come from our personal experiences and from published data from previous studies.

The populations studied by previous studies may not be comparable to your population. There may be medical, age, gender, or ethnic differences that need to be considered before the data presented are accepted as applicable to your population.

The magnitude of the risk can be biased. There are two types of error, known as availability and compression bias.

- *Availability bias* is also known as exposure bias or publication bias. This results in an overestimation of risk due to overexposure and increased publicity associated with a rare but catastrophic event. When rare events are sensationalized in the media, the perception of risk associated with it increases. Its perceived frequency is also increased.

  The general public are increasingly worried about terrorism, but the chance of being involved in a terrorist attack is very low. As these events command high-profile media coverage, the perceived risk is greatly exaggerated. Similarly, airline accidents command dramatic and sensational media coverage which increases public anxiety. However, car travel is vastly more dangerous in terms of fatalities per kilometer traveled.

  Common events are, by definition, less dramatic, and are therefore perceived to occur less frequently.

- *Compression bias* occurs because in many cases we do not know exactly how frequently something occurs. Usually there will be a range of probabilities, and this range may be vast for rarer events. Patients tend to overestimate small risks and underestimate large ones. To use the above example here, compression bias causes the risk of dying in a car crash to be underestimated, but the risk of dying in a plane crash to be overestimated.

Risk severity

This may be thought of as a combination of the actual probability and the weight or perceived impact that the event may have on the patient. Therefore this entity is subjective. The worst outcomes – death or permanent disability – will have great impact on the way the risk is perceived, even if the probability is low.

A mathematical concept used in the past in an attempt to analyze the process of risk perception was to compare different risks using an expectation value [6]. This is only of use, however, if a numerical value can be assigned to severity:

$$\text{Expectation value} = \text{Probability} \times \text{Severity}$$

This is an oversimplification of the processes involved in risk perception and evaluation. For example, risks with a very low probability but high severity, e.g. death or disability, are perceived worse than risks with a higher probability and less-severe outcome, even though they have the same expectation value.

- An example of events with the same expectation value: if people are offered the choice of being given £5000 or of winning £10 000 on the toss of a coin, the majority will choose the £5000 certainty rather than the uncertain alternative. This has been interpreted as evidence that, if possible, people will try to avoid risk and uncertainty.

Vulnerability

Vulnerability is the extent to which people believe an event could happen to them, or alternatively it is the degree of immunity one possesses to a risk. Generally we tend to exhibit unrealistic optimism and a feeling of immunity or invincibility, so people tend not to behave cautiously. Feeling invulnerable, we underestimate or downgrade our own risk but overestimate the risk to others.

- For example, one might fear more the catastrophic but rare risk of nuclear accident than the common but minor risk of passive smoking.

Controllability

As we like to be in control of things that affect us, the possibility of something happening that cannot be controlled tends to magnify the perceived severity of the risk. The perception of being in control or having choice downgrades the perceived severity of the risk [4].

- Risky pastimes, e.g. skiing, diving, parachuting, etc., all have major risks associated with the undertaking of that activity, including death. The individuals involved are aware of the risk, but because they are in some control of their outcome, they perceive the risk to be lower. The likelihood of accepting higher risk is greater when people have the choice whether to participate.
- Involuntary or imposed risks are significantly less acceptable and incite resentment.

Familiarity

Repeated exposure to a risk induces overconfidence and familiarity. This in turn desensitizes us to the risks present. On the contrary, unfamiliar risks incite a much greater degree of fear and dread. This is known as miscalibration bias.

Acceptability

This is another very subjective issue. Individual attitudes resulting from upbringing, class, ethnic, religious and cultural background can significantly affect the concept of acceptability or nonacceptability of the risk.

Characteristics of the hazard affect the acceptability including how severe, transient, controllable, familiar, and how vulnerable or immune the patient perceives themselves to be.

Risk comparison may help the patient reach a conclusion as to the acceptability of a risk. This is achieved by comparing the risk in question with an alternative event more familiar to the patient that has a similar numerical level of risk. This shows them that they have accepted similar risks in the past.

There are many other variables incuding the trust the patient has in the team responsible for his/her care and any support network, including family, that are close to the patient.

Framing effect or framing bias

This is how the presentation of the risk information can affect risk perception.

- It is well recognized that differences in the presentation of risk information can strongly affect the perception of risk in both lay people and doctors, and thereby influence decision-making [7].

- The order in which clinicians discuss advantages and disadvantages of treatment may have an impact on a patient's perception and final decision.
- Emphasizing positive aspects before discussing risks may be more likely to persuade an individual to accept a particular treatment.
- A therapy reported to be 60% effective would be evaluated more favorable than one with a 40% likelihood of failure, although the two statements mean the same thing.
- Similarly, a treatment with a 10% mortality will be more positively perceived if phrased as having a 90% chance of survival.

This is called positive framing.

- One study [8] compared the way in which a treatment option for cholesterol-lowering and hypertension was presented to patients. Relative risk reduction, absolute risk reduction, number needed to treat, average gain in disease-free years, and stratified gain in disease-free years were the methods compared. Relative risk reduction was the most likely to persuade patients to agree to treatment, whereas the number needed to treat was the least persuasive.

Communicating risk levels

As the assessment of risk and therefore the prediction of risk is not an exact science it is almost impossible to convey an accurate picture of what an individual's clinical risk actually is. There is no way of translating population risk data into specific data for an individual [9].

The range of probabilities when expressing risk can be large, due to the lack of accurate data and due to patient individuality and variability. This leaves us with the difficult issue of trying to be as accurate as we can, but also communicating this to the patient in a way that is best understood. When several orders of magnitude are covered by the range, integer logarithmic scales are often used as a way of presenting information in a manageable format for the patient.

- Examples of logarithmic scales in everyday use are the Richter scale for earthquake magnitude, the pH scale for hydrogen ion concentration and the decibel scale for sound intensity.
- Logarithmic scales may be helpful to some people, but they simply replace very large numbers with smaller ones, sometimes with the effect of overestimating very small risk.
- By substituting a word or a descriptive phrase instead of a number, Calman's verbal scale [3] and the community cluster classification [4] go some way to being more meaningful to the layperson (Table 1.1). It is quite easy to visualize one person in a street where you live, or one person in a small town compared with one person in a large city.

Other analogies more meaningful to the layperson have been sought. The UK Lotto, formerly UK National Lottery, and the probability of winning has been used [10].

3 balls	1 in 57
4 balls	1 in 1032
5 balls	1 in 55 491
5 balls + bonus	1 in 2 330 636
6 balls	1 in 13 983 816

Table 1.1 Risk scales

Risk level 1 in ...	Calman's verbal scale	Calman's descriptive scale	Community cluster
1–9	Very high		
10–99	High	Frequent, significant	Family
100–999	Moderate		Street
1000–9999	Low	Tolerable, reasonable	Village
10 000–99 999	Very low		Small town
100 000–999 999	Minimal	Acceptable	Large town
1 000 000–9 999 999	Negligible	Insignificant, safe	City

Number needed to treat (NNT)

This is a concept introduced by Laupacis *et al.* in 1988 [11]. It is a method used to compare the efficacy of treatments and is calculated from the reciprocal of the absolute risk reduction. In other words, it is the number of patients needed to be treated for one patient to benefit.

- It has been used to compare analgesics and a league table has been drawn up. This has been helpful to clinicians as NNT is said to convey both statistical and clinical significance [12]. Paracetamol (acetaminophen) and ibuprofen have NNTs of 3.6 and 2, respectively, and are therefore effective, whereas codeine has a rather poor in comparison NNT of 18.

This concept has evolved when looking at risk to number needed to harm (NNH) and if you do not treat (IYDT). The same principle calculates the number of patients needed to treat before one patient suffered the adverse effect in question.

- The higher the NNH, the safer the treatment.

IYDT gives a number of patients that treatment is withheld from before an adverse incident occurs.

- If we withhold thrombolytic agents from 20 patients with an acute myocardial infarction, 1 will die [13].

An extension into anesthetic practice would be the number needed to monitor (NNM) to prevent one anesthetic-related death.

- This number may be very high, but is worthwhile to preserve the safety of anesthesia [14].

Whilst trying to communicate risk to a patient, it must be remembered that what is actually perceived may not be the same as that which was intended. Differing knowledge base and past personal experience may result in the two people essentially "coming from opposite directions" and misunderstandings should be expected and predicted. As there are clearly many methods of trying to convey actual levels of risk to our patients, it is likely that their ability to understand is very variable, and more than one approach may well be required for many patients.

If booklets are used as a way of conveying information, it must be remembered that factual information is not the only thing that is communicated. The patient will respond on an emotional level, too, and this is all too often neglected by doctors. It could be that this is because we fail to appreciate the importance, or are not comfortable with the way the patient might be feeling.

What is high risk?

When evaluating risk we have already said it is difficult to convey a probability in terms that mean something to the layperson. Using an actual number may be misleading too.

- When asked, 85% of the population thought they had a better than average sense of humor.
- Many patients, however, are disturbed to learn that 49% of doctors show below-average performance.

We need to find a way to give a meaning to a number. When a likely risk, or a numerical probability, is displayed directly alongside a series of day-to-day events corresponding to the same probability of occurring, then the impact is greater and has some relevant meaning [14]. Figure 1.1 shows this as a risk ladder.

- A risk level of 1 in 100 000 has been deemed *acceptable* [4] and a risk level of 1 in 1 000 000 is deemed *safe*.
- The risk of death by road traffic accident in the UK in a year 1 is 8000 – a risk which a large proportion of us take every day on our way to and from work. This corresponds to a risk level less than 1 in 1000, which is deemed *tolerable* or *reasonable*. [3]
- There are those that do not believe that any degree of risk is universally acceptable [2].
- When evaluating risk perception, we have already seen that there are numerous subjective criteria to be considered alongside the numerical magnitude of risk.

When considering overall risk, one must consider the baseline risk and then add on, or superimpose, the relevant additional risk to reach the real risk.

- For example, we all have a risk of dying every day. This baseline risk increases as we get older. Any other risk of premature death such as smoking or murder needs to be added to the baseline to see the actual risk of death for that day.
- In anesthesia, the number given as baseline for death under anesthesia is 1 in 185 000. We all know that this is an artificial figure, as people are not generally given anesthetics without some operation or procedure also happening to them.
- The risk of death after surgery is much greater than this figure because the surgery, the patient, the surgeon and anesthetist all have a little extra risk to add on.
- The extra risk may not always be quantifiable, but will be additive.
- The more closely we can form a personalized estimate of risk for an individual, the more the gap between population-based data and the subjective experience of the patient will narrow and the more informed that patient's decision will be [15].

7

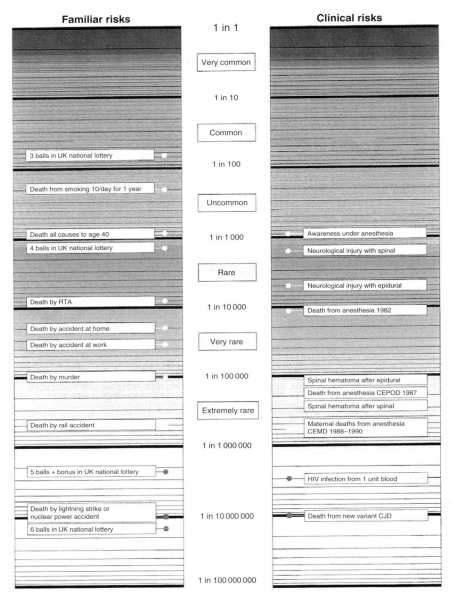

Figure 1.1 Risk ladder.

Relative and absolute risk

These two terms can be used solely or together to convey risk. When used solely, the relative risk of an event can be very misleading.

- If the absolute risk of an event occurring is very small, say 1 in 1 000 000, then this is often perceived quite correctly as a very unlikely occurrence. If the absolute risk were 2 in 1 000 000, then most observers would still perceive the risk as very unlikely.

- When described in terms of relative risk, we can say that the risk has doubled, or is twice as likely, or has increased by 100%. All of these terms tend to be more alarming and likely to result in the perception of a greatly increased risk.

This is a method the media use frequently to overdramatize a story.

- A very good example of this is the risk of venous thrombo-embolism (VTE) whilst taking a "low dose" third-generation oral contraceptive pill (OCP) [16]. The press revealed accurate but misleading relative risk figures without adequately stressing the absolute risk.
- This was further compounded by the general public, and many medical professionals, not having extra information to put these figures into context.
- The actual risk of VTE when pregnant is higher again, and the risk to someone neither pregnant nor on the OCP does not equal zero.

	Incidence of VTE per million women per year	Mortality; deaths per million women per year
No oral contraceptive	50	0.5
2nd generation OCP	150	1.5
3rd generation OCP	300	3.0
Pregnancy	600	6.0

Risk–benefit analysis

In the UK, the Department of Health has issued guidance on consent to examination and treatment [17]. It makes two main points.

- Firstly, the person taking consent should ideally be the person who is to perform the procedure.
- Secondly, patients should be given sufficient information before deciding to give their consent.

It goes on to say that the patient should be given as much information as they reasonably need to make their decision, and it should be given in a form that they can understand, or their consent may be invalid.

However, just how much information is enough will be different from patient to patient, and clinical judgment must be used. If the patient decides either verbally or nonverbally that they do not want this information, then it must be documented clearly in the medical notes.

We have moved from a concept of "the reasonable doctor" where the doctor knew what was best for the patient and decided what the patient needed to be told, to the concept of "the reasonable patient".

- Doctors are now expected to give much more information as a matter of course so the patient is empowered fully to decide what happens to them, but is this always in the patients' best interests?
- Although patients have the power to make decisions about their healthcare, it brings with it a significant amount of responsibility that many patients simply do not want or cannot deal with.

- Furthermore, the giving of information, some of which will have negative implications, may well frighten a patient just at the time when they are looking for reassurance and comfort.
- Is it justifiable that we scare our patients so that we can satisfy ourselves that we have disclosed all the risks?

The subject of consent throws into conflict two important ethical principles: autonomy (the individual having the right to determine what happens to them), and beneficence (the obligation for doctors to do only good for the patient). Doctors may exercise "therapeutic privilege" which allows us to withhold certain information if it is deemed that it would be contrary to the patient's best interests, cause harm to the patient, or could deter the patient from proceeding with a therapeutic procedure considered essential. All risks discussed and those not discussed, with the reasons for not doing so, should be documented in the patient's notes [18].

The "reasonable" patient who is fully informed may sometimes turn out to be an "unreasonable" patient.

- Patients sometimes choose the option that the doctor would not choose for them [19]. If a patient states a preference for a procedure that increases the risks for the patient (e.g. a patient requesting a general anesthetic for an elective cesarean section instead of a spinal technique), does this mean the patient has made a wrong choice?
- Should the anesthetist accept the decision and proceed whilst managing the extra risk, or should the anesthetist have the right to refuse to treat them on the grounds that they are putting themselves at unnecessary extra risk?

When making an assessment of risk acceptability, there needs to be a complete assessment of all the risks and benefits.

- Perception of the advantages of an event versus the disadvantages of the hazards associated with the event are personal to each individual.
- This is an unpredictable process and it is often surprising what patients are prepared to accept in terms of high risk for what might appear to be little gain.
- Conversely, some individuals will refuse treatment that is likely to have a positive outcome because of fears about something we perceive to be quite trivial.
- Our duty is to be as honest and as accurate with the information we have and allow the patient time to perform their own individual risk–benefit analysis.
- Depending on the urgency, this process can take months and sometimes even years.

The mnemonic BRAN offers a useful way of approaching this analysis. This covers the Benefits and Risks associated with a course of action. It also prompts us to think of Alternative treatments and what would happen if Nothing were done.

What are the Benefits?
- Identify the benefits.
- Assess the likelihood of benefit.
- Assess the perceived value of the benefit.
- How soon could benefit occur?
- Is the benefit permanent or temporary?

What are the Risks?
- Identify the risks.
- Assess the likelihood or probability of risk.
- Assess the perceived magnitude of the risk.
- How soon could the risk occur?
- Is the risk permanent or temporary?

What are the Alternatives?
- Are there alternative courses of action?
- Is there a new treatment on the horizon?
- Is there a less efficacious, but more acceptable, alternative?

What if you do Nothing?
- Remember *primum non nocere* – firstly do no harm.
- In the modern era with medical and surgical advances pushing the boundaries of what is achievable, it must not be forgotten that although we may be able to undertake a course of action, it does not always mean that we should.

The BRAN mnemonic may be useful in anesthetic practice to help direct discussion and thought – however, one must know what the risks are before it can be applied to individual patients.

What are the risks ?

When patients present for surgery, there are a number of potential hazards with risks associated. These risks can be divided into categories:

- risks associated with a hospital admission;
- risks associated purely with the anesthetic; and
- risks associated with the proposed surgery.

The degree of risk associated with all of the above will vary from patient to patient depending on a number of factors. These include whether the surgery is elective or emergency, and whether the patient has any premorbid conditions (chronic disease, obesity, etc.) or any lifestyle habits (smoking cigarettes or drinking alcohol) that may increase the risk involved. These are known as patient factors.

There are some risks present during an anesthetic irrespective of what the proposed surgery is. Not all of these risks are down to anesthesia. A significant risk is delivered by the surgery and by the patient themselves, which the anesthetist partly has a hand in managing.

Risks associated with a hospital admission

Appropriately trained staff

- The aviation industry is one that the medical profession looks to frequently and is compared to when it comes to errors, accidents and near misses. The training systems in place within the aviation industry do not focus solely on the captain, but include the crew and the whole corporation. All are encouraged to spot potential problems before they occur, and an open reporting system which does not apportion blame on an individual, but looks at the system itself and how it can be improved, has certainly increased airline safety [20].

- A rigorous critical incident reporting system is needed to record and subsequently investigate any incident that causes patient harm as well as the near misses that may have caused harm. This type of reporting system is only effective if all incidents and near misses are reported. This will only occur if the reporter does not fear blame as a repercussion for bringing the incident to light. This "no blame" culture is gradually becoming accepted as part of the culture in the UK NHS following the example of AIMS (Anaesthetic Incident Monitoring Study) already in place in Australia. This will allow thorough investigation of trends that could have led to a patient incident before it actually does. A system such as this will give more junior members of a team a voice, anonymously if necessary, so that a more complete picture can be built up and a more thorough assessment of the systems at fault can be made. This will ensure that more robust systems are in place and the patient journey through their hospital stay will be a safer one.
- The UK National Confidential Enquiry into Perioperative Deaths (NCEPOD) has identified the importance of training and adequate experience for medical staff. This applies equally to the Operating Room (OR) staff and nursing staff on the wards.
- Studies have shown that the training, experience and competence of the team have an effect on outcome. The team includes all the staff from the surgeon, anesthetist and OR team through to the nurses, physiotherapists and rehabilitation team involved in postoperative care and follow-up clinics.
- Although the volume for surgeons may be important, it has been shown that a high-volume hospital may compensate partially for low-volume surgeons [21].
- It is known that "board-certified" trauma surgeons improve the outcome following major trauma [22].
- It is also known that trained specialists improve the outcome of septic shock in intensive care units (ICU) [23].
- The outcome following colon cancer surgery varies significantly between surgeons, and it has been recommended that this surgery should only be carried out by specialist surgeons. A paper from the US supporting this [21] described a low-volume surgeon as doing 5 or fewer cases per year (this was the majority) and a high-volume surgeon doing more than 10 cases per year. In the UK, there are few surgeons undertaking this surgery that would fall into the low-volume group. Many would do more than 10 per month.
- Surgeons have been extensively studied, but not so the anesthetist. There have been few studies that have effectively shown the role of the anesthetist to have any effect on risk and outcome. One study looking at coronary artery bypass surgery showed that the only nonpatient-related factors influencing outcome were cardiac bypass time and the anesthetist [24].

Timing of surgery

NCEPOD in the UK has shown that surgery performed at night, when staff are more likely to be fatigued, is more hazardous and contributes to increased mortality [25].

- In the period between 1997 and 2003, there was an increase from 37 to 60% of emergency surgery being performed during the daytime in the week.
- This change has contributed to a reduction in adverse incidents [26].
- Since more of these high-risk operations are performed during the day, it also follows that a greater proportion of them are conducted by consultant surgeons and anesthetists.

Availability of equipment

- The absence of basic equipment, such as standard monitoring (pulse oximetry, ECG, BP, capnography) will contribute to an increased risk of hazard to the patient.
- Specialist equipment, such as ultrasonography for placement of central venous lines, may not be available, as the cost of such items may be prohibitive for some less well funded departments.

The work and recommendations of NCEPOD in the UK are explored in more detail in Chapter 2.

Risks associated with the anesthetic

- General anesthesia is easy to achieve, but is characterized by uncertainty and unpredictability.
- Its mechanisms, the mode of action of some of the drugs, and cause-and-effect relationships are incompletely understood.
- The constantly changing physiological status of the patient and the superimposed disturbances due to surgery create a potentially hazardous state for the patient.
- The process of anesthesia has been compared with the aviation industry in that it demonstrates high dynamism, time pressure, uncertainty, complex human–machine interactions and risk.
- Because the rare events are catastrophic (a plane crash or an anesthetic-related death), both of these professions have developed mechanisms for safety promotion. Anticipating complications and dealing with them prior to any potential untoward incident has become second nature.

Death is the complication both anesthetists and patients fear most, whether it results from surgical complications or directly as a result of the anesthetic.

There are four main reasons why deaths occur during anesthesia.

1. Anesthetist error – in the UK, the risk is 1 in 185 000 [27].
2. Surgeon error – this is entirely down to the expertise of the surgeon and the degree of difficulty of the procedure. Mortality rates for each operation can be tailored to each individual patient by the surgeon preoperatively at the time of taking consent.
3. Life-threatening unexpected anaphylactic reactions.
4. Patient factors – death is more likely if the patient is older, if the surgery is emergency surgery, if the patient is already extremely unwell, or if the operation is on the heart, lungs, bowel or major vascular surgery.

More than 90% of deaths that occur perioperatively are not directly caused by the anesthetic [28].

It is generally accepted that anesthesia is safer now than it was 30 years ago, and the report by the US Institute of Medicine, *To Err is Human: Building a Safer Health Care System,* supports this [29].

- The committee states that anesthesia-related deaths have fallen from 2 per 10 000 anesthetics to 1 in 2–300 000 anesthetics over this time period.
- Going back even further to the period of 1948–52, there are data to suggest that deaths where anesthesia was "a very important contributing factor" showed a rate of 1 in 1560 anesthetics [30].
- Comparing these mortality figures is not an exact science as the nature of surgical patients and the operations performed upon them have also changed. More complex procedures are now performed more frequently on sicker, more elderly patients [31].
- The risks for American Society of Anesthesiologists (ASA) 1 and 2 patients are likely to be predominantly iatrogenic, with anesthesia still contributing to serious adverse events and avoidable deaths.

Giving patients information leaflets specific to their surgery and their anesthetic, and by seeing them preoperatively in specifically designed clinics, helps to allay some common misconceptions and also gives the medical team an opportunity to impress upon the patient some of the rarer, but more serious risks.

- In 2004, the UK Royal College of Anaesthetists launched a project whereby they looked at 14 of the most commonly asked questions about adverse incidents [32].
- A website was launched and information leaflets were written to help with this. The subjects are:
  - nausea and vomiting;
  - sore throat;
  - shivering;
  - damage to the teeth, lips or tongue;
  - damage to the eyes during general anesthesia;
  - postoperative chest infection;
  - becoming confused after an operation;
  - awareness during general anesthesia;
  - serious allergy during an anesthetic (anaphylaxis);
  - nerve damage associated with an operation under general anesthesia;
  - nerve damage associated with a spinal or epidural injection;
  - nerve damage associated with a peripheral nerve block;
  - equipment failure; and
  - death or brain damage.

Some of these are covered in other chapters. Others are out of the remit of this text (being covered in the main anesthesia textbooks).

Risks associated with the surgery

- The number of deaths identified each year by the NCEPOD in the UK has changed very little between 1989 and 2003 [33, 34].

- Approximately 3 000 000 surgical procedures are performed every year in the UK, and 20 000 patients will die as a result of undergoing this surgery [35].

- The mortality rates in the UK are slightly higher than for similar patients in the USA [36].

- In the UK, there are 0.6 critical care beds per 10 000 patients compared to 4.4 per 10 000 patients in the USA.

- There are data showing that more patients should go to a critical care bed postoperatively rather than a general ward bed. Those that do go to a general ward bed but subsequently require escalation of care often cannot access a critical care bed simply because there is not one available without the added risk of an out-of-hospital transfer [37, 38].

- There is currently a plan to expand critical care (both ICU and high dependency unit (HDU)) bed numbers in the UK for the postoperative care of surgical patients in the hope that mortality rates will decrease. Unfortunately the financial implications of this will undoubtedly impede, or limit, the expansion of this facility.

- In the UK, there is a population of high-risk patients that amounts to 12.5% of surgical admissions. This population accounts for 83.8% of deaths. These high-risk surgical patients have an in-hospital mortality rate of 12.3% relating to advanced age, comorbidities and complex surgery often performed as an emergency [39].

- Clearly some procedures carry more risk than others. Emergency surgery carries greater risk than elective. No two patients present the same level of risk even though they might be undertaking the same procedure. Some more specific operations are discussed in more detail in later chapters.

Patient factors

- Many patient factors are beyond the control of the anesthetist. Some are beyond the control of the patient also!

- Any of the following factors may have an influence on the degree of risk and the likelihood of an adverse outcome.

- We may be able to modify some of these factors, with the help of the patient. This requires early access to the patient and a means by which the patient may be educated. This may take the form of preoperative clinics where advice and support may be given or specific leaflets prepared for the proposed procedure.

Gender

- The well-known issues of gender and its influence directly on cardiovascular risk are discussed in the cardiovascular risk chapter.

- Females tend to recover from anesthesia quicker than males. When the differences in baseline characteristics, duration and extent of surgery and anesthetic drug administration were adjusted for, it was found that females had a higher bispectral index (BIS) score intraoperatively, woke up quicker and were discharged from the postanesthesia care unit

(PACU) sooner than males. This study speculates than females are therefore less sensitive to the hypnotic effects of anesthetic drugs than males [40].

- Females have significantly better outcomes including mortality and recurrence rates from melanomas [41].
- The incidence of septic shock requiring intensive care is significantly less in females [42]. No differences were noted in outcome, however.
- Males have a higher incidence of infection following trauma [43].
- Females have a worse outcome following IPPV in the ICU setting, but this is less of a predictor than age, Acute Physiology score and Chronic Health Evaluation (APACHE) scores or presence of Acute Respiratory Distress Syndrome (ARDS) [44].
- Females have a worse outcome following vascular surgery [45].

Age

Age is discussed as a cardiovascular risk factor in a later chapter and also in the chapter on the elderly patient.

Obesity and malnutrition

These problems are discussed in Chapter 10.

Smoking, alcohol and recreational drugs

These problems are discussed in Chapter 11.

Race

This is an area that is poorly understood and difficult to investigate. It is a highly sensitive issue and any actual or perceived differences may be seen to reflect prejudice or the ability to access medical care.

There are, however, observed differences in ethnic incidences for some disease processes.

- Differences in drug responses have long since been recognized in the treatment of hypertension.
- Race has not been identified as an anesthetic risk factor.
- A number of studies in North American negroes have shown a worse outcome for endometrial cancer [46] and a more aggressive disease process with a worse outcome in prostate cancer [47].

Genetic predisposition

The understanding of genetic factors affecting risk of sepsis or cardiac prognosis is poor. It is almost certain that the inflammatory process and the response to infection is at least in part genetically predetermined.

- A genetic predisposition to high levels of angiotensin-converting enzyme is associated with reduced survival following the diagnosis of cardiac failure [48]. This may have implications for cardiac reserve and the response to the physiological stress of surgery and the perioperative period.

Chronic disease and clinical conditions

Of all organ systems, disease of the cardiovascular system is the most important factor associated with perioperative risk and poor outcome. This is discussed in some detail in relevant chapters.

There are some other clinical conditions that predict high perioperative risk:

- leaking abdominal aortic aneurysm,
- an unstarved patient with difficult intubation for emergency surgery,
- the emergency obstetric patient for cesarean section,
- fractured neck of femur,
- end-stage renal disease,
- emergency intracranial surgery,
- myopathic conditions,
- malignant hyperthermia,
- hereditary mastocystosis,
- latex allergy.

Thankfully, many of these conditions are rare.

References

1. Royal Society. *Risk Assessment: Report of a Royal Society Working Party*. London, Royal Society, 1983.

2. Keeney RL. Understanding life-threatening risks. *Risk Anal* 1995; **15**: 627–37.

3. Calman KC. Cancer: science and society and the communication of risk. *Br Med J* 1996; **313**: 799–802.

4. Calman KC, Royston HD. Risk language and dialects. *Br Med J* 1997; **315**: 939–42.

5. Bogardus ST, Holmboe E, Jekel JF. Perils, pitfalls and possibilities in talking about medical risk. *J Am Med Assoc* 1999; **281**: 1037–41.

6. Broadbent DE. Psychology of risk. In: Cooper MG, ed. *Risk: Man-made Hazards to Man*. Oxford, Clarendon Press, 1985.

7. Malenka DJ, Baron JA, Johansen S, *et al.* The framing effect of relative and absolute risk. *J Gen Intern Med* 1993; **8**: 543–8.

8. Hux JE, Naylor CD. Communicating the benefits of chronic preventative therapy: does the format of efficacy data determine patients' acceptance of treatment? *Med Decision Making* 1995; **15**: 152–7.

9. Edwards A, Prior L. Communication about risk – dilemmas for general practitioners. *Br J Gen Prac* 1997; **47**; 739–42.

10. Barclay P, Costigan S, Davies M. Lottery can be used to show risk (letter). *Br Med J* 1998; **316**: 124.

11. Laupacis A, Sackett DL, Roberts RS. An assessment of clinically useful measures of the consequences of treatment. *N Engl J Med* 1988; **318**: 1728–33.

12. Cook RJ, Sackett DL. The number needed to treat: a clinically useful measure of treatment effect. *Br Med J* 1995; **310**: 452–4.

13. Brassey J. IYDT vs NNT. *Bandolier* 1997; **37**: 8.

14. Adams AM, Smith AF. Risk perception and communication: recent developments and implications for anaesthesia. *Anaesthesia* 2001; **56**: 745–55.

15. Smith A, Adams A. *Risk Communication and Anaesthesia. Raising the Standard: Information for Patients*. London, The Royal College of Anaesthetists.

16. McPherson K. Third generation oral contraception and venous thromboembolism. *Br Med J* 1996; **312**: 68–9.

17. Department of Health. *Good Practice in Consent Implementation Guide: Consent to Examination or Treatment*. London, DoH, 2001.

18. Smith R. The discomfort of patient power (editorial). *Br Med J* 2002; **324**: 497–8.

19. General Medical Council. *Seeking Patients' Consent: The Ethical Considerations*. London, General Medical Council, 1998; 7.

20. Helmreich RL. On error management: lessons from aviation. *Br Med J* 2000; **320**: 781–5.

21. Harmon JW, Tang DG, Gordon TA, *et al.* Hospital volume can serve as surrogate for surgical volume for achieving excellent outcomes in colorectal resection. *Ann Surg* 1999; **230**: 404–11.

22. Rogers FB, Simons R, Hoyt DB, *et al.* In-house board-certified surgeons improve outcome for severely injured patients: a comparison of two university centers. *J Trauma* 1993; **34**: 871–5.

23. Reynolds HN, Haupt MT, Thill-Baharozian MC, *et al.* Impact of critical care physician staffing on patients with septic shock in a university hospital medical intensive care unit. *J Am Med Assoc* 1988; **260**: 3446–50.

24. Merry AF, Ramage MC, Whitlock RM, *et al.* First-time coronary artery bypass grafting: the anaesthetist as a risk factor. *Br J Anaesth* 1992; **68**: 6–12.

25. Campling EA, Devlin HB, Hoile RW, *et al. Who Operates When. The Report of the National Confidential Enquiry into Perioperative Deaths 1996/7*. London, NCEPOD, 1997.

26. Cullinane M, Gray AJG, Hargreaves CMK, *et al. Who Operates When II*. London, NCEPOD, 2003.

27. Buck N, Devlin HB, Lunn JN, eds. *The Report of the Confidential Enquiry into Peri-Operative Deaths 1987*. London, The Nuffield Provincial Hospitals Trust/King's Fund, 1987.

28. Department of Health. NHS performance indicators, February 2002.

29. Committee on Quality of Health Care in America IOM. *To Err is Human: Building a Safer Health Care System*, edited by Kohn L, Corrigan J, Donaldson M. Washington, National Academy Press, 1999; 241.

30. Beecher HK, Todd DP. A study of deaths associated with anesthesia and surgery. Based on a study of 599518 anesthesias in ten institutions 1948–1952 inclusive. *Ann Surg* 1954; **140**: 2–35.

31. Cooper J, Gaba DM. No myth: anesthesia is a model for addressing patient safety. *Anesthesiology* 2002; **97**: 1335–7.

32. Risk information leaflets. Royal College of Anaesthetists, London, 2006. www.rcoa.ac.uk

33. Campling EA, Devlin HB, Lunn JN. *Report of the National Confidential Enquiry into Peri-Operative Deaths*. London, NCEPOD, 1990.

34. Cullinane M, Gray AJ, Hargraves CM, *et al. The 2003 Report of the National Confidential Enquiry into Peri-Operative Deaths*. London, NCEPOD, 2003.

35. Improving Surgical Outcomes Group. *Modernising Care for Patients Undergoing Major Surgery: Improving Patient Outcomes and Increasing Clinical Efficiency*. London, 2005. http://www.reducingthelengthofstay. org.uk/doc/isog_report.pdf

36. Bennett-Guerrero E, Hyam JA, Shaefi S, *et al.* Comparison of P-POSSUM risk-adjusted mortality rates after surgery between patients in the USA and the UK. *Br J Surg* 2003; **90**: 1593–8.

37. National Confidential Enquiry into Perioperative Deaths. *The 2002 Report of the National Confidential Enquiry into Perioperative Deaths*. London, NCEPOD, 11 November 2002.

38. National Confidential Enquiry into Perioperative Deaths. *Changing the Way We Operate: The 2001 Report of the National Confidential Enquiry into Perioperative Deaths*. London, NCEPOD, 3 December 2001.

39. Pearse R, Harrison D, James P, *et al.* Identification and characterisation of the high-risk surgical population in the United Kingdom. *Critical Care* 2006; **10**: R81.

40. Buchanan F, Myles P, Leslie K, *et al.* Gender and recovery after general anaesthesia combined with neuromuscular blocking drugs. *Anesth Analg* 2006; **102**: 291–7.

41. Stidham KR, Johnson JL, Seigler HF. Survival superiority of females with melanoma. A multivariate analysis of 6383 patients exploring the significance of gender in prognostic outcome. *Arch Surg* 1994; **129**: 316–24.

42. Wichmann MW, Inthorn D, Andress HJ, *et al.* Incidence and mortality of severe sepsis in surgical intensive care patients: the influence of patient gender on disease process and outcome. *Int Care Med* 2000; **26**: 167–72.

43. Offner PJ, Moore EE, Biffl WL. Male gender is a risk factor for major infections after surgery. *Arch Surg* 1999; **134**: 935–8.

44. Kollef MH, O'Brien JD, Silver P. The impact of gender on outcome from mechanical ventilation. *Chest* 1997; **111**: 434–41.

45. Norman PE, Semmens JB, Lawrence-Brown M, *et al.* The influence of gender on outcome following peripheral vascular surgery: a review. *Cardiovasc Surg* 2000; **8**: 111–15.

46. Connell PP, Rotmensch J, Waggoner SE, *et al.* Race and clinical outcome in endometrial carcinoma. *Obstet Gynecol* 1999; **94**: 713–20.

47. Moul JW, Douglas TH, McCarthy WF, *et al.* Black race is an adverse prognostic factor for prostate cancer recurrence following radical prostatectomy in an equal access health care setting. *J Urol* 1996; **155**: 1667–73.

48. Andersson B, Sylven C. The DD genotype of the angiotensin-converting enzyme gene is associated with increased mortality in idiopathic heart failure. *J Am Coll Cardiol* 1996; **28**: 162–7.

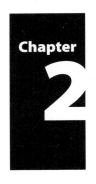

Chapter 2

Lessons from anesthetic audits and epidemiological studies

R. Sharma, C. Dunkley and I. McConachie

There has been intense interest in recent years in identifying the common causes of morbidity and mortality in anesthesia and surgery. The aims of these often national and international projects are to identify areas of concern in anesthetic practice, learn lessons from mistakes and form strategies for prevention.

International pioneers

- In Great Britain, efforts were made by the Association of Anaesthetists of Great Britain and Ireland (AAGBI) in 1982 to investigate perioperative mortality in an anonymous and confidential way [1]. Following this, the AAGBI initiated the first Confidential Enquiry into Peri Operative Deaths (CEPOD) [2]. This evolved into the National Confidential Enquiry into Peri Operative deaths (NCEPOD). Today the expanded and renamed National Confidential Enquiry into Patient Outcome and Death (NCEPOD) examines deaths in hospital within 30 days of surgery in England, Wales and Northern Ireland reported to it by local reporters.

  Much of this chapter focuses on the efforts of NCEPOD and, as such, applies in particular to patient care in the UK. However, much of this discussion may also be relevant to clinicians practising in other countries. The whole NCEPOD endeavor arguably stands as a shining example to the world of large-scale, systematic, structured audit and, as such, merits discussion in some detail.

- Similar efforts are made in Australia, where government-supported special committees collect data about anesthetic-related deaths and produce triennial reports. These reports, now national, were preceded by reports in New South Wales since the 1960s.

- The American Society of Anesthesiologists (ASA) Closed Claims Project is a structured evaluation of adverse anesthetic outcomes collected from the closed anesthesia malpractice insurance claim files of more than 35 professional liability companies throughout the United States. It was started in 1984 by the American Society of Anesthesiologists (ASA) to identify the causes of adverse anesthetic outcome, improve patient safety and prevent patient harm.

Anesthesia-related mortality

Although mortality is a well-defined end point for anesthesia-related risk, it is rare and therefore difficult to study. Prospective studies to look at the incidence of anesthetic mortality would require large patient numbers probably recruited from many centers. There have been several large, retrospective studies in the past examining mortality associated with anesthesia. Two common features of these studies are:

- anesthesia-related mortality has decreased, and
- the main causes of death remain broadly the same.

Anesthesia for the High Risk Patient, ed. I. McConachie. Published by Cambridge University Press.
© Cambridge University Press 2009.

The risk of death in the perioperative period directly due to anesthesia has declined in modern times, but the overall incidence of death following surgery has remained either unchanged or decreased less rapidly. Thus anesthesia as a causation of perioperative death is now very uncommon, but may still be identified as a contributory factor in a larger number of cases.

It is important when examining perioperative mortality to consider the many advances in resuscitation and organ support in recent years. Therefore, intraoperative death is extremely uncommon, with the vast majority of perioperative deaths either:

- occurring in ICU some days later despite various intraoperative catastrophes, or
- occurring as a result of late complications or poor mobilization.

The definition of perioperative death as used by NCEPOD, i.e. death within 30 days of surgery, therefore seems much more useful than either intraoperative death or death within 24 h.

In recent years, many large, national audit organizations have focused on anesthetic morbidity due to the gratifying reductions in anesthetic mortality. In addition, NCEPOD has expanded its remit in the UK to include other aspects of poor patient care and outcome.

International studies on anesthesia-related mortality

- In 1982, the Association of Anaesthetists of Great Britain and Ireland (AAGBI) undertook a study in five regions in the UK to identify mortality which occurred within six days of surgery [1]. Out of an estimated 1 147 362 operations, overall perioperative mortality was 0.53%. Anesthesia contributed to the death in less than 1 in 10 000 operations. This incidence had decreased to 1 in 185 086 anesthetics by 1987 when the first national CEPOD was performed [2].

- Kawashima *et al.* surveyed the incidence of perioperative mortality and cardiac arrest during anesthesia over a five-year period (1994–1998) in 2 363 038 anesthetic cases [3]. Anesthesia-related mortality was approximately 1:48 000. Cardiac arrest due to anesthesia occurred in 1:10 000 procedures.

- Braz *et al.* retrospectively studied 53 718 anesthetic cases over 9 years in Brazil between 1996 and 2005 [4]. The incidence of anesthesia-related cardiac arrest was 3.35:10 000. The incidence of anesthesia-attributed cardiac arrest was 1.86:10 000. All anesthesia-related cardiac arrests were related to airway management and medication administration.

- Arbous *et al.* published a study from the Netherlands in 2001 reporting the incidence of mortality towards which anesthesia contributed as 1 in 7143 procedures and as the only cause in 1:124 000 procedures [5].

- Lienhart *et al.* published a survey of anesthesia-related mortality in France for the year 1999 [6]. They quoted an incidence of 0.69 in 100 000 for deaths totally due to anesthesia, and 4.7 in 100 000 incidence for the deaths partially due to anesthesia. Airway management, postoperative respiratory complications, intraoperative hypotension and anemia leading to postoperative myocardial ischemia and infarction were important causes of death.

- The 2000–2002 triennial report of the Australia and New Zealand College of Anaesthesia reported 137 deaths related to anesthesia out of 1988 reported deaths [7]. This incidence was similar to that reported in their previous triennial report. Of these deaths, 20% were considered unavoidable. An important concern of this report was that 20% of the deaths happened in ASA 1–2 patients. During 2000–2002, an estimated 7.65 million anesthetics were administered. Thus, the approximate anesthesia-related mortality was 1 in 56 000 anesthetics.

- Hove *et al.* [8] retrospectively analyzed the deaths related to anesthesia from 1996 to 2004 from closed claims registered with the Danish Patient Insurance Association. There were 1256 compensation cases related to anesthesia. They reported a total of 24 deaths within 3 months of an anesthetic procedure. Six deaths were due to respiratory events such as difficult intubation or ventilation and aspiration, and four deaths each were due to drug error, equipment failure, central venous line placement and regional anesthesia.
- NCEPOD and the ASA Closed Claims projects will be considered in more detail.

NCEPOD

Since 1990, NCEPOD has produced numerous reports. Deaths in hospital within 30 days of surgery in England, Wales and Northern Ireland are reported to NCEPOD by local reporters. A selective or random sample is studied in more detail by sending questionnaires to the surgeons and anesthetists involved in the case. Since the introduction of Clinical Governance in the UK in April 1999, participation in these confidential enquiries has become a mandatory requirement for clinicians in the UK NHS. The NCEPOD Clinical Coordinators, together with the advisory groups for anesthesia and surgery, review the completed questionnaires and the aggregated data to produce a final report. NCEPOD does not attempt to collect denominator data or calculate mortality figures. NCEPOD also has suggested a consistent approach to differentiating and defining elective and nonelective operations (Table 2.1) which has been revised recently.

Table 2.1 Current NCEPOD classification

Existing	Proposed
EMERGENCY	IMMEDIATE – Life-saving
	IMMEDIATE – Other
URGENT	URGENT
SCHEDULED	EXPEDITED
ELECTIVE	ELECTIVE

Definitions:

IMMEDIATE – immediate life-, limb- or organ-saving intervention: resuscitation simultaneous with intervention. Normally within minutes of decision to operate.

(A) Life-saving

(B) Other, e.g. limb- or organ-saving

URGENT – intervention for acute onset or clinical deterioration of potentially life-threatening conditions, for those conditions that may threaten the survival of limb or organ, for fixation of many fractures and for relief of pain or other distressing symptoms. Normally within hours of decision to operate.

EXPEDITED – patient requiring early treatment where the condition is not an immediate threat to life, limb or organ survival. Normally within days of decision to operate.

ELECTIVE – intervention planned or booked in advance of routine admission to hospital. Timing to suit patient, hospital and staff.

Reproduced courtesy of NCEPOD, UK.

Data submitted to the Department of Health as Hospital Episode Statistics are used to calculate NHS Performance Indicators. The Performance Indicators for 1998/99 [9] reveal:

- 32 956 deaths in hospital within 30 days of an operative procedure;
- 24 920 after emergency surgery and 8036 after nonemergency surgery;
- a total of 2.3 million procedures were undertaken (of which 26% were emergencies);
- a mortality rate of 1.4% after emergency surgery;
- a mortality rate of 0.5% after nonemergency surgery;
- death occurs within 5 days of an operation in almost half of the patients reported.

The most recent UK national figures from 2002 show a reduction of 5.4% in the mortality following nonelective admissions and a reduction of 4.6% in the mortality rate following elective admissions [10]. One should note that the definition of procedures used for NHS Performance Indicators is not directly comparable to the definitions used by NCEPOD.

ASA Closed Claims Project

The ASA Closed Claims Project is a structured evaluation of adverse anesthetic outcomes collected from the closed anesthesia malpractice insurance claim files of more than 35 professional liability companies throughout the United States. It was started in 1984 by the ASA to improve patient safety, prevent patient harm and reduce anesthesia personnel liabilities. This may be considered an easy and cost-effective way of data collection to investigate the major causes of anesthetic injury and death in comparison to retrospective studies. However, it has its own limitations.

- It does not provide a denominator (number of anesthetics given) for calculating the risk of anesthetic injury or death.
- Not all anesthetic injuries or deaths may lead to a claim, hence the anesthetic injury data in the closed claims do not represent a random sample of all the anesthetic injuries. Hence the results of the closed claims project may not be valid in all anesthetic injuries or deaths.
- Individual injury data are collected by insurance companies and may be incomplete, making it difficult to assess the causes of anesthetic injury.

Currently, there have been 7328 claims in the database. These claims were reviewed at the respective insurance company by independent anesthetists using a standard data collection form to assess the standard of anesthetic care, which was judged as appropriate, inappropriate or difficult to judge. They were further reviewed by the project investigators and staff to increase the consistency of the review. Claims were referred to a second or a third anesthetist investigator for further review if initial reviews were challenged. A recent closed claims analysis [11] of 6750 claims from 1975 to 2000 shows that the percentage of claims for death or permanent brain damage has decreased from 39% in 1975 to 1985 to 27% in 1986–2000. The two main causes of brain damage or death have been respiratory events (28% of total claims, with inappropriate care in 64%) and cardiovascular events (28% of total claims, with inappropriate care in 28%) in 2000. Medication, equipment and central, neuroaxial block related events, made up 9%, 6% and 6%, respectively, of the total claims, and inappropriate care was identified in 50–57% of these cases. The most common respiratory events leading to injury were difficult intubation, inadequate oxygenation/ventilation, esophageal intubation and early extubation. The cardiovascular events were pulmonary embolism, inadequate fluid, stroke, hemorrhage and myocardial infarction.

Causes of anesthetic-related mortality

Various studies have also examined the causes of deaths while enumerating them. These causes can be broadly divided into patient factors, surgical factors, anesthetic factors, equipment failure and organizational factors. The principal causes of the deaths have not changed over a period of time. In addition to causes already identified from some of the studies discussed above, the following have been shown to be relatively common features, especially in the NCEPOD reports:

Patient factors
- ASA 3–5,
- old age,
- multiple co-morbidities.

Surgical factors
- Urgent or emergency surgery.

Anesthetic factors
- inadequate preoperative assessment and resuscitation,
- airway and ventilation-related problem,
- drug errors, adverse effects,
- lack of supervision of trainees,
- lack of experience,
- inadequate vigilance,
- fatigue.

Resource factors
- No availability of HDU/ ICU facility, equipment, monitors,
- equipment failure.

Recommendations to decrease anesthesia-related mortality and morbidity

In general, most of the NCEPOD recommendations represent nothing more than common sense and good clinical practice. However, sadly many of the recommendations have required repeating in subsequent reports.

NCEPOD has broadly classified its recommendations for best clinical practice under various subheadings.

Facilities

- Individual clinicians' efforts to provide the level of care they know is required for the high-risk surgical patient is often frustratingly thwarted by lack of facilities. NCEPOD has helped identify these shortcomings.
- One of the major lessons to be learnt is that to provide the highest quality of care for these patients, acute surgical services may need to be concentrated in fewer well-staffed and resourced hospitals [12].

- A dedicated emergency operating room (OR) and recovery should be staffed and available 24 h a day. The aim should be to deal with emergency cases during the working day and avoid out-of-hours operating on nonessential cases.
- There should be easy access to a High Dependency Unit and Intensive Care Unit on a single site.
- An Orthopedic Trauma OR operating during the day with senior staff is recommended [13].
- Elderly patients should not have to wait more than 24 h (once fit) for operation [14]. When a decision to operate is taken, there should be a commitment by the clinicians and adequate facilities available to provide appropriate critical care postoperatively.
- Local protocols should be in place to ensure immediate access to blood products.
- CT scanning and neurosurgical consultation should be available in any hospital receiving trauma patients [13].
- A fiberoptic laryngoscope should be available with trained and nominated staff able to use it.
- Children's services should be concentrated to avoid occasional practise. Local arrangements should be in place for the skilled transport of critically ill children when appropriate.
- Surgeons and anesthetists should not undertake occasional pediatric practise. Consultants who do undertake responsibility for the care of children must keep up-to-date and competent in the management of children.
- An arbitrator/co-ordinator should exist to ensure emergency cases are prioritized appropriately and emergency OR space is utilized efficiently.

Personnel

It is clear that the high-risk surgical patient should be directly cared for by experienced senior anesthetic and surgical members of staff. This recommendation has been one of the cornerstones of the NCEPOD reports over the years.

(International readers should understand that, historically in the UK, trainee anesthetists often directly administered anesthesia to emergency patients without direct consultant supervision. This may seem inappropriate and surprising to many from other countries where direct consultant attendance at cases is the norm. Pressure from NCEPOD and other bodies has increasingly changed this practice in the UK.)

- It may on occasion be appropriate or unavoidable that consultants cannot be directly involved in patient care. At the very least, the consultant has a vital role in providing advice, support and making crucial decisions.

There are a number of reasons why senior help may not be requested for the high-risk patient:

- insufficient experience of junior staff to identify the at-risk patient;
- inability to recognize personal limitations;
- lack of familiarity with local procedures;
- practical barriers to communication;
- poor understanding of personal limits of responsibility.

Although these are mainly personal shortcomings, senior clinicians should ensure that the system within their hospital is robust enough to ensure these individual limitations do not compromise patient safety and good practice.

Supervision

- Trainees should not undertake anesthesia or surgery in children without advice.
- Junior trainees should have suitable supervision by consultants.
- Ensure local guidelines are in place so trainees are clear when to ask for help.
- National or regional guidelines may be preferable to avoid confusion when trainees rotate between hospitals.

Communication

- Staff (including consultants) must be aware of their limitations and work in an environment where they are encouraged to, and are comfortable with, asking for help.
- Anesthetists should be consulted as opposed to informed about cases.
- Encourage a team approach between surgeons, anesthetist and physicians for complex cases.
- Ensure there is adequate communication between specialties and between grades of staff within a specialty.
- Who to call, when to call and how to call for help should be easily available and clearly understood.

Staff availability

- All staff covering emergencies should be free from other commitments and easily available.
- Emergency OR sessions should be staffed by consultants.

Locums and Non Consultant Career Grade (NCCG) anesthetists and surgeons

- Ensure NCCG doctors within the hospital are aware of their role and limit of responsibility. They should have equal access to supervision, involvement in audit, and opportunities for continued professional development.
- Supervising consultants should be aware of the abilities of locum doctors before appointment.
- Extra effort and vigilance is required to ensure that locums are appraised of local guidelines and afforded the same degree of supervision and support as other members of staff. The UK Royal College of Anaesthetists provides guidance on the level of supervision of doctors in training. It complements the statement from the Clinical Negligence Scheme for Trusts (CNST), which increases the statutory requirement to ensure that doctors taking up post in a new hospital are adequately trained and competent to fulfill the role for which they have been employed. There is now a requirement for supervisors to list the technical skills that new doctors are expected to perform and, in turn, for the new doctor to indicate their competence to perform the

specific tasks. A supervised training program must rectify any deficiencies in initial or continuing competence.

Preoperative assessment and preparation

In the time period that NCEPOD has issued reports, the profile of patients dying within 30 days of their operation has changed [15]. Patients are more likely to be older, to have undergone an urgent operation, to be of poorer physical status, and to have a co-existing cardiovascular or neurological disorder.

- Adequate preoperative assessment and preparation for OR is vital in the management of the high-risk surgical patient.

- The management of the patient at this time will greatly influence the subsequent outcome of the operation, and it is crucial that appropriate care is given and appropriate decisions made to prevent avoidable morbidity and mortality.

- The decision to operate and when not to operate should be made by consultants. It is important that there is direct communication between the consultant surgeon and the anesthetist and that decisions are made jointly.

- NCEPOD has frequently referred to the problem of operations being performed on moribund patients or where the objective of surgery is unclear. These patients clearly need a consultant evaluation and a sensitive but honest approach to the patient and relatives. All too often hasty decisions to opt for surgery are made without fully considering their ramifications.

- If the decision to operate or not is contra to that of the patient or relatives, having a mechanism to allow discussion with consultant colleagues from the same or allied specialty can be invaluable in reassuring the patient and relatives that an appropriate decision has been made.

- NCEPOD has emphasized the need to provide junior members of staff with guidance on when to ask for help. NCEPOD has highlighted the inadequacies and inconsistencies of the ASA classification if used as an assessment tool [15]. The ASA classification may not, on its own, be an adequate trigger for alerting inexperienced doctors to a high-risk patient. NCEPOD suggested that the use of the P-POSSUM score might be more appropriate and encouraged [14].

- The importance of avoiding rushing patients to OR before adequate resuscitation is a recurring theme of NCEPOD. Emergency patients invariably require appropriate fluid resuscitation prior to OR. In some patients this can be safely undertaken on the ward. In other patients, particularly the elderly, this may require a critical care environment and appropriate invasive monitors.

- Poor understanding of fluid management especially in the elderly is often cited as a contributing factor in NCEPOD cases [14].

- The use of preoperative critical care services for resuscitation and preoperative preparation may well avoid the need for lengthy postoperative critical care. However, in the UK and other countries, finding a critical care bed preoperatively in many hospitals may be impossible. The ability to utilize OR recovery beds prior to surgery and the development of critical care outreach services may be a short-term solution to this problem.

- Whatever the particular local solution, it is important to have a mechanism in place to allow patients to be adequately resuscitated in an appropriate environment by knowledgeable staff.

- Starting a high-risk case without first identifying adequate critical care facilities post-operatively is to be avoided. Consultation with colleagues who control these beds at the earliest opportunity is essential. It is not always easy to identify those patients that require HDU care. NCEPOD has called for simple, nationally agreed criteria to help assess the need for HDU and ICU care.

- Over the time period of NCEPOD, the percentage of patients with co-existing medical disorders has increased from 89% to 94% [15]. Cardiac disorders have increased from 54% to 66%. NCEPOD suggests that echocardiography should be available and used more widely in preoperative assessments [15]. For complex medical disorders, the advice of a specialist physician may be invaluable. NCEPOD would like to see hospitals develop an organizational structure to allow prompt medical review should it be required [15].

- Thromboembolic complications continue to be a major cause of morbidity and mortality. CEPOD has recognized this in all its reports and highlighted the inconsistent nature of prophylactic measures. It recommends the development of guidelines and clear definition of responsibility for implementing prophylactic measures. The guidelines need to be audited regularly to ensure compliance and efficacy. Individuals dealing with high-risk patients in the preoperative period should be aware of the importance of thromboembolic prophylaxis.

Audit

NCEPOD recognizes that audit can be a useful tool locally to help improve the management of high-risk surgery. There is a lack of consistency in the participation in audit both between hospitals and within surgical specialities and anesthesia.

Of cases sampled for NCEPOD 2000 [15], one-third of deaths were subsequently reviewed in a formal audit setting by anesthetists, and three-quarters of deaths were reviewed by surgeons. This was unchanged from previous reports.

In an effort to improve local practice, NCEPOD recommends:

- improved access to notes, especially of deceased patients;

- more post-mortem examinations;

- better communication between pathologists and clinicians;

- regular Morbidity and Mortality review meetings. Ideally these should be multidisciplinary meetings to enhance the working relationships of surgeon, anesthetist and physician; and

- ensure all members of staff participate equally in the audit.

In the light of public concern over organ retention following post-mortem examination, there is rightly greater rigor now required for the consent to post-mortem examination. Details of the consent process are beyond the scope of this chapter. The Department of Health in the UK has published guidance on consent for post-mortem examinations [16]. In this guidance, they echo the recommendations from NCEPOD in emphasizing the importance of post-mortem examination to improving clinical care and maintaining standards.

Have these studies and reports resulted in change of practice?

The ASA Closed Claims Project has arguably played a part in various important changes in practice [17]:

- active management recommendations for spinal anesthesia-induced hypotension in order to reduce myocardial infarctions;
- recommendations to use pulse oximetry and end tidal CO_2 monitors after identification that respiratory events such as difficult intubation/ventilation and esophageal intubation were major causes of death and brain damage. Whether this helped to decrease the respiratory events as a cause of injury from 68% in 1975–1985 down to 28% in 1986–2000 is difficult to prove; and
- the development of difficult intubation guidelines by the ASA and their impact on decreasing the respiratory cause of deaths awaits evaluation.

NCEPOD is seen as a positive influence amongst many UK anesthetists. It has been helpful in negotiating better facilities and staffing levels with hospital management. It has also helped anesthetists to improve their clinical practice, supervision and communication. Derrington [18] performed a postal survey to find out the effect NCEPOD has had on clinical practice in the UK. Of the 100 consultant anesthetists who were contacted, 72% responded. Although the sample was small, 74% of respondents said that NCEPOD influenced their own clinical practice by:

- increased responsibility and involvement in patient care, supervision of locums and trainees; and
- increased communication and discussion with surgical colleagues.

Eighty per cent of respondents said that NCEPOD recommendations have been useful in:

- introducing local guidelines or protocols, for example in pediatric anesthesia;
- rationalizing emergencies to avoid night-time operating;
- matching grade of anesthetists with complexity of case; and
- thromboembolic prophylaxis.

Eighty per cent of the respondents felt that NCEPOD has been useful in improving essential services, staff or equipment during negotiations with management. Careful reading of the reports reveal that fewer of the sampled patients are anesthetized or operated on by trainees. Many of the oft-repeated recommendations regarding timing of surgery, and not operating "out of hours" have been implemented or encouraged in many hospitals. However, a retrospective study of over 5000 emergency operations [19] in a university hospital has shown that, between 1997 and 2004, the annual volume of emergency cases performed increased significantly. Despite increased daytime and evening operating availability, the absolute number of cases performed at night remained constant over the period of the study (but the proportion of the emergency workload that took place after midnight decreased significantly). A small but consistent volume of complex cases (chiefly laparotomies and complex vascular cases) will still require emergency surgery after midnight.

Since the first NCEPOD report it is clear that the rate of change is often slow. Many of the lessons continue to be repeated and are not always heeded. There can be many reasons for this, e.g. underfunding, financial restrictions, money-saving measures, anesthetic manpower problems, and changes in trainee doctors' work time and training. Both hospital managers and clinicians need commitment backed up with resources to implement changes in practice. In their introduction to the 2000 report, Ingram and Hoile state "We believe that future change will depend on money, manpower, mentality and mentoring" [15].

Further reading

ASA Closed Claims Project website: www.asaclosedclaims.org.

Lunn JN. The history and achievements of the National Confidential Enquiry into

Perioperative Deaths. *J Qual Clin Pract* 1998; **18**: 29–35.

NCEPOD website: www.ncpod.org.uk.

References

1. Lunn JN, Mushin WW. *Mortality Associated with Anaesthesia*. London, Nuffield Provincial Hospitals Trust, 1982.

2. Buck N, Devlin HB, Lunn JN. *Report on the Confidential Enquiry into Perioperative Deaths*. London, Nuffield Provincial Hospitals Trust, The Kings Fund Publishing House, 1987.

3. Kawashima Y, Takahashi S, Suzuki M, *et al.* Anaesthesia-related mortality and morbidity over a 5-year period in 2,363,038 patients in Japan. *Acta Anaesthesiol Scand* 2003; **47**: 809–17.

4. Braz LG, Módolo NS, do Nascimento P, *et al.* Perioperative cardiac arrest: a study of 53,718 anaesthetics over 9 yr from a Brazilian teaching hospital. *Br J Anaesth* 2006; **96**: 569–75.

5. Arbous MS, Grobbee DE, van Kleef JW, *et al.* Mortality associated with anaesthesia: a qualitative analysis to identify risk factors. *Anaesthesia* 2001; **56**: 1141–53.

6. Lienhart A, Auroy Y, Péquignot F, *et al.* Survey of anaesthesia-related mortality in France. *Anesthesiology* 2006; **105**: 1087–97.

7. Gibbs N, Borton C. *Safety of Anaesthesia in Australia – A Review of Anaesthesia Related Mortality 2000–2002*. Melbourne: Australian and New Zealand College of Anaesthetists, 2006.

8. Hove LD, Steinmetz J, Christoffersen JK, Moller A, Nielsen J, Schmidt H. Analysis of deaths related to anaesthesia in the period 1996–2004 from closed claims registered by the Danish Patient Insurance Association. *Anesthesiology* 2007; **106**: 675–80.

9. www.performance.doh.gov.uk/ nhsperformanceindicators/indicators 2000.htm

10. www.performance.doh.gov.uk/ nhsperformanceindicators/hlpi2002/index. html

11. Cheney FW, Posner KL, Lee LA, Caplan RA, Domino KB. Trends in anaesthesia-related death and brain damage: a closed claims analysis. *Anesthesiology* 2006; **105**: 1081–6.

12. Ingram GS. The lessons of the National Confidential Enquiry into Perioperative Deaths. *Ballières Clin Anaesthesiol* 1999; **13**: 257–66.

13. Campling EA, Devlin HB, Hoile RW, Lunn JN. *The Report of the National Confidential Enquiry into Perioperative Deaths 1992/1993*. London, NCEPOD, 1995.

14. Extremes of Age. *The 1999 Report of the National Confidential Enquiry into Perioperative Deaths*. London, NCEPOD, 1999.

15. Then and Now. *The 2000 Report of the National Confidential Enquiry into Perioperative Deaths*. London, NECPOD, 2000.

16. Elam G. *Consent to Organ and Tissue Retention at Post Mortem Examination and Disposal of Human Materials*. London, Department of Health, December 2000.

17. Derrington MC, Gallimore S. The effect of the National Confidential Enquiry into Perioperative Deaths on clinical practice – report of a postal survey of a sample of consultant anaesthetists. *Anaesthesia* 1997; **52**: 3–8.

18. Faiz O, Banerjee S, Tekkis P, *et al.* We still need to operate at night! *World J Emerg Surg* 2007; **2**: 29.

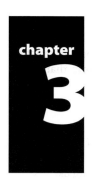

Assessment of cardiovascular risk

N. Moreland and A. Adams

The significance of cardiovascular disease

- Coronary artery disease is a complex inflammatory process influenced by both genetic and environmental factors, the progression and outcome of which can be modulated in many ways [1].
- Cardiac complications pose a significant risk to patients undergoing major noncardiac surgery.
- The prevalence of cardiovascular disease increases with age, and the proportion of the population over the age of 65 is steadily increasing.
- Coincidentally, this is the age group in which the largest number of surgical procedures is performed.
- In 1977, the overall perioperative risk of cardiac death or major cardiac complications (nonfatal myocardial infarction [MI], pulmonary edema or ventricular tachycardia) in patients aged over 40 years was 5.8% [2].
- In 1995 a more selective review was done looking at MI and cardiac death [3]. To summarize: if a patient has cardiac disease, they are at higher risk of having a perioperative acute cardiac event.
- The ideal approach is to institute appropriate investigations to ascertain the risk, and then commence therapeutic measures so as to minimize the risk [4].

Pathophysiology

Physiological factors associated with surgery predispose to myocardial ischemia which is more pronounced in patients with underlying coronary disease. These include volume shifts and blood loss, enhanced myocardial oxygen demand from elevations in heart rate and blood pressure secondary to stress from surgery, and an increase in platelet reactivity [5].

The mechanisms for poor outcome include the following.

- *Myocardial ischemia*: tachycardia, hypertension and increased oxygen demand of the myocardium coupled with the decreased coronary filling time and increased myocardial wall tension causes reduced coronary blood flow leading to myocardial ischemia which may progress to infarction. An alternative route to infarction is increased shear stress on atherosclerotic plaques causing increased likelihood of rupture leading to coronary thrombosis, which may completely occlude a vessel, resulting in infarction.
- *Poor cardiopulmonary physiological reserve*: when the heart and lungs fail to deliver adequate oxygen to fulfill the demands of the tissues then this is known as shock,

Anesthesia for the High Risk Patient, ed. I. McConachie. Published by Cambridge University Press.
© Cambridge University Press 2009.

which will be manifest in the organ systems in terms of organ failure. A study measuring the pH of gastric mucosa in preoperative patients due to undergo major surgery has shown that those with pH < 7.35 had an increase in mortality [6]. It has been hypothesized that gastric mucosa pH could be an indicator of decreased gut perfusion due to poor cardiopulmonary physiological reserve. Some organs are more vulnerable than others, but if this state remains then all organs will fail, resulting ultimately in multi-organ dysfunction syndrome (MODS) and eventually death. This process and its potential modification perioperatively are further explored in Chapter 5.

Risk stratification

Grading or stratifying patients into incremental levels of risk serves several purposes.

- Given that the risk of a perioperative cardiac event increases in line with increasing degrees of cardiac disease, it is useful to be able to more accurately predict what the risk is.
- To facilitate meaningful conversation around the time of consent.
- To identify those who need support with lifestyle risk-reduction strategies (weight loss, smoking cessation).
- To identify those would benefit from medical optimization.
- To identify those that may benefit from revascularization (coronary bypass surgery, coronary stenting, or angioplasty).
- Patients with mildly symptomatic and those with occult, asymptomatic ischemic heart disease (IHD) need to be recognized as they too have an increased perioperative risk.

Clinical factors associated with increased cardiac risk

Advanced age

- Elderly patients have a shorter life expectancy.
- Elderly patients have higher rates of treatment-related risks.
- Age increases the likelihood of coronary artery disease (CAD).
- The mortality of acute MI increases dramatically in the aged.
- Intraoperative and perioperative MI has a higher mortality in the aged.
- UK NCEPOD data show the peak age for death within 30 days of surgery is 70–74 in males and 80–84 in females.
- The problems of the elderly patient are discussed in Chapter 15.

Gender

- Premenopausal women have a lower incidence of CAD.
- CAD occurs up to 10 years later in women than in men [7].
- Diabetic women have an equivalent risk to nondiabetic men of the same age.
- The mortality rate post acute MI is greater for women. This is likely to be explained by older age and diabetes mellitus [8].

Table 3.1 Canadian Cardiovascular Society angina scale. Adapted from [10].

Grade	Activity
I	Ordinary physical activity does not cause angina (e.g. walking or climbing stairs). Angina occurs only with strenuous physical exertion.
II	Slight limitation of ordinary activity (e.g. angina occurs on walking, climbing stairs, in cold, in wind, under emotional stress).
III	Marked limitation of ordinary physical activity (e.g. angina occurs during gentle walking or climbing one flight of stairs).
IV	Inability to carry out any physical activity without anginal symptoms. Angina may be present at rest.

Coronary artery disease (CAD)

- The natural progress of CAD is one of increasing myocardial ischemia and gradual decline in functional capacity as a consequence.
- This can happen over a period of years, or it may occur suddenly as a coronary vessel becomes occluded due to a ruptured plaque and subsequent thrombosis.
- Previous history of acute MI, coronary artery bypass graft (CABG), coronary angioplasty, or coronary angiography showing coronary artery stenosis are all indicators of ongoing CAD.
- Patients with a previous history of MI have an increased risk of further MI, the risk being graded according to the time interval since the MI [9].

Time since MI > 6 months	Risk of further MI	5%
3–6 months		15%
< 3 months		37%

- Current management of MI or unstable angina provides for risk stratification during convalescence in patients who have not been fully revascularized. If a stress test does not indicate ischemia or myocardium at risk, the likelihood of reinfarction after noncardiac surgery is low. A positive stress test is usually an indication for revascularization.

One method of grading the degree of ischemia is with the Canadian Cardiovascular Society angina scale [10] as shown in Table 3.1.

The asymptomatic patient with CAD

- Asymptomatic disease is very often missed as there are no symptoms to enquire about. One must keep a high index of suspicion if there are any other predictors of risk or general risk factors.
- Some patients remain symptomless because they are functionally limited for other reasons. Arthritis, peripheral vascular disease causing claudication and other musculo-skeletal problems often interfere with the clinician's ability to assess function.

These symptomless patients who are suspected of having CAD demand further investigation.

Noninvasive techniques should be performed before progressing to more invasive techniques. Further investigation is only worthwhile if the patient is likely to be a candidate for revascularization if the investigation proves positive.

The information required by testing is:

- How much of the myocardium is critically perfused?
- How much stress is required to produce ischemia?
- What is the left ventricular function?
- Is the patient on optimum medical therapy?

Pulmonary disease

Hypoxemia, hypercapnia, acidosis and increased work of breathing will all lead to further deterioration of an already compromised cardiopulmonary system. Pulmonary risk and assessment are discussed in Chapter 6.

Hypertension

- Moderate hypertension is not an independent risk factor for perioperative cardiovascular complications. Therefore, there is no need to delay surgery for mild or moderate hypertension with no metabolic or cardiovascular abnormalities [11].
- Poorly controlled hypertension causes intraoperative swings in blood pressure and ECG evidence of ischemia. This has been shown to be a factor in postoperative cardiac morbidity.
- Effective preoperative blood pressure (BP) control reduces the incidence of perioperative ischemia, so usual antihypertensive medication should be continued during the perioperative period, blood pressure permitting.
- Hypertension is associated with CAD.
- Although hypertension is diagnosed from a series of BP readings taken in a nonstressful setting, a single elevated reading preoperatively does correlate with a more labile BP intraoperatively.
- Causes of secondary hypertension should be sought, if suspected, to rule out renal artery stenosis, pheochromocytoma, coarctation of the aorta or hyperaldosteronism.
- Severe diastolic hypertension (>110 mmHg) should be controlled before surgery when possible. The risk of delaying surgery needs to be weighed against the benefit of medical optimization.
- If urgent or emergency surgery is essential, beta blockade can achieve rapid control and a degree of intraoperative stability, and so reducing the number and duration of perioperative ischemic episodes.

Congestive heart failure (CHF)

- Has been identified in numerous studies as a predictor of poor outcome in noncardiac surgery [12].
- Validated clinical signs include the presence of a third heart sound and bibasal inspiratory crackles in the lungs.
- The etiology of the CHF is important; CHF of ischemic origin carries a greater significance and greater risk than that caused by hypertension [13].

- Brain natriuretic peptide (BNP) is released from the ventricles and is well established as a marker for the presence of CHF. Recently, elevated levels of BNP have been shown to be a predictor of poor outcome following major surgery [14].

Cardiomyopathy

- Hypertrophic obstructive cardiomyopathy poses significant problems. As suggested by the name, outflow obstruction with catastrophic consequences is a possibility. A reduction in blood volume, decreased systemic vascular resistance, and increased venous capacitance can lead to reduced left ventricular (LV) volume, causing a reduction in stroke volume.
- Other cardiomyopathies need to be treated with caution. The cause of the cardiomyopathy and how the pathophysiology affects the cardiac function need to be assessed and understood. The patient's overall functional capacity is a good indicator of risk.
- The commonest complications suffered by these patients are CHF and arrhythmias.

Valvular heart disease

With all murmurs one needs to know:

- Is the murmur organic or simply a physiological flow murmur?
- Is the murmur significant?
- Is it a valve lesion or a septal defect?
- What is the severity of the valve disease, if present?
- Is endocarditis prophylaxis required?
- Is an echo required?

Patients with mechanical prosthetic valves will need endocarditis prophylaxis when undergoing any procedure likely to cause a bacteremia. They also need careful management of the coagulation status.

Symptomatic stenotic lesions
- Symptomatic stenotic lesions are associated with severe perioperative CHF or shock and often require surgical repair or replacement prior to surgery to reduce any further cardiac risk.
- Severe aortic stenosis poses the most significant risk and elective noncardiac surgery should be postponed until the patient can be fully assessed [12].
- Those patients that refuse valve surgery or are deemed not to be candidates for valve surgery will have at least a 10% mortality if noncardiac surgery is carried out [15].
- Mitral stenosis, although rare, increases the risk of CHF. Percutaneous balloon valvuloplasty or open repair may reduce perioperative risk [16].
- Stenotic lesions of the mitral valve reduce filling of the left ventricle during diastole leading to pulmonary congestion and subsequently CHF. Avoidance of tachycardia helps to minimize this effect.
- If emergency noncardiac surgery is required, then balloon valvuloplasty may help reduce the operative risk [17].

Symptomatic regurgitant valve disease

- Regurgitant valve disease is usually better tolerated than stenotic disease. Monitoring and medical therapy may help stabilize symptoms preoperatively.

- Definitive treatment is by open repair if possible or by valve replacement if repair is not deemed feasible. This may be done after noncardiac surgery if reasonable LV function is preserved.

- In severe aortic regurgitation slow heart rates increase the time the heart is in diastole and therefore increase the volume of regurgitation. Moderate tachycardia reduces the diastolic time and in turn reduces the amount of regurgitation.

- In severe mitral regurgitation the patient may benefit from afterload reduction and diuretics to produce hemodynamic stability.

Arrhythmias and conduction abnormalities

- Significant arrhythmias are defined as high-grade atrioventricular block, sustained ventricular tachycardia, nonsustained ventricular tachycardia in the presence of underlying heart disease, and supraventricular arrhythmias with an uncontrolled ventricular rate.

- Both ventricular and supraventricular arrhythmias have been identified as independent risk factors for coronary events in the perioperative period [12]. They are likely to be significant because they reflect the presence of underlying serious cardiopulmonary disease, drug toxicity, or metabolic abnormality.

- The presence of any new cardiac arrhythmia in the perioperative period should raise the suspicions of the clinician to ongoing cardiac ischemia or infarction, metabolic derangements or drug toxicity.

- Sustained atrial fibrillation or flutter may require electrical or pharmacological cardioversion. Beta blockers, calcium channel blockers or digoxin may be used to control the ventricular response, beta blockers being the most effective usually and digoxin the least [18]. Beta blockers are also the most likely of the drugs to result in conversion back to sinus rhythm [19].

- Almost half of all high-risk patients have premature ventricular ectopics or runs of unsustained asymptomatic ventricular tachycardias. The presence of these is not associated with an increase in MI or cardiac death [20].

- Perioperative beta blocker therapy has been shown to reduce the incidence of arrhythmias in the perioperative period [21].

- Patients that require temporary pacing perioperatively are those with symptomatic atrioventricular blocks, complete heart block, or tri-fascicular block [22].

- Bundle branch blocks do not seem to increase the risk of perioperative cardiac complications [23].

Permanent pacemakers and implantable cardioverter-defibrillators (ICDs) [24]

Metabolic derangements, anti-arrhythmic and other drugs may affect the pacing and sensing thresholds of the device. Volatile anesthetic agents do not seem to affect pacing thresholds [25].

There is a possibility of interference in the operating theatre affecting the function of pacemakers and ICDs. Electric current generated most commonly from electrocautery may be sensed by the device.

Electrocautery may be monopolar or bipolar.

- *Bipolar* operates with much lower energy levels and current only passes from one pole of the bipolar forceps to the other. The potential for adverse interactions with a pacemaker is very low.
- *Monopolar* electrocautery uses much higher energy levels and current passes through the patient from the cautery device to an indifferent plate attached to the patient. More current is passed through the patient whilst monopolar cautery is being used, and interactions are more likely if the current passes near to the pacemaker, or if the plane of current is in line with the pacemaker wires.

The effects of any interaction could include:

- temporary or permanent resetting to a backup pacing mode,
- temporary or permanent inhibition of pacemaker output,
- an increase in pacing rate activation of the rate-responsive sensor,
- ICD firing due to activation by electrical noise, and
- myocardial injury at the lead tip that may lead on to failure to sense or pace.

During the preoperative assessment of a patient with an implanted cardiac device there are a number of questions that need to be answered.

1. What was the original indication for having the device?
2. Is the patient pacemaker-dependent?
3. When was the most recent check done on its function?
4. Exactly what type of device is present, and what is it programmed to do?

Prior to major surgery, where large amounts of electrocautery are expected, the device should have the defibrillator function switched off and the pacing function should be programmed to ventricle or dual-chamber fixed pacing.

Placing a magnet over the device has been advocated in the past, but may have varied effects depending on the type of device. Many pacemakers will default to a pre-prescribed back-up rate if disabled by a magnet. With all devices advice should be sought from the cardiologist responsible for its ongoing care, and following surgery the patient should have their device rechecked and, if necessary, re-programmed.

Diabetes mellitus (DM)

- Diabetes mellitus increases both the likelihood and extent of CAD.
- Myocardial ischemia and infarction are more likely to be silent with diabetes mellitus [26].
- Older patients with DM are more likely to develop congestive cardiac failure (CCF) postoperatively than those without DM [27].

Peripheral vascular disease and cerebrovascular disease

Patients with underlying vascular disease have an increased risk of perioperative cardiac complications for two reasons.

- They constitute a selected population with a high incidence of significant CAD. This is because the risk factors are the same (e.g. DM, smoking, hyperlipidemia).
- In addition, left ventricular systolic dysfunction (ejection fraction <40%) is five times more common in patients with peripheral vascular or cerebrovascular disease [28].
- Symptoms suggestive of CAD may not be revealed due to the physical limitations imposed by peripheral vascular disease (PVD).
- The presence of PVD is more important as a predictor of cardiac events than the actual vascular operation to be performed [13].

Renal disease

Renal disease is a major independent risk factor for postoperative cardiac complications [29].

Creatinine clearance has been used to predict postoperative complications [30]. This is a better measure of renal function than creatinine levels alone, as it takes into consideration the age and weight of the patient also.

Scoring systems and risk indices

These multi-variable analyses identify combinations of factors, generally based upon routine clinical information and laboratory tests, used to estimate the risk of cardiac complications. Certain factors identified as predictors of increased risk are weighted according to their individual significance. Such risk stratification is most critical for patients in the intermediate risk group.

The ideal scoring system would be:

- simple to use,
- highly sensitive,
- highly specific high positive predictive value, and
- cheap and easily repeatable.

American Society of Anesthesiologists (ASA) status [31]

This classification of physical status was originally introduced in 1941 with seven classes. It was revised to five classes in 1963 (Table 3.2). ASA 6 (a declared brain-dead patient whose organs are being removed for donor purposes) was later introduced.

Important points to note in the ASA classification:

- it stratifies patients by simple assessment of physical status,
- no expensive tests or clinical resources are required, and
- there can be considerable observer variability of patients' physical status

Table 3.2 The ASA classification.

ASA class	Definition	Pooled mortality (%)
I	Healthy	0–0.3
II	Mild systemic disease with no functional limitation	0.3–1.4
III	Severe systemic disease with functional limitation	1.8–5.4
IV	Severe systemic disease – constant threat to life	7.8–25.0
V	Moribund patient – unlikely to survive 24 h with or without operation	9.4–57.8
E	Suffix added to denote emergency operation	

Important points not taken into account are:

- age – some add an extra grade for ages >75,
- complexity of operation,
- duration of operation, and
- whether the disease process is incidental or associated to the current illness.

Wolters *et al.* [32] investigated the ASA classification along with perioperative risk factors to see if any predictions could be drawn regarding postoperative outcome and complications. Factors seen to correlate with increasing ASA class included:

- intraoperative blood loss,
- duration of operation,
- duration of postoperative ventilation,
- postoperative wound and urinary tract infections,
- length of ICU and hospital stay,
- rates of pulmonary and cardiac complications, and
- in-hospital mortality.

The variables found to be most important for predicting complications were a high ASA class, having a major operation, and having an emergency operation.

Many retrospective studies and a couple of prospective studies have demonstrated a correlation between ASA and perioperative mortality – justifying the use of ASA as a crude predictor of patient outcome.

Goldman's Cardiac Risk Index [12]

Goldman and colleagues took 1001 surgical patients and allocated a point value to 9 different clinical risk factors. Four risk classes were defined on the basis of the total points scored. The Goldman cardiac risk index is shown in Table 3.3.

Although this index is easy to use, it has some limitations.

- It was developed from data originating in the 1970s, and as such it does not reflect modern practice in anesthesia, medicine, or surgery.
- The study population contained few vascular patients, and as such its application to that subset of patients is unproven.

Table 3.3 The Goldman cardiac risk index. Adapted from [12].

History			
Age > 70		5 points	
Pre-operative MI within 6 months		10 points	
Physical examination			
S3 gallop or increased JVP > 12 cm H_2O		11 points	
Significant valvular aortic stenosis		3 points	
ECG			
Rhythm other than sinus		7 points	
VPBs > 5/min at any time		7 points	
General medical status — one or more		3 points	
$PO_2 < 60$ or $PCO_2 > 50$ mmHg			
Serum K < 3.0 or $HCO_3 < 20$ mmol l^{-1}			
Urea > 18 mmol l^{-1} or Cr > 240 mcmol l^{-1}			
Abnormal AST			
Chronic liver disease or debilitation			
Operation			
Intraperitoneal, intrathoracic, aortic		3 points	
Emergency		4 points	
Total points possible		53 points	
Group	*Score*	*Complications (%)*	*Deaths (%)*
I	0–5 points	0.7	0.2
II	6–12 points	5	1.5
III	13–25 points	11	2.3
IV	26–53 points	22	56

- The study group contained only elective cases.
- The index overestimated the incidence of cardiac morbidity in Class IV patients undergoing noncardiac surgery.
- The index underestimated the risk in Class I and II patients undergoing aortic surgery.

In 1986, Detsky *et al.* published a modification to this risk index: The Modified Cardiac Risk Index [33]. It incorporated a number of other clinical conditions, namely:

- Canadian Cardiovascular Society angina Classes III and IV,
- unstable angina, and
- history of pulmonary edema.

Since then, other authors have suggested the inclusion of further investigations, such as coronary perfusion scans or dobutamine stress echocardiography, as a means of improving the sensitivity and specificity of the test.

Revised Goldman Cardiac Risk Index

The Revised Cardiac Risk Index was introduced by Lee *et al.* [29] in 1999. This index, looking at the risk of major cardiac complications, was derived from a population of 4000 patients undergoing nonemergency, noncardiac surgery.

Six independent predictors of major cardiac complications were used in combination to stratify patients into four classes.

- High-risk type of surgery (includes any intraperitoneal, intrathoracic or suprainguinal vascular procedures).
- History of IHD (previous MI or a positive exercise test, current complaint of chest pain considered to be cardiac in origin, use of nitrate therapy, or ECG with pathological Q waves; do not count prior coronary revascularization unless one of the other criteria for IHD is present).
- History of CHF.
- History of cerebrovascular disease.
- Diabetes mellitus requiring treatment with insulin.
- Preoperative serum creatinine >2.0 mg dl^{-1} (177 mcmol l^{-1}).

The rate of major cardiac complications (MI, pulmonary edema, ventricular fibrillation or primary cardiac arrest, or complete heart block) was assessed according to the number of predictors [34]:

- no risk factors = 0.4% (95% CI 0.1–0.8),
- one risk factor = 1.1% (95% CI 0.5–1.4),
- two risk factors = 4.6% (95% CI 1.3–3.5),
- three risk factors = 9.7% (95% CI 2.8–7.9).

Patients with no or one risk factor accounted for 75% of the population, and had an overall risk of 1.5% of developing a major cardiac complication.

Patients with two risk factors accounted for 18% of the population, and had an overall risk of 4.6% of developing a major cardiac complication.

Patients with three or more risk factors accounted for 7% of the population, and had an overall risk of 9.7% of developing a major cardiac complication.

The advantages of this index over earlier scoring systems include:

- only six prognostic factors are involved,
- simple variables,
- dependent on presence or absence of conditions rather than estimating disease severity,
- less reliant on clinical judgment,
- could easily be incorporated into preoperative evaluation forms.

The disadvantages of this system are:

- it is not applicable to emergency surgery,
- it is not applicable to lower-risk populations,
- it may not be as reliable for pre-selected high-risk populations, such as patients undergoing major vascular surgery.

APACHE systems – Acute Physiology and Chronic Health Evaluation

APACHE II and III are scoring systems used widely in ICUs. They are not suitable as preoperative risk prediction tools as the score needs to be generated from 12 physiological variables taken from the first 24 h of care. It also incorporates age and previous health status.

POSSUM

Physiological and Operative Severity Score for the enUmeration of Mortality and Morbidity (POSSUM) was developed in 1991 by Copeland *et al.* [35] for audit purposes. The idea was to adjust the risk of a surgical procedure based on the patient's physiological condition, and therefore allow more accurate comparison of units (or individuals') performance. Originally 62 physiological parameters were investigated and multi-variate analysis was used to find the most powerful predictors. This was reduced to 12 physiological variables and 6 operative severity score factors. It is reliant on outcome for the final score. With this in mind, it is therefore not suitable for preoperative risk prediction.

- It is, however, becoming more widely used in the UK, as surgical culture moves more towards outcome measures and providing the patient with as much information as possible to make informed consent.
- It is used as a means of comparing hospitals for audit purposes.
- The risk-adjusted prediction is becoming an essential tool for comparing a unit's performance for clinical governance reviews.
- The score may overpredict mortality in low-risk patients.
- It does not predict mortality accurately for ruptured aortic aneurysms [36].
- POSSUM is better than APACHE II in predicting mortality in high-dependency unit (HDU) patients [37].
- In colorectal surgery, the predicted mortality with POSSUM accurately reflects actual mortality [38].

POSSUM used an exponential analysis and as previously mentioned did overpredict mortality in a subset of patients, especially very low-risk patients. In an effort to counteract this effect, the original POSSUM equation was modified leading to the Portsmouth predictor equation for mortality (P-POSSUM) utilizing the same physiological and operative variables. This method used linear analysis. The P-POSSUM model still overpredicts mortality in low-risk groups, but is a better "fit" than POSSUM. There have also been reports that mortality in different surgical specialities may be overpredicted. This has led some to produce speciality-specific POSSUM, such as V-POSSUM for use in elective vascular surgery.

Comparison of scoring systems

- 2035 patients referred for medical consultation before elective or urgent noncardiac surgery were scored with the ASA, Goldman, Detsky and Canadian Cardiovascular Society indices. Myocardial infarction, unstable angina, acute pulmonary edema, or death occurred in 6.4% of patients. The prediction of cardiac complications was better than chance, but no index was significantly superior [39].

- 16 227 patients were studied [40]. Within 4 weeks of operation, 215 died. Both indices correlated significantly with perioperative mortality, the ASA grade showing a closer correlation. The combination of the two scores increased the accuracy of prediction of perioperative mortality.

Individual clinician-based patient assessment

- This is a clinical philosophy that is gaining increasing acceptance as a valid alternative to the use of rigid risk scoring systems and guidelines.
- It relies on the history, physical examination and acquired clinical experience to identify potential markers of increased risk.
- The difference between this approach and the use of scoring systems is that clinicians have a unique ability to integrate the numerous other factors surrounding the patients' presentation for surgery that contribute to perioperative risk, but would be impossible to quantify and validate in a scoring system.
- The result is a clinician-based assessment of risk that is specifically tailored to each individual patient. Diagnostic testing and risk-reduction strategies are then *selectively* instigated, according to this experience, where clinical and financial resources permit.
- Clinician-based judgment strategies are thus adaptable to individual clinical situations, rather than rigidly applying an index score alone when estimating perioperative risk.
- This philosophy maintains that risk scoring systems and guidelines are most useful, therefore, only as guides for inexperienced clinicians.

American College of Cardiologists/American Heart Association Guidelines

In 2007 the American College of Cardiologists and the American Heart Association (ACC/ AHA) revised their guidelines first produced in 1980. A task force comprising of experts in all related fields was set up to examine current practice and evaluate the most up-to-date literature. Subsequent to this, updated guidelines relating to cardiovascular disease and procedures were published [41].

- The original guidelines reflected the failings of the scoring systems and were designed to provide central, evidenced-based advice as a strategy to reduce litigation claims for suboptimal preoperative management in the USA.
- They were also an attempt to rationalize the increasing demand for expensive risk stratification tests being requested as part of routine preoperative assessments.
- The overriding theme of these guidelines is that revascularization is rarely necessary to simply lower the risk of surgery. It should not usually be undertaken unless there are clear indications for revascularization according to the guidelines for treatment of MI and acute coronary syndrome (ACS).
- The purpose of the preoperative evaluation is to assess the patient's current medical status, make recommendations regarding the evaluation, management, and risk of cardiac problems over the entire perioperative period; also to provide a clinical risk profile of the patient.

- No test should be performed unless it is likely to influence the patient treatment, either by changing the surgical procedure to be performed, or by instigating a change in medical treatment so as to optimize the patient's condition, thereby reducing the perioperative risk.

- High-risk patients should be identified and a plan can then be drawn up for not just perioperative management, but for postoperative management too. It may be evident that an elective stay in ICU or HDU for more intensive monitoring and management is appropriate.

General approach to the patient

The guidelines are aimed at evaluating the patient undergoing noncardiac surgery who is at risk of perioperative cardiac morbidity or mortality. Those at highest risk are those with known CAD and those with symptoms or signs suggestive of CAD. The asymptomatic over the age of 50 requires further scrutiny of their history and physical examination in order to ascertain whether there are any indicators of increased risk present as directed by the Revised Cardiac Risk Index [29].

- In a study of patients that were thought of as having an increased cardiac risk, 146 patients were sent for a cardiological opinion. In only 3.4% of patients did the consultation reveal a new finding that would have an effect on the perioperative outcome [42].

- In the emergency setting, our evaluation of the cardiovascular system may be more rudimentary, encompassing vital signs, volume status, hematocrit, electrolytes, renal function, urine analysis and ECG.

History

CAD or comorbidity associated with CAD should be concentrated upon.

- Specifically, the history should identify unstable coronary syndromes, prior angina, recent or past MI, CCF, significant arrhythmias and valve disease.

- The functional capacity of the patient should be ascertained. This has been shown to correlate well with oxygen uptake by treadmill testing [43]. Patients with good functional status have a lower risk of cardiac complications.

- Functional status can be expressed as metabolic equivalents. 1 MET is defined as 3.5 ml oxygen uptake/kg/min. This is the resting oxygen uptake in a sitting position.

Perioperative cardiac risk and long-term risk is increased if a patient cannot achieve at least a 4 MET demand. Various activity scales allow the clinician to determine a patient's functional capacity [44]. Table 3.4 shows METs appropriate for different levels of activities.

More accurate estimations of metabolic equivalents can be made from the Duke activity index [45] in Table 3.5.

Another method of classifying functional capacity for those patients with known cardiac disease is the New York Heart Association (NYHA) classification [46] as shown in Table 3.6.

- Poor functional capacity may not necessarily have a cardiac cause. It may have a respiratory cause, or be caused by peripheral vascular disease or musculoskeletal disease, such as arthritis in the lower limbs.

Table 3.4 METs for different activities. Adapted from [44].

Can take care of self such as eat, dress or use toilet	(1 MET)
Can walk up a flight of steps or a hill	(4 METs)
Can do heavy work around the house, such as scrubbing floors or moving heavy furniture	(4–10 METs)
Can participate in strenuous sports such as swimming, tennis, football, basketball and skiing	(>10 METs)

Table 3.5 The Duke activity index. Adapted from [45].

Activity	Weighting	MET value
Poor		
Walk indoors around the house	1.75	<4
Do light work around the house – strip and make a bed	2.70	
Take care of self – eating, dressing, bathing	2.75	
Intermediate		
Walk one or two blocks on the flat	2.75	4–7
Do moderate housework – sweeping, vacuuming or carrying shopping	3.50	
Do garden work – raking leaves, weeding or mowing the lawn	4.50	
Having sexual relations	5.25	
Climb a flight of stairs or walk uphill	5.50	
Play golf, bowling, dancing, football	6.0	
Good		
Go swimming, play tennis, skiing	7.5	>7
Run a short distance at 5 mph	8.0	
Do heavy housework – scrubbing floors, lifting/moving heavy furniture	8.0	

- The combination of good functional status, absence of known cardiovascular disease, and a low score on one of the multi-factorial risk indices questionnaires is associated with a very low rate of major complications even in patients undergoing major vascular surgery.

Physical examination

The examination of the cardiovascular system should include an assessment of vital signs (BP in both arms), carotid pulse contour and bruits, jugular venous pressure and pulsations, auscultation of the lungs, precordial auscultation and palpation, abdominal palpation and examination of the extremities for edema and vascular integrity. The presence of an implanted pacemaker or defibrillator should also be noted.

The history and physical examination are the most important aspects of assessing the patient's status and therefore risk. Further investigations or tests can be planned following the relevant findings.

Table 3.6 New York Heart Association (NYHA) classification. Adapted from [46].

Class	Description
I	Patients with cardiac disease but without resulting limitation of physical activity due to fatigue, palpitations, dyspnea or angina
II	Patients with cardiac disease resulting in slight limitation in physical activity
III	Patients with marked limitation of physical activity
IV	Patients with cardiac disease who are unable to carry out any physical activity without discomfort. Symptoms of angina or heart failure may be present at rest

Clinical predictors of coronary risk

The ACC/AHA guideline summary describes clinical predictors of increased perioperative cardiovascular risk (MI, heart failure and death) [44].

Major predictors that require intensive management and may lead to delay or cancellation of the operative procedure unless emergent:

- acute MI (within 7 days) in patients with evidence of important ischemic risk as determined by symptoms or noninvasive testing;
- recent MI (within 8–30 days) in patients with evidence of important ischemic risk as determined by symptoms or noninvasive testing;
- unstable angina;
- severe angina (Canadian Cardiovascular Society class III or IV); may include patients with stable angina who are usually sedentary;
- decompensated heart failure;
- high-grade atrioventricular block;
- symptomatic ventricular arrhythmias in patients who have underlying heart disease;
- supraventricular arrhythmias with a poorly controlled ventricular rate;
- severe heart valve disease.

Intermediate predictors that warrant careful assessment of current status:

- mild angina pectoris (Canadian Cardiovascular Society class I or II);
- previous MI as determined from the history or the presence of pathologic Q waves;
- compensated heart failure or a prior history of heart failure;
- diabetes mellitus, particularly in patients who are insulin-dependent;
- reduced renal function, which is defined as a serum creatinine $> 2.0 \, \text{mg} \, \text{dl}^{-1}$ ($177 \, \text{mcmol} \, \text{l}^{-1}$) or a $> 50\%$ increase above normal baseline concentration.

Minor predictors that have not been proven to independently increase perioperative risk. Patients with minor predictors do not usually require any further noninvasive testing.

- Advanced age.
- Abnormal ECG (left ventricular hypertrophy, left bundle branch block, ST-T abnormalities).

- Rhythm other than sinus rhythm (e.g. atrial fibrillation).
- Low functional capacity (e.g. inability to climb one flight of stairs with a bag of shopping).
- History of stroke.
- Uncontrolled systolic hypertension.

Surgical risk

The type and timing of surgery significantly affects the risk of perioperative cardiac complications. The 2002 ACC/AHA guidelines stratify the risk by procedure [44].

High-risk procedure → 5% risk of cardiac death or non-fatal MI:

- emergent major operations, particularly in elderly patients;
- aortic and other major vascular surgery;
- peripheral arterial surgery;
- anticipated prolonged surgical procedures associated with large fluid shifts and/or blood loss.

Intermediate risk procedure → 1–5% risk:

- carotid endarterectomy;
- head and neck surgery;
- intraperitoneal and intrathoracic surgery;
- orthopedic surgery;
- prostate surgery.

Low-risk procedure → < 1% risk:

- endoscopic procedures;
- superficial procedures;
- cataract surgery;
- breast surgery.

Emergency surgery → 2–5 times the risk [47].

Low-risk procedures are usually short, with minimal fluid shifts, while higher-risk operations tend to be prolonged with large fluid shifts and greater potential for postoperative myocardial ischemia and respiratory depression.

Noninvasive tests to stratify cardiovascular risk

12-Lead electrocardiogram (ECG)

A resting ECG is a helpful baseline piece of information. It may show signs of acute ischemia or previous ischemia. Presence of Q waves, both extent and magnitude, are a crude estimate of LVEF and a predictor of long-term mortality [48]. LV hypertrophy or ST segment depression or elevation have been associated with increased incidence of cardiac complications. It may reveal an underlying conduction defect or arrhythmia. Patients who should have an ECG are:

- those with at least one risk factor, and are undergoing a vascular procedure (Class I recommendation);
- those with a recent history of chest pain or an ischemic equivalent who are considered to be at intermediate or high risk and are scheduled for an intermediate to high-risk procedure (Class I recommendation);
- asymptomatic patients with diabetes mellitus (Class IIa recommendation);
- patients who have undergone previous coronary revascularization (Class IIb recommendation);
- asymptomatic men above age 45 and asymptomatic women above age 55 who have two or more risk factors for atherosclerosis (Class IIb recommendation);
- may be reasonable in patients with one risk factor who are undergoing an intermediate-risk operative procedure (Class IIb recommendation); and
- patients who have had prior hospital admission for cardiovascular disease (Class IIb recommendation).

Although the ideal time prior to surgery that an ECG should be obtained is unknown, it is generally agreed that if the disease process is stable then within 30 days of surgery is acceptable.

Ambulatory electrocardiographic monitoring

This allows a 24 h monitor of the ECG, measuring the variables throughout the patient's daily routine. It can also be a way of capturing electrical evidence of transient or unpredictable symptoms.

This is not a good test to further stratify a high-risk patient [49].

Assessment of left ventricular function

- Should be assessed in patients with dyspnea of unknown origin (Class IIa recommendation).
- Should be assessed in patients with prior history of CHF if not assessed in the previous 12 months or if symptoms are deteriorating (Class IIa recommendation).
- There is no need to re-assess patients with cardiomyopathy if the symptoms are stable (Class IIb recommendation).

The methods available for assessment of LV function are radionuclide angiography, echocardiography and contrast ventriculography.

Poor LV function preoperatively correlates well with postoperative CHF and death, especially so in critically ill patients. The same does not correlate well to prediction of ischemic events postoperatively [50].

Stress testing

Many patients with coronary artery disease will have a relatively normal looking resting 12-lead ECG. Maybe up to 50% of patients with single vessel coronary artery disease will have a normal looking ECG even whilst undergoing gentle to moderate exercise [51]. However, it is how the heart behaves under stress that is much more important to us. What is the functional capacity of the heart? Just how ischemic does it become, and under what degree of stress does this occur? How well does the myocardium recover?

These questions may be answered by putting the heart under some degree of stress in a controlled environment. There are a number of ways of achieving this effect.

Patients who should be considered for stress testing are:

- those with active cardiac conditions (ACS, CHF, arrythmias, severe valve disease) (Class I recommendation);

- those having vascular surgery if they have 3 or more risk factors or if their functional capacity is reduced below 4 METs (Class IIa recommedation); and

- those with 1 or 2 risk factors and poor functional capacity (less than 4 METs) who are due to undergo at least intermediate-risk surgery (Class IIb recommendation).

There are a number of ways in which we can stress the heart, and it will depend on some patient factors and local resources as to which modality is used. Physical exercise is used if the patient is able and they have an ECG which is amenable to this form of study.

Exercise stress testing

The commonest form of exercise stress testing is on a treadmill following the Bruce protocol. This is a standardized exercise test, gradually becoming more difficult over a period of time. The ECG and hemodynamic responses are analyzed. If the patient already has an abnormal ECG (e.g. left bundle branch block, LV hypertrophy with "strain" pattern, or digitalis effect) then it is difficult to interpret this test and an alternative method of assessing myocardial ischemia should be used. This test does, however, give a good estimation of the functional capacity of the patient.

Becoming more popular is the cardiopulmonary exercise testing (CPX) regime. This combines exercise, usually in the form of a bicycle to pedal, but it can be modified so patients can use their arms to perform the exercise, especially so in patients with musculoskeletal limitations. This modality not only analyzes the ECG, but also utilizes spirometry and analyzes inspired and expired gases from the lungs. This gives us much more useful information than the standard treadmill test. It is not yet available in most institutions, certainly across the UK.

Nonexercise Stress Testing

The two commonest techniques in current practise are the dodutamine stress echocardiogram and the intravenous dipyridamole/adenosine myocardial perfusion imaging with both thallium-201 and technetium-99 m. When compared, these two modalities were both able to detect moderate-to-large defects, and these were the defects that predict postoperative MI and death [52].

- Dobutamine stress echocardiography has become the method of choice for pharmacological stress testing coupled with ultrasound imaging. This modality allows visualization of the myocardium under stressful conditions. Wall motion abnormalities can be directly observed and quantified in relation to the supplying blood vessels. Fixed and reversible defects are also visualized. Atropine may be incorporated to enhance the chronotropic effect. Studies have shown that wall motion abnormalities at low ischemic threshold and at less than 60% of maximum age-related heart rate is a predictor of adverse events in both the long and short term postoperatively [53, 54].

- Radionuclide perfusion imaging shows areas of the myocardium with perfusion defects. It shows fixed defects and defects that appear when the myocardium is stressed. Fixed defects tend not to be predictive of untoward perioperative cardiac events, unlike reversible defects. Reversible defects of increasing size tend to predict increasing perioperative risk [55]. Fixed defects tend to be more likely to predict long-term cardiac events [56].

- In those patients not deemed suitable for dobutamine stress transthoracic echocardiography, dobutamine stress magnetic resonance imaging has been used successfully to identify myocardial ischemia [57].
- Patients that can be shown to have inducible myocardial ischemia are at a 20% risk of an adverse cardiac event compared to 2% in those who do not have inducible ischemia [58].
- Approximately 15% of those patients tested by pharmacological stress testing of any form reveal a positive test [59].

Invasive testing

Coronary angiography is part of the preoperative investigations required by the cardiologist and the cardiothoracic surgeon when deciding what form of revascularization is indicated: angioplasty, stent insertion, or coronary artery bypass surgery.

- This is an investigation usually reserved for the patients who have positive results from the above selection of investigations and are therefore, by definition, extremely high-risk for an adverse cardiac event.
- They must also fulfill the criteria for coronary revascularization independently of their need for noncardiac surgery.

Preoperative revascularization

Prophylactic coronary revascularization in patients with asymptomatic CAD before major noncardiac surgery has no benefit, whether by percutaneous coronary intervention (PCI) or coronary artery bypass grafting (CABG) [60, 61].

CABG or PCI prior to noncardiac surgery are indicated according to the ACC/AHA 2004 guidelines [62].

CABG

Class I indications for CABG:

- patients with stable angina who have significant left main coronary artery stenosis (level A evidence);
- patients with stable angina who have 3 vessel disease. There is greater benefit if LVEF is less than 0.5 (level A evidence);
- patients with stable angina who have 2 vessel disease with significant proximal LAD stenosis and either LVEF less than 0.5 or demonstrable ischemia on noninvasive testing (level A evidence);
- patients with high-risk unstable angina or non-ST segment elevation MI (level A evidence); and
- patients with acute ST elevation MI (level A evidence).

In summary, patients who are found to have prognostic high-risk coronary anatomy and in whom long-term outcome would likely be improved by CABG should undergo revascularization prior to undergoing elective vascular surgery or intermediate- to high-risk noncardiac surgery.

PCI

- There is currently no proven benefit in performing prophylactic PCI in patients with Canadian Cardiovascular Society class III angina [63, 64].

- Preoperative PCI (angioplasty or stent insertion) should be limited to those who have unstable CAD who would be eligible for revascularization according to the ACC/AHA guidelines for PCI and CABG [62, 64]. In those patients where emergency noncardiac surgery was imminent, then balloon angioplasty or bare metal stenting should be considered.

- Following balloon angioplasty the noncardiac surgery should be performed within 8 weeks as restenosis of the angioplasty site rates increase after that. However, having said that, performing the noncardiac surgery too soon after PCI may also be hazardous. Arterial recoil or acute thrombosis tends to occur in the first few hours to days following angioplasty. The recommended timing, therefore, for a noncardiac surgical procedure to be performed is 2–4 weeks following angioplasty [65].

Coronary artery stents and noncardiac surgery

Since first described in 1977 there have been some important developments in the field of percutaneous coronary intervention (PCI), initially with balloon angioplasty alone, and now in combination with coronary stent insertion [66]. There are currently two types of stent being deployed: bare metal stents (BMS) and drug-eluting stents (DES).

- Re-stenosis following neointimal hyperplasia complicates BMS in 12–20% of cases, commonly in the first 3–6 months [67]. DES were designed to prevent re-stenosis by eluting a substance that inhibits smooth muscle proliferation and neointimal hyperplasia within the stented segment [68]. The re-stenosis rate was cut to 5% [69].

- The use of DES expanded rapidly and by 2004 one study showed that in the USA 80% [70] of stents were DES, and worldwide almost 6 million patients had a DES implanted [71]. Currently, DES are coated with either sirolimus or paclitaxel.

- Stent thrombosis is usually a significant clinical event and is a potentially devastating complication carrying a 50% MI risk and a 20% mortality [72]. The overall stent thrombosis rate after 4-year follow up is 3% and did not differ between BMS and DES [73].

- Patients with stents therefore are put on various combinations of anti-platelet medication [74]. Clopidogrel and aspirin are currently recommended; the aspirin is for life, and the clopidogrel depends on the stent, and is still much debated.

- Premature cessation of these drugs is the largest risk factor for stent thrombosis [75]. This risk is greatest for those patients with a recently implanted stent that is poorly endothelialized, or those that have had a recent acute coronary syndrome (ACS) [76].

- There have been a number of studies that show that noncardiac surgery within 2 weeks of BMS placement is the most high-risk period for stent thrombosis, and the risk is much reduced after a period of 6 weeks has lapsed [77, 78]. Some studies recommend 4 weeks delay [79, 80].

Table 3.7 Management approach to patients with previous PCI. Adapted from [41].

Balloon angioplasty	<14 days	Delay elective/nonurgent surgery
	>14 days	Proceed to surgery with aspirin
Bare metal stent	<30–45 days	Delay elective/nonurgent surgery
	>30–45 days	Proceed to surgery with aspirin
Drug-eluting stent	<365 days	Delay elective/nonurgent surgery
	>365 days	Proceed to surgery with aspirin

- The combination of stopping anti-platelet therapy and the hypercoagulable perioperative state and a poorly endothelialized stent leads to a high risk of acute stent thrombosis, which is associated with considerable morbidity and mortality [75, 76].
- Clopidogrel and aspirin have a synergistic effect [81], and the effect of not stopping these drugs for cardiac surgery is the increased risk of bleeding and a greater need for blood product transfusion [82].
- There is hardly any evidence for noncardiac surgery that shows increased deep bleeding, except for bruising and ooze at the wound edges [83].
- There needs to be a complete assessment of the patient's hemorrhagic risk balanced against the thrombotic risk.
- There should be consultation between surgeon, anesthetist, cardiologist and maybe hematologist.

The short-acting glycoprotein IIb/IIIa agent tirofiban has been used in conjuction with unfractionated heparin as a method of maintaining low thrombosis risk whilst allowing the clopidogrel to be stopped perioperatively so as to reduce the risk of intraoperative hemorrhage. There are various regimens being used with the disadvantage of requiring the patient to be admitted to hospital for a number of days preoperatively [84]. It is usually acceptable to continue aspirin throughout the perioperative period.

A summary of management approach to patients with previous PCI who are due to undergo noncardiac surgery [41] is shown in Table 3.7.

Perioperative optimization of medical therapy

This more common alternative to revascularization is discussed in Chapters 4 and 5.

Emergency surgery

Occasionally a patient may present for emergency life-saving noncardiac surgery, but is also at very high risk of perioperative MI. This may be because they have already had a recent MI, because there is no time to optimize their medical management, or because they have severe 3-vessel coronary artery disease or critical left main stem disease requiring revascularization. There is no proven way of reducing the very high risk involved in this scenario. There have been a number of case reports describing the use of the intra-aortic balloon pump (IABP) for such patients [85, 86].

The IABP, first introduced in 1962, is a device usually inserted via the femoral artery which allows a balloon to be positioned in the aorta.

- During diastole the balloon is inflated, leading to an increase in the aortic diastolic pressure.
- This in turn leads to an augmentation of the coronary artery blood flow, resulting in an increase in myocardial oxygen supply without an increase in myocardial workload.
- In systole the balloon is deflated and this leads to a reduction in aortic root pressure.
- This produces a reduction in the afterload.
- In turn, this reduction in LV workload decreases the oxygen consumption of the LV and increases the cardiac output.

This procedure is not without its complications. Limb ischemia, thromboembolic events, rest pain, femoral artery dissection and false aneurysm formation have all been described.

Perioperative myocardial infarction

- The incidence varies according to the underlying patient risk.
- There is no standard diagnostic criteria for perioperative MI after noncardiac surgery. The diagnosis is made more difffcult as only 14% of patients have chest pain and only 53% have any sign or symptom at all [87].
- The ECG and biomarkers of cardiac damage (troponins) play an important role, alongside a high index of suspicion.
- Patients with a perioperative MI have an increased in-hospital stay and longer-term mortality.

Given that the symptoms are atypical and sometimes not present at all, the only way of detecting many postoperative MIs, and subsequently predicting a greater long-term mortality, would be to do serial troponin levels and serial ECG for 3 days after surgery. This is not a common practice [87].

Further reading

Fleisher LA, Beckman JA, Brown KA, *et al*. ACC/AHA Task Force. ACC/AHA 2007 Guidelines on Perioperative Cardiovascular Evaluation and Care for Non-Cardiac Surgery. A Report of the American College of Cardiology/American Heart Association Task Force on Practice Guidelines. *Circulation* 2007; **116**: e418–99.

References

1. Ross R. Atherosclerosis – an inflammatory disease. *N Engl J Med* 1999; **340**: 115–26.

2. Goldman L, Caldera D, Nussbaum S, *et al*. Multifactorial index of cardiac risk in non-cardiac surgical procedures. *New Engl J Med* 1977; **297**: 845.

3. Mangano DT, Goldman L. Pre-operative assessment of patients with known or suspected coronary disease. *New Engl J Med* 1995; **333**: 1750.

4. Devereaux PJ, Goldman L, Cook DJ, *et al*. Perioperative cardiac events in patients undergoing non-cardiac surgery: a review of the magnitude of the problem, the pathophysiology of the events and methods to estimate and communicate risk. *CMAJ* 2005; **173**: 627.

5. Wong T, Detsky A. pre-operative cardiac risk assessment for patients having peripheral vascular surgery. *Ann Intern Med* 1992; **116**: 743.

6. Poeze M, Takala J, Greve JWM, Ramsay G. Pre-operative tonometry is predictive for mortality and morbidity in high-risk surgical patients. *Int Care Med* 2000; **26**: 1272–81.

7. Castelli WP. Epidemiology of coronary heart disease: the Framingham study. *Am J Med* 1984; **76**: 4–12.

8. Becker RC, Terrin M, Ross R, *et al.* and the Thrombolysis in Myocardial Infarction Investigators. Comparison of clinical outcomes for women and men after acute myocardial infarction. *Ann Intern Med* 1994; **120**: 638–45.

9. Shah KB, Kleinman BS, Rao TLK, *et al.* Angina and other risk factors in patients with cardiac diseases undergoing non-cardiac operations. *Anesth Analg* 1990; **70**: 240–7.

10. Campeau L. Grading of angina pectoris. *Circulation* 1976; **54**: 522–3.

11. Howell SJ, Sear JW, Foëx P. Hypertension, hypertensive heart disease and perioperative cardiac risk. *Br J Anaesth* 2004; **92**: 570–83.

12. Goldman L, Caldera DL, Nussbaum SR, *et al.* Multifactorial index of cardiac risk in non-cardiac surgical procedures. *N Engl J Med* 1977; **297**: 845–50.

13. Eagle KA, Brundage BH, Chaitman BR, *et al.* Guidelines for peri-operative cardiovascular evaluation for non-cardiac surgery: an abridged version of the report of the American College of Cardiologists/American Heart Association Task Force on Practice Guidelines. *J Am Coll Cardiol* 1996; **27**: 910–48.

14. Cuthbertson BH, Amiri AR, Croal BL, *et al.* Utility of B-type natriuretic peptide in predicting perioperative cardiac events in patients undergoing major non-cardiac surgery. *Br J Anaesth* 2007; **99**: 170–6.

15. Raymer K, Yang H. Patients with aortic stenosis: cardiac complications in non-cardiac surgery. *Can J Anaesth* 1998; **45**: 855–9.

16. Reyes VP, Raju BS, Wynne J, Stephenson, *et al.* Percutaneous balloon valvuloplasty compared with open surgical commissurotomy for mitral stenosis. *N Engl J Med* 1994; **331**: 961–7.

17. Roth RB, Palacios IF, Block PC. Percutaneous aortic balloon valvuloplasty: its role in the management of patients with aortic stenosis requiring major non-cardiac surgery. *J Am Coll Cardiol* 1989; **13**: 1039–41.

18. Farshi R, Kistner D, Sarma JS, Longmate JA, Singh BN. Ventricular rate control in chronic atrial fibrillation during daily activity and programmed exercise: a crossover open-label study of five drug regimens. *J Am Coll Cardiol* 1999; **33**: 304–10.

19. Balser JR, Martinez EA, Winters BD, *et al.* Beta-adrenergic blockade accelerates conversion of postoperative supraventricular tachyarrhythmias. *Anesthesiology* 1998; **89**: 1052–9.

20. Mahla E, Rotman B, Rehak P, *et al.* Perioperative ventricular dysrhythmias in patients with structural heart disease undergoing non-cardiac surgery. *Anesth Analg* 1998; **86**: 16–21.

21. Bayliff CD, Massel DR, Inculet RI, *et al.* Propranolol for the prevention of postoperative arrhythmias in general thoracic surgery. *Ann Thorac Surg* 1999; **67**: 182–6.

22. ACC/AHA guidelines for implantation of cardiac pacemakers and anti-arrhythmia devices: a report of the American College of Cardiology/American Heart Association Task Force on Assessment of Diagnostic and Therapeutic Cardiovascular Procedures (Committee on Pacemaker Implantation). *J Am Coll Cardiol* 1991; **18**: 1–13.

23. Dorman T, Breslow MJ, Pronovost PJ, *et al.* Bundle-branch block as a risk factor in noncardiac surgery. *Arch Intern Med* 2000; **160**: 1149–52.

24. Practice advisory for the perioperative management of patients with cardiac rhythm management devices: pacemakers and implantable cardioverter-defibrillators: a report by the American Society of Anesthesiologists Task Force on Perioperative Management of Patients with Cardiac Rhythm Management Devices. *Anesthesiology* 2005; **103**: 186–98.

25. Zaidan JR, Curling PE, Craver JM Jr. Effect of enflurane, isoflurane, and halothane on pacing stimulation thresholds in man. *Pacing Clin Electrophysiol* 1985; **8**: 32–4.

26. Alpert JS, Chipkin SR, Aronin N. Diabetes mellitus and silent myocardial ischemia. *Adv Cardiol* 1990; **37**: 279–303.

27. Charlson ME, MacKenzie CR, Gold JP, Ales KL, Topkins M, Shires GT. Risk for post-operative congestive heart failure. *Surg Gynecol Obstet* 1991; **172**: 95–104.

28. Kelly R, Staines A, Mac Walter R, *et al.* The prevalence of treatable left ventricular systolic dysfunction in patients who present with non-cardiac vascular episodes. A case-control study. *J Am Coll Cardiol* 2002; **39**: 219.

29. Lee TH, Marcantonio ER, Mangione CM, *et al.* Derivation and prospective validation of a simple index for prediction of cardiac risk of major non-cardiac surgery. *Circulation* 1999; **100**: 1043.

30. Kertai MD, Boersma E, Bax JJ, *et al.* Comparison between serum creatinine and creatinine clearance for the prediction of post-operative mortality in patients undergoing major vascular surgery. *Clin Nephrol* 2003; **59**: 17–23.

31. ASA. New classification of physical status. *Anaesthesiology* 1963; **24**: 111.

32. Wolters U, Wolf T, Stutzer H, Schroder T. ASA classification and peri-operative variables as predictors of post-operative outcome. *Br J Anaesth* 1996; **77**: 217–22.

33. Detsky AS, Abrams HB, Forbath N, *et al.* Cardiac assessment for patients undergoing non-cardiac surgery. A multifactorial clinical risk index. *Arch Int Med* 1986; **146**: 2131–4.

34. Devereaux PJ, Goldman L, Cook DJ, *et al.* Rate of cardiac death, non-fatal MI, and non-fatal cardiac arrest according to the number of predictors. *CMAJ* 2005; **173**: 627.

35. Copeland GP, Jones D, Waiters M. POSSUM: a scoring system for surgical audit. *Br J Surg* 1991; **78**: 355–60.

36. Lazarides MK, Arvanitis DP, Drista H, *et al.* POSSUM and APACHE II scores do not predict the outcome of ruptured infra-renal aortic aneurysms. *Ann Vasc Surg* 1997; **11**: 155–8.

37. Jones DR, Copeland GP, de Cossart L. Comparison of POSSUM with APACHE II for prediction of outcome from a surgical high-dependency unit. *Br J Surg* 1992; **79**: 1293–6.

38. Sagar PM, Hartley MN, Mancey-Jones B, *et al.* Comparative audit of colo-rectal resection with the POSSUM scoring system. *Br J Surg* 1994; **81**: 1492–4.

39. Gilbert K, Larocque BJ, Patrick LT. Prospective evaluation of cardiac risk indices for patients undergoing noncardiac surgery. *Ann Intern Med* 2000; **133**: 356–9.

40. Prause G, Ratzenhofer-Comenda B, Pierer G, *et al.* Can ASA grade or Goldman's cardiac risk index predict peri-operative mortality? A study of 16,227 patients. *Anaesthesia* 1997; **52**: 203–6.

41. Fleisher LA, Beckman JA, Brown KA, *et al.* ACC/AHA Task Force. ACC/AHA 2007 Guidelines on Perioperative Cardiovascular Evaluation and Care for Non-Cardiac Surgery. A Report of the American College of Cardiology/American Heart Association Task Force on Practice Guidelines. *Circulation* 2007; **116**: e418–99.

42. Katz RI, Camino L, Vitkun SA. Pre-operative medical consultations: impact on peri-operative management and surgical outcome. *Can J Anaesth* 2005; **52**: 697–702.

43. Hlaty MA, Boineau RE, Higginbotham MB, *et al.* A brief self-administered questionnaire to determine functional capacity (the Duke Activity Status Index). *Am J Cardiol* 1989; **64**: 651–4.

44. Eagle KA, Berger PB, Calkins H, *et al.* ACC/AHA guideline update for peri-operative cardiovascular evaluation for non-cardiac surgery – executive summary: a report of the American College of Cardiology/ American Heart Association Task Force on Practice Guidelines (Committee to update the 1996 Guidelines on Peri-operative Cardiovascular Evaluation for Non-cardiac Surgery). *J Am Coll Cardiol* 2002; **39**: 542.

45. Nashef SA. Patient selection and risk stratification. In: Mackay JM, Arrowsmith JE, eds. *Core Topics in Cardiac Anaesthesia.* London: Greenwich Medical Media. 2004; 97–100.

46. American Heart Association. 1994 Revisions to classification of functional capacity and objective assessment of patients with diseases of the heart.

47. Mangano D. Peri-operative cardiac morbidity. *Anesthesiology* 1990; **72**: 153.

48. Crow RS, Prineas RJ, Hannan PJ, *et al.* Prognostic associations of Minnesota Code serial electrocardiographic change classification with coronary heart disease mortality in the Multiple Risk Factor Intervention Trial. *Am J Cardiol* 1997; **80**: 138–44.

49. Fleisher LA, Rosenbaum SH, Nelson AH, Jain D, Wackers FJ, Zaret BL. Preoperative dipyridamole thallium imaging and ambulatory electrocardiographic monitoring as a predictor of perioperative cardiac events and long-term outcome. *Anesthesiology* 1995; **83**: 906–17.

50. Kertai MD, Boersma E, Baxx JJ, *et al.* A meta-analysis comparing the prognostic accuracy of six diagnostic tests for predicting perioperative cardiac risk in patients undergoing major vascular surgery. *Heart* 2003; **89**: 1327–34.

51. Chaitman BR. The changing role of the exercise electrocardiogram as a diagnostic and prognostic test for chronic ischaemic heart disease. *J Am Coll Cardiol* 1986; **8**: 1195–210.

52. Beattie WS, Abdelnaem E, Wijeysundera DN, *et al.* A meta-analytic comparison of preoperative stress echocardiography and nuclear scintigraphy imaging. *Anesth Analg* 2006; **102**: 8–16.

53. Day SM, Younger JG, Karavite D, *et al.* Usefulness of hypotension during dobutamine echocardiography in predicting perioperative cardiac events. *Am J Cardiol* 2000; **85**: 478–83.

54. Kertai MD, Boersma E, Bax JJ, *et al.* Optimizing long-term cardiac management after major vascular surgery: role of beta-blocker therapy, clinical characteristics, and dobutamine stress echocardiography to optimize long-term cardiac management after major vascular surgery. *Arch Intern Med* 2003; **163**: 2230–5.

55. Bigatel DA, Franklin DP, Elmore JR, *et al.* Dobutamine stress echocardiography prior to aortic surgery: long-term cardiac outcome. *Ann Vasc Surg* 1999; **13**: 17–22.

56. Lette J, Waters D, Cerino M, *et al.* Preoperative coronary artery disease risk stratification based on dipyridamole imaging and a simple three-step, three-segment model for patients undergoing non-cardiac vascular surgery or major general surgery. *Am J Cardiol* 1992; **69**: 1553–8.

57. Shaw LJ, Eagle KA, Gersh BJ, *et al.* Meta-analysis of intravenous dipyridamole-thallium-201 imagin (1985–1994) and dobutamine echocardiography (1991–1994) for risk stratification before vascular surgery. *J Am Coll Cardiol* 1996; **27**: 787–98.

58. Nagel E, Lehmkuhl HB, Bocksch W, *et al.* Non-invasive diagnosis of ischemia-induced wall motion abnormalities with the use of high-dose dobutamine stress MRI: comparison with dobutamine stress echocardiography. *Circulation* 1999; **99**: 763–70.

59. Fleisher LA, Rosenbaum SH, Nelson AH, Jain D, Wackers FJ, Zaret BL. Preoperative dipyridamole thallium imaging and ambulatory electrocardiographic monitoring as a predictor of perioperative cardiac events and long-term outcome. *Anesthesiology* 1995; **83**: 906–17.

60. Mason JJ, Owens DK, Harris RA, Cooke JP, Hlatky MA. The role of coronary angiography and coronary revascularization before non-cardiac vascular surgery. *JAMA* 1995; **273**: 1919–25.

61. McFalls EO, Ward HB, Moritz TE, *et al.* Coronary artery revascularization before elective major vascular surgery. *N Engl J Med* 2004; **351**: 2795–804.

62. Eagle KA, Guyton RA, Davidoff R, *et al.* ACC/AHA 2004 guideline update for coronary artery bypass graft surgery: a report of the American College of Cardiology/ American Heart Association Task Force on Practice Guidelines (Committee to Update the 1999 Guidelines for Coronary Artery Bypass Graft Surgery). *Circulation* 2004; **110**: e340–e437.

63. Poldermans D, Schouten O, Vidakovic R, *et al.* A clinical randomized trial to evaluate the safety of a noninvasive approach in high-risk patients undergoing major vascular surgery: the DECREASE-V Pilot Study. *J Am Coll Cardiol* 2007; **49**: 1763–9.

64. Smith SC, Feldman TE, Hirshfield JW, *et al.* ACC/AHA/SCAI 2005 guideline update for percutaneous coronary intervention: a report of the American College of Cardiologists/ American Heart Association Task Force on Practice Guidelines (ACC/AHA/SCAI Writing Committee to Update the 2001 Guidelines for Percutaneous Coronary Intervention). *J Am Coll Cardiol* 2006; **47**: e1–121.

65. Brilakis ES, Orford JL, Fasseas P, *et al.* Outcome of patients undergoing balloon angioplasty in the two months prior to non-cardiac surgery. *Am J Cardiol* 2005; **96**: 512–4.

66. Smith SC Jr, Feldman TE Jr, Hirshfeld JW, *et al.* ACC/ AHA/ SCAI 2005 guideline update for PCI: a report of the American College of Cardiology/ American Heart Association Task Force on Practice Guidelines (ACC/AHA/SCAI

Writing Committee to Update 2001 Guidelines for PCI). *Circulation* 2006; **113**: e166–286.

67. Ellis SG, Bajzer CT, Bhatt DL, *et al.* Real-world bare metal stenting: identification of patients at low or very low risk of 9-month coronary revascularisation. *Catheter Cardiovasc Interv* 2004; **63**: 135–40.

68. Costa MA, Simon DI. Molecular basis of re-stenosis and drug-eluting stents. *Circulation* 2005; **111**: 2257–73.

69. Colombo A, Iakovou I. Drug-eluting stents: the new gold standard for percutaneous revascularisation. *Eur Heart J* 2004; **25**: 895–7.

70. Kandzari DE, Roe MT, Ohman EM, *et al.* Frequency, predictors, and outcomes of drug-eluting stent utilization in patients with high-risk non-ST segment elevation acute coronary syndromes. *Am J Cardiol* 2005; **96**: 750–5.

71. Shuchman M. Trading re-stenosis for thrombosis? New questions about drug-eluting stents. *N Engl J Med* 2006; **355**: 1949–52.

72. Cutlip DE, Baim DS, Ho KK, *et al.* Stent thrombosis in the modern era: a pooled analysis of multi-center coronary stent clinical trials. *Circulation* 2001; **103**: 1967–71.

73. Mauri L, Hsieh WH, Massaro JM, *et al.* Stent thrombosis in randomized clinical trials of drug-eluting stents. *N Engl J Med* 2007; **356**: 1020–9.

74. Investigators TP-P. Inhibition of the platelet glycoprotein IIb/IIIa receptor with tirofiban in unstable angina and non-Q-wave myocardial infarction. *N Engl J Med* 1998; **338**: 1488–97.

75. Iakovou I, Schmidt T, Bonizzoni E, *et al.* Incidence, predictors, and outcome of thrombosis after successful implantation of drug-eluting stents. *JAMA* 2005; **293**: 2126–30.

76. McFadden EP, Stabile E, Regar E, *et al.* Late thrombosis in drug-eluting coronary stents after discontinuation of antiplatelet therapy. *Lancet* 2004; **364**: 1519–21.

77. Reddy PR, Vaitkus PT. Risks of noncardiac surgery after coronary stenting. *Am J Cardiol* 2005; **95**: 755–7.

78. Sharma AK, Ajani AE, Hamwi SM, *et al.* Major noncardiac surgery following coronary stenting: when is it safe to operate? *Cathet Cardiovasc Interv* 2004; **63**: 141–5.

79. Wilson SH, Rihal CS, Bell MR, *et al.* Timing of coronary stent thrombosis in patients treated with ticlopidine and aspirin. *Am J Cardiol* 1999; **83**: 1006–11.

80. Berger PB, Bell MR, Hasdai D, *et al.* Safety and efficacy of ticlopidine for only 2 weeks after successful intracoronary stent placement. *Circulation* 1999; **99**: 248–53.

81. Payne DA, Hayes PD, Jones CI, *et al.* Combined therapy with clopidogrel and aspirin significantly increases the bleeding time through a synergistic antiplatelet action. *J Vasc Surg* 2002; **35**: 1204–9.

82. Yende S, Wunderink RG. Effect of clopidogrel on bleeding after coronary artery bypass surgery. *Crit Care Med* 2001; **29**: 2271–32.

83. Vicenzi MN, Meislitzer T, Heitzinger B, Halaj M, Fleisher LA, Metzler H. Coronary artery stenting and non-cardiac surgery – a prospective outcome study. *Br J Anaesth* 2006; **96**: 686–93.

84. Broad L, Lee T, Conroy M, *et al.* Successful management of patients with a drug-eluting coronary stent presenting for elective non-cardiac surgery. *Br J Anaesth* 2007; **98**: 19–22.

85. Masaki E, Takinami M, Kurata Y, Kagaya S, Ahmed A. Anesthetic management of high-risk cardiac patients undergoing noncardiac surgery under the support of intra-aortic balloon pump. *J Clin Anesth* 1999; **11**: 342–5.

86. Shayani V, Watson WC, Mansour A, Thomas N, Pickleman J. Intra-aortic balloon counterpulsation in patients with severe cardiac dysfunction undergoing abdominal operations. *Arch Surg* 1998; **133**: 632–6.

87. Devereaux PJ, Goldman L, Yusuf S, *et al.* Surveillance and prevention of major perioperative ischemic cardiac events in patients undergoing noncardiac surgery: a review. *CMAJ* 2005; **173**: 779–88.

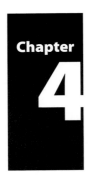
Perioperative use of cardiac medications in the high-risk patient

C. Railton

The perioperative management of medications remains one of the most problematic and controversial areas of perioperative medicine. The area is filled with recommendations based on expert opinion and information based on small clinical studies that are in many cases flawed, and open to much criticism. The most recent American College of Cardiology (ACC) and the American Heart Association (AHA) guidelines [1] and two recent reviews have been published offering guidelines for the perioperative management of nonanesthetic medications in noncardiac surgery [2, 3].

- Traditionally, all medications were held at the time of anesthesia and surgery for fear that the natural reflexes of physiology would be blunted and result in catastrophe for the patient.
- However, starting in the early 1980s, practice changed to where most cardiovascular medications are continued at the time of surgery to improve cardiovascular stress tolerance [4].
- The change in practice was not dictated by clinical research, but opinion.
- More recently, an evidence-based approach towards medication management has started to be employed.
- However, many physicians still use opinion to guide therapy given the quality of information available.

The goal of the perioperative physician should be to:

- continue or start beneficial medications, and
- hold or stop harmful medications.

Despite the simplicity of these goals, putting them into practice is difficult. The information that follows is not an exhaustive review of the literature, but more of a highlight of important papers and an approach to making sense of a controversial area of perioperative medicine.

Beta-blockade

Despite being one of the most researched areas of perioperative medication management, the answer to the question of whether perioperative beta-blockade is beneficial still remains elusive.

- The three largest studies of perioperative beta-blockade were done using atenolol [5, 6] and bisoprolol [7].
- All three studies were able to show short-term protective effects of beta-blockade on vascular patients.

Anesthesia for the High Risk Patient, ed. I. McConachie. Published by Cambridge University Press.
© Cambridge University Press 2009.

- The paper of Mangano *et al.* [5] has been heavily criticized and often discounted.
- Many other papers have been published in this area with mixed results.
- Meta-analysis has not helped, as explained by Devereux *et al.* [8] because not enough cases have been examined in the literature to draw statistically meaningful conclusions from the published studies for the population at large.

In an attempt to answer the question of whether perioperative beta-blockade is cardioprotective, the large Perioperative Ischemic Events Trial (POISE) was undertaken to study the effects of an extended-release metoprolol preparation on perioperative outcomes [9]. Preliminary results of the POISE trial were released at the November 2007 meeting in Orlando Florida (see www.theheart.org/article/826435). The multi-center study randomized patients to extended-release metoprolol (4174) subjects or placebo (4174) subjects. The trial did show a reduction in the number of nonfatal myocardial infarctions (OR 0.70, $P = 0.0007$)*, but there was an unexpected increase in perioperative total mortality (OR 1.33, $P = 0.03$)* and stroke (OR = 2.17, $P = 0.005$)* in the treatment group of the study. Preliminary study results have met with mixed opinion and the study methodology has been questioned. The results of the study question the current ACC/AHA recommendation to start patients on a beta-blocker prior to surgery.

The current recommendation regarding beta-blocker therapy is that only high-risk patients are likely to benefit from therapy [10]. The most recent guidelines regarding perioperative beta-blockade have been revised to reflect this opinion [1, 11].

- The general recommendation in the guidelines is to continue beta-blocker therapy in patients already taking beta-blockers, especially in those patients with the following medical conditions: angina, symptomatic arrhythmias, hypertension or other ACC/AHA class I guideline indications.
- Beta-blockade is indicated in patients with coronary heart disease undergoing vascular surgery.
- Beta-blockade is indicated in high cardiac risk patients with more than one clinical risk factor undergoing vascular surgery
- Beta-blockade is indicated in patients with coronary heart disease or more than one clinical risk factor undergoing major or intermediate surgery.
- For patients with multiple risk factors or in whom ischemic heart disease is identified and are undergoing major surgery, perioperative beta-blockade is likely to be beneficial.
- The benefit of beta-blockade is uncertain in patients with a single risk factor or no risk factors undergoing vascular or intermediate surgery.
- Beta-blockers should not be used in patients with absolute contraindications to beta-blockade.

The choice of beta-blocker does appear to affect outcomes.

- Redelmeier *et al.* [12] published a paper based on research using the database at the Institute for Clinical Evaluative Sciences in Toronto. They argued that the half-life of the beta-blocker used determines the effectiveness in the prevention of postoperative

---

* 95% confidence intervals not available.

myocardial infarction. They compared over 37 000 patients; the postoperative outcomes of patients taking metoprolol (half-life 3 h) were compared to the postoperative outcomes of patients taking atenolol (half-life 9 h) at the time of surgery. They found that patients on atenolol, the longer half-life drug had fewer myocardial events than the patients taking metoprolol (atenolol 2.5% versus metoprolol 3.5%, $P < 0.001$).

- The dosing of the beta-blocker also appears to have an effect on outcome as demonstrated by Feringa *et al.* [13] showing a dose–response effect in 272 vascular surgery patients in cardioprotection as assessed by serial troponin T measurements and long-term outcome. The most common beta-blocker used in the study was bisoprolol 67% (half life 9–12 h) although atenolol (5%, half-life 9 h) and metoprolol (15%, 3–4.5 h) were also included.

The earliest papers in the area of beta-blockade largely focused on the benefits that heart rate control had on coronary perfusion and cardiac ischemia. Beta-blockade can be used to successfully prevent cardiac ischemia by rate control as assessed by Holter monitoring [14].

Beta-blockers cannot be abruptly stopped because the resulting withdrawal syndrome predisposes patients to increased rates of myocardial infarction and stroke [15]. This was largely discovered when patients had adverse events when their beta-blockers were held awaiting surgery in the early 1970s. Most physicians are reluctant to continue or start a negative inotrope or chronotrope in a patient postoperatively who is hypotensive, placing a patient chronically on beta-blockers at risk of withdrawal syndrome and at increased risk of myocardial infarction or worse.

In summary, the data regarding perioperative beta-blockade remain controversial. The things to keep in mind in the perioperative time period for management are:

- if a patient is on a beta-blocker, continue the beta-blocker;
- if a patient has demonstrated ischemia on preoperative testing or multiple risk factors for cardiac ischemia, consider starting a beta-blocker [1, 11];
- it seems likely that only the highest-risk patients will receive the most benefit, especially in large surgeries;
- the choice of beta-blocker does seem to matter, with longer half-life beta-blockers possibly providing more benefit;
- heart rate control appears to be the most beneficial effect of beta-blockade in the perioperative setting;
- dosing matters, and benefit appears to be dose-related, with the highest dosed patients having the smallest changes in laboratory markers of ischemia;
- above all, for patients chronically taking beta-blockers, do not stop them abruptly in the perioperative period, because of the risk of developing adverse events due to beta-blocker withdrawal syndrome.

Renin–angiotensin blockade

In contrast to beta-blockade, this is an area of perioperative medication management where very little is known. It has been long-established that patients are heavily dependent on the renin–angiotensin system under anesthesia [16]. Controversy exists whether angiotensin converting enzyme inhibitors (ACE) and angiotensin receptor blocking agents (ARB) should be held at the time of surgery.

It has been long-established that blockade of the renin–angiotensin system by ACE inhibitors or ARB agents is associated with intraoperative hypotension [17]. For this reason, many physicians believe that these classes of medications should be held perioperatively. However, other physicians have countered that the beneficial effects of afterload reduction, cardiac remodeling, and possible antioxidant effects of ACE inhibitors and ARBs justifies their continuation at the time of surgery. There appears to be disagreement among physicians with respect to perioperative management of medications that blockade the renin–angiotensin system.

Two published case-control studies examining the effects of ACE inhibitors on postoperative outcome exist.

- The first study published was by Sear et al. [18] who used health region registry data to study the effects of intercurrent medical therapy on cardiac death rates in elective and emergency surgery patients. The study had problems matching control patients, and only eight patients taking ACE inhibitors were identified; and due to small numbers and problems matching, only simple odds ratios could be calculated. The odds ratio for increased risk of death for ACE-exposed patients undergoing elective surgery was 0.19, but was not statistically significant. The odds ratio calculated by Sear et al. for ACE-exposed patients undergoing emergency surgery was 1.18, $P = 0.0032$, but a 95% confidence interval could not be calculated.

- The second published study by Kurzencwyg et al. [19] used hospital cost computing systems to study abdominal aortic aneurysm (AAA) patients exposed to many classes of medications. They examined 223 consecutive cases and identified 24 deaths (11 elective repair and 13 emergency repair for ruptured aneurysm). They reported that ACE inhibitor exposure showed a statistically nonsignificant trend towards protection, odds ratio 0.09, CI_{95} (0.01–1.31), $P = 0.08$. However, it does not seem reasonable to compare emergency AAA repair subjects to elective subjects due to large differences in expected mortality. The surgical factors in emergency AAA repair are likely to dominate medical factors.

- In an abstract, Railton et al. [20] reported a study of 874 elective AAA repair patients. They reported that ACE/ARB-exposed patients were at higher risk of death within 30 days of surgery: ACE/ARB-exposed patients 21/347 (6%) versus unexposed 11/527 (2%), odds ratio 2.869, CI_{95} 1.36–6.06, $P = 0.044$. Multi-variate logistic analysis was done to account for the effects of underlying medical conditions, age, renal function, and medication exposures and the corrected odds ratio increased to 3.080, CI_{95} 1.278–7.424, $P = 0.012$. ACE inhibitor and ARB exposure were identified as independent predictors for death within 30 days of AAA repair. Separating the effects of the medication from the disease for which it was prescribed is especially problematic. Further analysis of this data set will perhaps clarify the results reported in the abstract.

- Corait et al. [21] have argued that the beneficial effects of renin–angiotensin blockade persist beyond the time when the medication is held.

- Comfère et al. [22] have shown that holding ACE inhibitors and ARB agents on the morning of surgery reduces the incidence of hypotension during the induction of anesthesia. The active metabolites of ACE inhibitors and ARBs can have very long half-lives and may persist in patients' systems for days.

- The recommendations of Goldstein et al. [2] seem to be prudent, which is to hold the medication for at least one dosage interval prior to surgery. This would at least reduce the amount of hypotension following the induction of anesthesia as reported by Comfère et al. [22].

In summary, very little is known about the benefits or risks associated with the continuation or stopping of ACE inhibitors and ARBs in the perioperative period. One should consider the following when making a decision regarding the management of ACE inhibitors and ARBs.

- Patients under anesthesia are heavily dependent on the renin–angiotensin system for the maintenance of blood pressure and volume regulation [16].
- Little is known about the possible risks associated with continuation of either class of medication.
- ACE inhibitor and ARB exposure is an independent risk factor for death within 30 days of surgery in vascular surgery patients [20].
- Exposure to ACE inhibitors and ARB agents is associated with hypotension following the induction of anesthesia.
- Holding a dose for at least 10 h or one dosing interval is associated with a reduction in the frequency of hypotension following the induction of anesthesia [22].
- It seems reasonable to assume that some of the benefits of long-term therapy will persist for a short period of time if the medication is held for the immediate perioperative period and then restarted shortly after surgery.

Calcium channel blockers

In contrast to the first two classes of medications examined, the perioperative use of calcium channel blockers (CaCB) is less controversial. More than 1000 papers have been published about the perioperative use of CaCB. However, very few of these papers have examined perioperative outcomes. In theory, the decrease in systemic vascular resistance (SVR), negative chronotropic effects, and prolongation of sinoatrial and arteriovenous (AV) node conduction would appear to be very dangerous when anesthetic agents are present.

- There have been case reports of intraoperative hypotension, and sudden death [23, 24].
- However, to date, no study has found any increase in risk due to perioperative CaCB administration.
- It has been shown that pretreatment with CaCB prior to the induction of anesthesia does result in a lower mean arterial pressure and less SVR in cardiac surgery patients [25].
- A potentiation of AV nodal block has been reported when inhalational anesthetics are used in patients chronically treated with CaCB [26, 27].
- However, the acute administration of CaCB under anesthesia has been reported to result in hypotension [28, 29].
- CaCB may also interact with nondepolarizing and polarizing neuromuscular blocking agents, resulting in prolonged neuromuscular blockade [30].

The studies of CaCB and anesthesia have been fairly small. Meta-analysis has recently been used to examine if there are any beneficial effects of perioperative use of CaCB.

Wijeysundera et al. studied both noncardiac (31) and cardiac surgery patients [32]. In noncardiac surgery, patients were exposed to a decrease in cardiac ischemia (relative risk (RR) 0.49, CI_{95} 0.30–0.80, $P = 0.004$), and a trend towards the reduction of myocardial infarction (RR 0.25, CI_{95} 0.05–1.18, $P = 0.08$), and a possible reduction in mortality (RR 0.40, CI_{95} 0.14–1.16, $P = 0.09$). Weijeysundera et al. [31] found in cardiac surgery patients that perioperative exposure to CaCB reduced MI (odds ratio [OR] 0.58, CI_{95} 0.37–0.91; $P = 0.02$), and ischemia (OR 0.53, CI_{95} 0.39 to 0.72; $P < 0.001$). Despite the reductions in myocardial infarction and ischemia, no decrease in mortality was observed.

Despite the theoretical risks and possible interactions with medications commonly used in anesthesia, there appears to be some reduction of postoperative adverse events in patients treated with CaCB. However, given the large sample sizes needed to show effect, it seems likely the benefit derived by individual patients is small. It seems that limited benefit would result from starting a patient perioperatively on CaCB.

In summary, the following should be considered when deciding to treat a patient on CaCB perioperatively.

- CaCB interact with inhaled anesthetic agents and neuromuscular blocking agents used in anesthesia.
- Patients chronically treated with CaCB show decreases in SVR and mean arterial pressure compared to controls.
- No harm has been reported in large studies of perioperative use of CaCB.
- Meta-analysis has shown some benefit towards reduction of ischemia, arrhythmias, myocardial infarction but not mortality.
- The expected benefits are small due to the large numbers of patients that need to be treated to show effects.
- It seems reasonable to continue patients chronically taking CaCBs, but not to start patients just prior to surgery.

HMG CoA reductase inhibitors

HMG CoA (hydroxymethylglutaryl-coenzyme A) reductase inhibitors – more commonly known as statins – have recently been examined for beneficial perioperative effects. The mechanism of any potential beneficial effects is not understood. The inhibition of cholesterol synthesis in the liver does not seem to be the likely mechanism. The role statins play in plaque stabilization and regression would seem to be more likely an explanation of the possible benefits. However, one must keep in mind that perioperative myocardial infarctions do not share a common pathophysiology with plaque rupture–artery occlusion infarctions.

- Durazzo *et al.* [33] were able to demonstrate a reduction in postoperative cardiac events in vascular surgery patients treated with short-term atrovastatin therapy.
- Le Manach *et al.* [34] have also shown how continuation of statin therapy reduced the risk of postoperative myonecrosis as assessed by Troponin I measurements. The relative risk reduction achieved by continuation of statin therapy was 5.5, CI_{95} 1.2–26.0, $P < 0.001$.
- The effect of statin withdrawal was studied by Schouten *et al.* [35], who found that statin discontinuation was associated with an increased risk of postoperative troponin release, myocardial infarction and nonfatal MI and cardiovascular death. They also found that an extended-release preparation of fluvastatin was associated with fewer cardiac events.
- Preoperative statin therapy has also been associated with decreased mortality following coronary artery bypass grafting [36].

No meta-analysis studies have as yet been published; however, two systematic reviews have been supportive of perioperative statin therapy [37, 38]. The recent ACC/AHA guidelines [1] also review some of the literature associated with perioperative statin use.

In summary, perioperative use of statins seems to afford some benefit to high-risk patients undergoing surgery. The following issues should be considered when making a decision for the management of HMG CoA Reductase Inhibitors.

- For patients chronically taking statins, the statins should be continued in patients scheduled for noncardiac surgery [1].
- There has only been one randomized study to show a risk reduction with the starting of statins perioperatively [33].
- The discontinuation of statins perioperatively is associated with an increase in risk of cardiac events [35].
- Statin use is reasonable in patients undergoing vascular surgery [1].
- Patients with at least one risk factor undergoing intermediate or major surgery should be considered for starting a statin preoperatively [1].
- Statins should be restarted as soon as possible following surgery [1].

Nitrates

The perioperative use of nitrates for the treatment of angina has raised concerns among some physicians that the use of such medications may lead to endothelial cell dysfunction and possibly worse postoperative outcomes. Despite obvious concerns that nitrates may predispose a patient towards developing postoperative complications, very little information is available.

- Sear et al. [18] used the data in the Oxford Linkage Study database to examine medication exposures in elective and emergency surgeries. They did find that after adjustment for the effects of age, cardiac disease and medication exposure, patients exposed to nitrates prior to elective surgery were at increased risk of death, corrected odds ratio 4.79 CI_{95} 1.00–22.72, $P = 0.049$. Nitrate exposure in emergency surgical patients was not associated with worse outcomes in the same study. The study of Sear et al. [18] does have some limitations due to problems matching controls subjects, which caused some cases not to be included in the analysis.
- My own research group has collected data on medication exposures and postoperative outcomes in vascular surgery patients. We reviewed 874 cases of elective open AAA repair and showed that 106/874 (12%) of patients were taking a nitrate preparation prior to surgery [39]. The uncorrected odds ratio for death within 30 days of surgery for patients exposed to nitrates was: odds ratio 1.076, CI_{95} 0.369–3.139, $P = 0.893$ [39].
- In both the studies of Sear et al. [18] and Railton et al. [39], it is unclear what type of nitroglycerin preparation was used: periodic use versus sustained-release formulations.
- Patients with symptomatic coronary artery disease use nitrates. Trying to parse out the effects of the coronary artery disease from the medication exposure is impossible with the information available at this time.

The simple approach for the perioperative management of nitrates in high-risk patients would be to advise the following.

- Patients should use nitrates as needed but should otherwise minimize use.
  - In many centers, nitroglycerin patches are discontinued prior to the induction of anesthesia and surgery.
  - There is no conclusive information available to help the perioperative physician know what to further advise patients.

Conclusion

The perioperative medication management is difficult and often an area of disagreement between anesthesiologists and internal medicine specialists. Trying to keep abreast of the latest information is challenging for physicians, and using an evidence-based approach is challenging when the quality of evidence is poor or quantity of information available is small. Large studies such as the DECREASE IV study (Fluvastatin and bisoprolol for the reduction of perioperative cardiac mortality and morbidity in high-risk patients undergoing non-cardiac surgery) may provide some answers.

References

1. Fleisher LA, Beckman JA, Brown KA, *et al.* ACC/AHA Guidelines on the Preoperative Cardiovascular Evaluation and Care for Noncardiac Surgery. A Report of the American College of Cardiology/American Heart Association Task Force on Practice Guidelines. *Circulation* 2007; **116**: e419–e488.

2. Goldstein S, Amar D. Pharmacotherapeutic considerations in anaesthesia. *Heart Disease* 2003; **5**: 34–48.

3. Pass SE, Simpson RW. Discontinuation and reinstitution of medications during the perioperative period. *Am J Health-Syst Pharm* 2004; **61**: 899–912.

4. Kim Y, Danchak M, MacNamara TE. Drug interaction and anaesthesia. *Clin Ther* 1987; **9**: 342–3.

5. Mangano DT, Layug EL, Wallace A, Tateo I. Effect of atenolol on mortality and cardiovascular morbidity after noncardiac surgery. Multicenter Study of Perioperative Ischemia Research Group. *New Engl J Med* 1996; **335**: 1713–20. (Erratum *New Eng J Med* 1997; **336**: 1039.)

6. Wallace A, Layug B, Tateo I. Prophylactic atenolol reduces postoperative myocardial ischemia. *Anesthesiology* 1998; **88**: 7–17.

7. Poldermans D, Boersma E, Bax JJ, *et al.* The effect of bisoprolol on perioperative mortality and myocardial infarction in high-risk patients undergoing vascular surgery. Dutch Echocardiographic Risk Evaluation Applying Stress Echocardiography Study Group. *New Engl J Med* 1999; **341**: 1789–94.

8. Devereux PJ, Salim U, Yang H, *et al.* Are the recommendations to use perioperative β-blocker therapy in patients undergoing noncardiac surgery based on reliable evidence? *CMAJ* 2004, **171**: 245–7.

9. www.clinicaltrials.gov/ct/show/ NCT00182039, 28 Sept, 2006. Principle investigator Devereux PJ, McMaster University, Hamilton, Ontario, Canada.

10. Lindenauer PK, Pekow P, Wang K, *et al.* Perioperative beta-blocker therapy and mortality after major noncardiac surgery. *New Engl J Med* 2005; **353**: 349–61.

11. Fleisher LA, Beckman JA, Brown KA, *et al.* ACC/AHA 2006 Guideline Update on Perioperative Cardiovascular Evaluation for Noncardiac Surgery: Focused Update on Perioperative Beta-Blocker Therapy – A Report of the American College of

Cardiology/American Heart Association Task Force on Practice Guidelines. *Anesth Analg* 2007; **104**: 15–26.

12. Redelmeier D, Scales D, Kopp A. Beta blockers for elective surgery in elderly patients: population based, retrospective cohort study. *BMJ* 2005; **331**: 932–8.

13. Feringa HHH, Bax J, Boersma E, *et al.* High-dose beta-blockers and tight heart rate control reduce myocardial ischemia and troponin T release in vascular surgery patients. *Circulation* 2006; **114** (Suppl I): I344–9.

14. Raby KE, Brull SJ, Timimi F, *et al.* The effect of heart rate control on myocardial ischemia among high-risk patients after vascular surgery. *Anesth Analg* 1999; **88**: 477–82.

15. Shammash JB, Trost JC, Gold JM, *et al.* Perioperative beta-blocker withdrawal and mortality in vascular surgery patients. *Am Heart J* 2001; **141**: 148–53.

16. Miller ED, Ackerly JA, Peach MJ. Blood pressure support during general anaesthesia in a renin-dependent state in the rat. *Anesthesiology* 1978; **48**: 404–08.

17. Colson P, Ryckwaert F, Coriat P. Renin angiotensin system antagonists and anaesthesia. *Anesth Analg* 1999; **89**: 1143–55.

18. Sear JW, Howell SJ, Sear M, *et al.* Intercurrent drug therapy and perioperative cardiovascular mortality in elective and urgent/emergent surgical patients. *Br J Anaesthesia* 2001; **86**: 506–12.

19. Kurzencwyg D, Filion KB, Pilote L, *et al.* Cardiac medical therapy among patients undergoing abdominal aortic aneurysm repair. *Ann Vasc Surg* 2006; **20**: 569–76.

20. Railton C, Belo S, Lam-McCullogh J. Perioperative renin–angiotensin and perioperative outcome. *Abstract number 44529*, Canadian Anaesthesia Society meeting, Calgary, 2007.

21. Corait P. Interactions between inhibitors of the renin angiotensin system and anaesthesia. *European Society of Anesthesiologists*, Refresher Courses, Gothenburg, 7 Apr, 2001.

22. Comfère T, Sprung J, Kumar MM, *et al.* Angiotensin system inhibitors in a general surgical population. *Anesth Analg* 2005; **100**: 636–44.

23. Lewis GB. Hemodynamic disturbances during anaesthesia in a patient receiving verapamil. *Br J Anaesthesia* 1987; **59**: 522–3.

24. Moller IW. Cardiac arrest following IV verapamil combined with halothane anaesthesia. *Br J Anaesthesia* 1987; **59**: 522–3.

25. Hess W, Meyer C. Haemodynamic effects of nifedipine in patients undergoing coronary artery bypass. *Acta Anaesthesiol Scand* 1986; **30**: 614–19.

26. Kates RA, Kaplan JA, Guyton RA, *et al.* Hemodynamic interactions of verapamil and isoflurane. *Anesthesiology* 1983; **59**: 132–8.

27. Brichard G, Zimmermann PE. Verapamil in cardiac dysrhythmias during anaesthesia. *Br J Anaesthesia* 1970; **42**: 1005–12.

28. Schulte-Sasse U, Hess W, Markschies-Hornung A, *et al.* Combined effects of halothane anaesthesia and verapamil on systemic hemodynamics and left ventricular myocardial contractility in patients with ischemic heart disease. *Anesth Analg* 1984; **63**: 791–8.

29. Schulte-Sasse U, Hess W, Markschies-Hornung A, *et al.* Cardiovascular interactions of halothane anaesthesia and nifedipine in patients subjected to elective coronary artery bypass surgery. *Thorac Cardiovasc Surg* 1983; **31**: 261–5.

30. Durant NN, Nuygen N, Katz RL. Potentiation of neuromuscular blockade by verapamil. *Anesthesiology* 1984; **60**: 298–303.

31. Wiejeysundera, DN, Beattie WS. Calcium channel blockers for reducing cardiac morbidity after noncardiac surgery: a meta-analysis. *Anesth Analg* 2003; **97**: 634–41.

32. Wiejeysundera, DN, Beattie WS, Rao V, *et al.* Calcium antagonists reduce cardiovascular complications after cardiac surgery: A meta-analysis. *J Am Coll Cardiology* 2003; **41**: 1496–505.

33. Durazzo AE, Machado FS, Ikeoka DT, *et al.* Reduction in cardiovascular events after vascular surgery with atorvastatin: A randomized trial. *J Vasc Surg* 2004; **39**: 967–75.

34. Le Manach Y, Godet G, Coriat P, *et al.* The impact of postoperative discontinuation or continuation of chronic statin therapy on

cardiac outcome following major vascular surgery. *Anesth Analg* 2007; **104**: 1326–33.

35. Schouten O, Hoeks SE, Welten GM, *et al.* Effect of statin withdrawal on frequency of cardiac events after vascular surgery. *Am J Cardiol* 2007; **100**: 316–20.

36. Collard CD, Body SC, Shernan SK, *et al.* Multicentre Study of Perioperative Ischemia (MCSPI) Research Group, Inc; Ischemia Research and Education Foundation (IREF) Investigators. Perioperative statin therapy is associated with reduced cardiac mortality after coronary bypass graft surgery. *J Thorac Cardiovasc Surg* 2006; **132**: 392–400.

37. Paraskevas KI, Liapis CD, Hamilton G, *et al.* Can statins reduce perioperative morbidity and mortality in patients undergoing non-cardiac vascular surgery? *Eur J Vasc Endovasc Surg* 2006; **32**: 286–93.

38. Kapoor AS, Kanji H, Buckingham J, *et al.* Strength of evidence for perioperative use of statins to reduce cardiovascular risk: A systematic review of controlled studies. *BMJ* 2006; **333**: 1149.

39. Railton C, manuscript in preparation.

Chapter 5

Pharmaco-physiological approaches to the high-risk surgical patient

M. Cutts

Introduction

The complexity of surgery and the average age of the population are increasing. Despite this, death rates following surgery are now low. Just a small percentage of patients undergoing surgery still carry most of the postoperative morbidity and mortality. Pearce *et al.* identified a high-risk surgical population who account for 12.5% of surgical procedures but for 80% of deaths [1].

Those most at risk are:

- the elderly: most deaths occur in patients over 60–70 years of age;
- those undergoing emergency surgery;
- those with co-existing disease such as cardiorespiratory disease or diabetes mellitus; and
- those undergoing high-risk surgical procedures.

Cause of death

The cause of death is most commonly from myocardial infarction (MI) or the gradual development of multiple organ failure (MODS). Almost half the deaths occur in the first 5 days postoperatively [2], with the median day of death being on the sixth postoperative day. The mechanisms of the development of MODS are still being elucidated. However, it is likely that it results from inflammatory cascades provoked by a multi-factorial etiology that may include any combination of:

- altered microcirculation causing tissue injury;
- ischemia–reperfusion injury;
- direct surgical or traumatic tissue injury;
- surgical stimulation of metabolic and endocrine processes;
- blood loss and fluid shifts causing regional and global hypoperfusion;
- anesthetic agents causing vasodilatation and altered regional blood flow; and
- splanchnic hypoperfusion – this may be especially important since splanchnic blood may amount to two-fifths of the blood volume. Damage to mucosal integrity and bacterial translocation may be important in initiating inflammatory cascades.

Many of these perioperative events have the potential to cause an imbalance between oxygen delivery and demand, be it local or global. This is especially likely to occur in the presence of reduced physiological reserve where cardiac index cannot rise to meet the demand placed by

Anesthesia for the High Risk Patient, ed. I. McConachie. Published by Cambridge University Press.
© Cambridge University Press 2009.

surgery. The tissue hypoxia that results may precipitate the systemic inflammatory response syndrome (SIRS) that may then progress on to MODS.

To reduce perioperative risk, we need to target those patients with limited physiological reserve undergoing surgery of sufficient physiological insult. The concern in the UK is that, of those patients identified retrospectively as being at high risk, only a small proportion were admitted to critical care areas [2]. This suggests lack of, or inappropriate, resource allocation. The challenge is to successfully identify patients at risk and ensure an appropriate level of care.

Identifying perioperative risk

(See also Chapter 3.)

Risk of cardiac death after major surgery has been defined by Goldman *et al.* [3], who examined 1001 patients undergoing noncardiac surgery. By multivariate discriminate analysis they identified nine correlates of life-threatening and fatal cardiac complications.

- The risk index so developed was later validated and modified by Detsky [4] (Chapter 3).
- In this scoring system, particular risk is attached to poor cardiac reserve in the form of congestive cardiac failure, aortic stenosis and precarious myocardial perfusion. This suggests that the patient's ability to meet the demands of surgery by maintaining, or increasing, perfusion and oxygen delivery is important in determining survival.

In support of this:

- Early work by Boyd *et al.* [5] suggested that in cardiac surgery, failure to raise post-operative cardiac index (CI) above $2.5\,l\,min^{-1}\,m^{-2}$ was associated with increased mortality rate.
- Clowes *et al.* [6] later showed that failure to increase cardiac output after thoracic surgery was associated with reduced survival.

The work of Goldman *et al.* looked specifically at the risk of perioperative cardiac events and death in terms of premorbid conditions. Shoemaker [7] also defined indicators of risk for perioperative death by correlating preoperative criteria with mortality rates (Table 5.1). This work identified both patient criteria and criteria relating to the type of surgery to be undertaken. They and others have subsequently used these criteria to identify and study high-risk patients.

More recent work has contributed further to our ability to evaluate perioperative risk.

- Perioperative risk has been correlated with (patient-reported) exercise tolerance. Limitation to climbing two flights of stairs or walking four blocks was associated with significantly increased risk [8].
- Preoperative studies of left ventricular function using radionuclide angiography, echo-cardiography, and contrast ventriculography have been used to assess perioperative risk. These hold the advantage that pharmacological stress to the left ventricle can be used to assess patients unable to exercise due to arthritis or claudication. This is further discussed in Chapter 3.
- Exciting work from Australia [9, 10] has developed the use of preoperative cardiopulmonary exercise (CPX) testing to create conditions of stress in order to detect cardiac insufficiency and stratify patients into high- or low-risk groups.

Table 5.1 Shoemaker's indicators of high risk.

Previous severe cardiorespiratory illness, e.g. acute myocardial infarction or chronic obstructive airways disease

Extensive ablative surgery planned for malignancy, e.g. gastrectomy, esophagectomy or surgery > 6 h

Multiple trauma, e.g. more than three organ injury, more than two systems, or opening two body cavities

Massive acute hemorrhage, e.g. more than eight units

Age above 70 years and limited physiological reserve of one or more organs

Septicemia (positive blood cultures or septic focus) WCC > 13, pyrexia to 38.3 for 48 h

Respiratory failure (Pa O_2 < 8 kPa on an FiO_2 > 0.4 or mechanical ventilation > 48 h

Acute abdominal catastrophe with hemodynamic instability (e.g. pancreatitis, perforated viscus, peritonitis, gastrointestinal bleed)

Acute renal failure (urea > 20 mmol l^{-1}, creatinine > 260 mmol l^{-1})

Late stage vascular disease involving aortic disease

Shock, e.g. MAP < 60 mmHg, CVP < 15 cm H_2O, urine output < 20 ml h^{-1}

CPX testing [9, 10]

- CPX testing is performed on a bicycle ergometer with a ramp protocol. The test takes less than an hour and is relatively inexpensive. Respiratory gases and ECG are monitored. Oxygen consumption and carbon dioxide production during the exercise are measured. Oxygen uptake as work increases is used to objectively assess cardiopulmonary performance.

- The principle is that oxygen consumption is dependent on oxygen delivery and this in turn is dependent on cardiopulmonary performance. When exercising, oxygen consumption is linearly related to cardiac output. The measurement of aerobic capacity is therefore a surrogate for the measurement of ventricular function.

- The most useful measurement made is the anerobic threshold. This occurs when aerobic metabolism, and therefore oxygen delivery, is inadequate, forcing anerobic metabolism to develop.

- This group has demonstrated a clear relationship between anerobic threshold and perioperative risk, allowing them to target critical care resources to those patients most in need.

- Specifically, an anerobic threshold below 11 ml min^{-1} kg^{-1} is associated with an increased perioperative risk. This, combined with myocardial ischemia occurring on ECG during the test, is associated with especially high risks. In contrast, very few perioperative cardiovascular deaths occur in those patients with anerobic thresholds of 11 ml min^{-1} kg^{-1} or above.

- This work serves to emphasize the importance of impaired physiologic reserve in determining a patient's ability to respond to the demands of surgery and survive. It will be interesting to see if efforts to improve reserve with a preoperative exercise program result in better survival.

Improving outcome

Having identified the high-risk patient, how do we then set about improving outcome? There are several potential strategies to consider.

Treatment of existing medical disease

The principle of treating treatable medical conditions such as hypertension, angina, diabetes, congestive cardiac failure and respiratory disease is well established in anesthetic practice.

- *Hypertension.* The evidence for reduction in perioperative risk by treating moderate degrees of hypertension preoperatively is actually limited. The studies cited previously have failed to identify hypertension as a significant independent risk factor. There is, though, evidence of increased intraoperative blood pressure fluctuation in hypertensive patients [11] and this may be associated with intraoperative cardiac ischemia [12]. Beta-blocking agents appear to be a good choice for control of perioperative hypertension, particularly in emergency surgery [12].

- *Angina and the role of coronary revascularization.* Normal cardiac medications (except perhaps ACE inhibitors which have a propensity to cause postinduction hypotension, as discussed in Chapter 4) should be continued perioperatively. A recent study [13] in patients with stable coronary artery disease (with greater than 70% stenosis in at least one coronary artery) and due to undergo major vascular surgery did not show any significant benefit to prior coronary revascularization (either operative or percutaneous). Coronary bypass grafting or percutaneous coronary intervention is further discussed in Chapter 3.

- *Diabetes and glycemic control.* Evidence in critically ill patients supports protocols for tight glycemic control even in nondiabetic patients. Survival rates are increased, whilst septic episodes, length of ventilation and length of critical care stay are reduced [14]. This study was performed in a predominantly postsurgical intensive care unit, so it would seem reasonable that the same might apply to the general surgical population, although as yet there is no definitive evidence. There is evidence to support postoperative tight glycemic control in diabetic cardiac surgery patients [15]. There is no evidence, though, for tight glycemic control intraoperatively, and the evidence from cardiac surgery patients suggests that this may in fact be detrimental [16].

- *Management of congestive cardiac failure.* Beta-blockers, ACE inhibitors and diuretics should be continued in the perioperative period. Diuretics and ACE inhibitors may be associated with hypovolemia and intraoperative hypotension, although specific detriment has not been demonstrated. Stopping beta-blockers perioperatively may be particularly dangerous, although because of potential for perioperative electrolyte disturbance, withholding of digoxin has been advised [17].

Resuscitation of presenting disease and cardiovascular optimization

Where time allows, attention should be directed to correcting electrolyte, metabolic and fluid balance. Intravenous fluids should be given preoperatively to prevent dehydration, particularly where there is a prolonged period of starvation or bowel preparation has been given.

- Debate continues as to the merits of colloid compared to crystalloid. This is discussed in Chapter 14. The evidence for these impacting on survival is lacking despite several randomized trials [18].

- There is much interest in the use of balanced solutions for resuscitation. Normal saline infusions cause hyperchloremic acidosis, whereas balanced solutions such as Hartmann's solution and Ringer's lactate do not. There is some evidence for improved hemostasis, renal function and gastric perfusion when these solutions are used, but influence on outcome has not been demonstrated [18].

- The use of albumin for fluid resuscitation has largely fallen into disrepute [19].
- There is considerable evidence to support "perioperative cardiovascular optimization". Using invasive monitoring, titrated fluids and inotropes are given in high-risk patients to achieve enhanced cardiovascular function in anticipation of the increased perioperative oxygen consumption created by the metabolic demands of surgery. The effects of anesthetic agents and surgical stress mean that the traditionally measured values such as heart rate, blood pressure, urine output and central venous pressure are inadequate to assess fluid volume filling. Instead, fluid challenges and inotropes are tailored to individuals to maximize flow variables such as stroke volume or cardiac output. An inability to respond by increasing cardiac output, and, thereby, oxygen delivery predisposes the tissues to inadequate perfusion with subsequent organ dysfunction. The evidence for perioperative cardiovascular optimization will be reviewed in the latter part of this chapter.
- Despite the overwhelming evidence in support of perioperative cardiovascular optimization, it has recently been suggested that a more fluid-restrictive regimen should be used in gastrointestinal surgery. This is discussed in Chapter 18.

Management of anemia

The influence of anemia on outcome and the risks and benefits of blood transfusion are discussed in Chapter 9.

Oral carbohydrate loading

- The metabolic effects of surgery include development of postoperative insulin resistance. This postoperative insulin resistance is reduced by a preoperative oral carbohydrate load [20].
- Preoperative oral carbohydrate loading can prevent surgery-induced immunodepression and this might reduce the risk of perioperative infectious complications [21].
- Preoperative oral carbohydrate loading may reduce length of stay and may reduce the length of time to return of bowel function in colorectal surgery [22], although numbers in this study were small.

Use of regional anesthesia

The use of central neuraxial anesthesia has been shown to result in better postoperative respiratory function [23] and many other qualitative improvements in the postoperative period. To date, however, there is little evidence to suggest that mortality rates or times to discharge are affected [24]. This subject is further discussed in Chapter 8.

Strategies to prevent myocardial events

Beta-blockers, nitrates, calcium channel blockers, alpha$_2$ antagonists and statins have all been used to try to reduce postoperative mortality. Increasing evidence for benefit lies with perioperative beta-blockade, and more recent evidence suggests a role for statins. The perioperative role of beta-blockers will be discussed later in this chapter and also in Chapter 4.

- Statins are used for their effect of lowering serum lipid concentrations. However they also have antioxidant, anti-inflammatory and plaque-stabilizing actions. They also improve endothelial function and reduce platelet aggregation. They have been shown to reduce cerebrovascular events and myocardial infarction when used long term in high-risk patients [25].

- Several studies in vascular and cardiac surgery have now shown increased cardiac risk where long-term statin therapy is interrupted postoperatively. There is also retrospective evidence to suggest that patients taking statins are at lower perioperative risk [26].

- There is no evidence to support the routine perioperative use of statins, although the DECREASE IV trial [27] is a large, ongoing study involving an estimated 6000 patients aiming to assess the effects of fluvastatin perioperatively.

- Small studies on the perioperative administration of clonidine for 4 days to patients at risk for coronary artery disease show a significant reduction in the incidence of perioperative myocardial ischemia and postoperative death [28].

The evidence for perioperative cardiovascular optimization

The perioperative cardiovascular changes seen in high-risk patients undergoing major surgery were characterized in the 1970s by Shoemaker's group.

- In 1973, they studied 98 patients undergoing major surgery and in variable levels of established shock. Comparing 67 survivors with 31 nonsurvivors, they were able to demonstrate significantly different hemodynamic changes in the days following surgery. Surviving patients had a higher cardiac index, higher oxygen delivery and higher oxygen uptake. These indices were much better predictors of mortality than the more traditionally used values of blood pressure and heart rate [29].

- Following this, the same group studied 220 high-risk patients, this time undergoing major elective and semi-elective surgery. In these patients they confirmed higher values of cardiac index, oxygen delivery and oxygen consumption in the survivors. From these findings, they postulated that if cardiovascular performance could be enhanced in high-risk patients to achieve the cardiac index and oxygen delivery values manifest by survivors, then overall survival rate could increase. They were able to suggest specific goals of cardiac index, $4.5 \, l \, min^{-1} \, m^{-2}$, oxygen delivery, $600 \, ml \, min^{-1} \, m^{-2}$, and oxygen consumption, $170 \, ml \, min^{-1} \, m^{-2}$, that they termed "supranormal values" [30].

- In a subsequent nonrandomized study of 100 patients, they either actively increased cardiovascular performance with fluids and inotropes aiming to achieve the above supranormal values, or in the control patients allowed cardiac index to remain between 2.8 and $3.5 \, l \, min^{-1} \, m^{-2}$. Mortality and complication rate were both reduced in the intervention group [31].

Several other nonrandomized studies confirmed these findings; however, it was not until the 1980s that further evidence was gained from properly randomized controlled trials.

- Firstly, in 1985, Shultz [32] studied 70 patients undergoing surgical repair of hip fractures. Half of the patients were monitored with pulmonary artery flotation catheters and managed with intravenous fluids and inotropes to enhance cardiac index and oxygen delivery to preset goals. The other half was managed conventionally. The intervention group had a significantly lower mortality rate by over 25%. It was unclear, however, whether the improvement was due to better monitoring or to enhanced oxygen delivery.

- Subsequently, in 1988, Shoemaker's group [33] published a randomized, controlled trial of 340 high-risk surgical patients. They recruited patients using their previously defined criteria for high risk. Control patients were managed conventionally, whereas the protocol group were given intravenous fluids, inotropes and vasodilators, aiming to achieve the supranormal values they had described previously. The protocol group had significantly lower mortality (4% vs. 33%, $p < 0.01$) and complication rates (1.3 vs. 0.4, $p < 0.05$).

- Another group, Berlauk et al. [34], published further data to support the use of perioperative optimization. In this study, 89 patients underwent peripheral vascular surgery under general anesthesia. Patients were randomized into three groups. One group received conventional management and the other two groups were monitored with a pulmonary artery catheter placed either 12 h before or immediately before surgery. In the latter two groups, the invasive monitoring was used to guide circulatory "tune up" with fluid loading, inotropes and vasodilators. Treatment was given to maintain pulmonary capillary wedge pressure of 8–15 mmHg, cardiac index $> 2.8 \, l \, min^{-1} \, m^{-2}$ and SVR $< 1100 \, dyne \, s^{-1} \, cm^{-5}$ pre- and intraoperatively. The study groups both had fewer intraoperative adverse events, less early graft thrombosis and lower postoperative cardiac morbidity.

- In 1992 and 1995, Shoemaker's group published two further randomized, controlled trials, this time in 67 and 125 patients with severe trauma [35, 36]. In patients treated to increase oxygen delivery to supranormal values, they found reduced organ failure, lower mortality rate, shorter stays in intensive care and shorter periods of ventilation.

- In a further randomized, controlled trial, Boyd [37] studied 107 patients at high risk as defined by Shoemaker's criteria. The majority of patients were admitted to intensive care preoperatively, although some were admitted postoperatively. All patients received conventional therapy with invasive monitoring, intravenous fluids, vasodilators and inotropes. The protocol group were managed in addition to deliberately increase oxygen delivery. Dopexamine was used to achieve goals of oxygen delivery of $> 600 \, ml \, min^{-1} \, m^{-2}$ with pulmonary capillary wedge pressure 12–14 mmHg and hemoglobin $> 12 \, g \, l^{-1}$. The result was a significantly lower mortality and complication rate (by 75% and 59%, respectively).

These impressive reductions in mortality and complication rates have not, however, been mirrored in some of the randomized trials that followed.

- Ziegler et al. [38] and Valentine et al. [39] both failed to show any significant benefit in terms of morbidity and mortality from optimization attempts in patients undergoing peripheral vascular surgery.

- In 2000, Takala et al. [40], in a multi-center randomized, controlled study of 412 patients undergoing major abdominal surgery, did not show any reduction in mortality using dopexamine at fixed doses of either a dose of $0.5 \, \mu g \, kg^{-1} \, min^{-1}$ or $2.0 \, \mu g \, kg^{-1} \, min^{-1}$.

It is likely that in at least some of these studies, the targeted populations were not at high enough risk and therefore were unlikely to show benefit from optimization strategies. Clearly the patients chosen for optimization protocols need to be selected with care. Further, in one of these studies [39] the intraoperative complication rate was actually increased in the optimized group. Optimization techniques should therefore be titrated with care to avoid inducing morbidity related to the therapy.

Another study by Wilson *et al.* [41] suggested an exciting dimension to the concept of perioperative optimization. In a randomized, controlled trial of 138 patients, they studied three high-risk groups undergoing surgery.

- The control group were managed conventionally and were admitted to intensive care only if deemed necessary. The other two groups were admitted preoperatively to intensive care and given goal-directed therapy with either adrenaline or dopexamine lasting for at least 12 h postoperatively.
- Both the treatment groups had a significantly improved survival rate, but only the dopexamine group saw a significant reduction in morbidity.

    This is particularly interesting because the dopexamine-treated group did not see an increase in cardiac index by as much as the adrenaline-treated group. The reduced morbidity was due to a reduction in sepsis and ARDS.

Dopexamine is a pure $beta_2$ agonist with very little $beta_1$ effect and no $alpha_1$ activity. Its inotropic effects result from inhibition of endogenous catecholamine re-uptake and from stimulation of baroreceptor reflexes. It reduces systemic and pulmonary vascular resistance and increases both renal and splanchnic blood flow. $Beta_2$ stimulation also brings about anti-inflammatory properties. It may be that this, together with improved splanchnic blood flow, both maintains mucosal barriers and attenuates the inflammatory cascade that leads to SIRS and MODS. In support of this, dopexamine has been shown to reduce inflammatory change in the upper gastrointestinal mucosa in high-risk surgical patients [42]. The role of catecholamines and their actions at different adrenoceptors on the immune system is explored fully in a review cited in further reading.

The specific benefits of dopexamine suggested in the study of Wilson *et al.* [41] are by no means universally accepted. It has been suggested [43] that the three treatment groups in the study were not comparable and that this may have led to some of the differences seen between the dopexamine- and adrenaline-treated groups. Certainly two subsequent studies using dopexamine did not see it fulfill expectations.

- The study of Takala *et al.* [40] described above used dopexamine at two fixed doses in a non goal-directed way. It may be that failure to goal-direct the inotropic therapy resulted in overtreatment of patients vulnerable to cardiac ischemia. The higher mortality rate seen in the group receiving the higher dose of dopexamine might support this idea, although the difference was not statistically significant.
- In 2003, Stone *et al.* [44] studied the effect of dopexamine at a fixed rate of $0.25 \, \mu g \, kg^{-1} \, min^{-1}$ in 100 patients undergoing major abdominal surgery for 24 h after commencement of surgery. They found no reduction to postoperative morbidity. This study was not designed to show differences in mortality rate. Also the patients in both the treatment and placebo groups had their cardiac output optimized using esophageal Doppler monitoring to guide appropriately titrated fluids. The resulting mortality rates were perhaps too low to show any additional benefit from the dopexamine.

Using goal-directed therapy has proved disappointing in lower-risk groups or when using fixed nontailored doses of inotropes. The last decade, however, has seen much work that has been strongly supportive of individually tailored goal-directed therapy. This is particularly so when more qualitative outcome measures are examined and when fluid therapy is used.

- Three studies of optimization either intraoperatively or started postoperatively in cardiac surgical patients showed reduced intensive care and hospital length of stay, reduced complications and reduced gastric hypoperfusion (measured by tonometric assessment of gastric intramucosal pH) [45–47].

- Two studies of intraoperative intravascular fluid volume optimization guided by esophageal Doppler ultrasonography in hip fracture found a reduction in time to medical fitness for discharge [48, 49].

- Four studies in major (nonvascular) abdominal surgery using intraoperative esophageal Doppler ultrasound-guided intravascular fluid optimization have shown reduced length of stay, reduced intensive care admissions, reduced postoperative nausea and vomiting, earlier return to normal bowel function, reduced complications, and reduced gastrointestinal morbidity [50–53].

- Pearse *et al.* in 2005 found reduced length of stay and reduced complications in general surgical patients optimized with fluids and inotropes starting in the postoperative period [54].

None of these studies were designed to be large enough to have the statistical power to show an effect on mortality, although meta-analyses including these studies do suggest an effect on perioperative mortality [55, 56]. The weight of evidence certainly supports the use of goal-directed fluid therapy for its reduction in morbidity and improved recovery rates. The bulk of earlier work also supports the further addition of inotropic support, where patients and surgery are of sufficiently high risk and the patient is able to tolerate it.

Intraoperative esophageal Doppler has been used in many of the recent goal-directed therapy studies with improved outcome, usually using a strategy of fluid challenges until there are only small or no further increases in stroke volume. Circulatory filling is then optimum. Reassessment and appropriate additional fluid challenges follow to maintain filling. Esophageal Doppler has several advantages over pulmonary artery catheters which have fallen somewhat into disrepute [57]; it does not require calibrating and is reasonably easy to use. Newer esophageal catheters are also well tolerated, allowing them to be used into the postoperative period in awake patients. There are several alternatives to the esophageal Doppler, such as thermodilution techniques from a central venous pressure and arterial catheter or plethysmography, none of which are as well-validated for perioperative optimization. Useful reviews of optimization monitoring techniques are available [18, 58].

Cardiovascular optimization in critical illness

Although there is good evidence to support the use of perioperative optimization in elective and semi-elective surgery, there is unfortunately little to support the pursuit of supranormal goals for oxygen delivery in patients who are already critically ill.

- Initial nonrandomized studies in patients with established septic shock [59] suggested that optimization might be of benefit; however, subsequent randomized controlled trials have not supported this.

- A randomized study of patients with septic shock by Tuchshmidt *et al.* [60] found a reduced mortality rate in optimized patients, but this was not significantly so.

- Other randomized studies [61–63] have all failed to show benefit from optimization. All of these studies had in common the recruitment of patients with established septic shock and/or organ failure.

Two interesting studies help to clarify the situation.

- Gutierrez *et al.* [64] examined pHi as an indicator of hypoperfusion at entry to their study. Those with a low pHi at entry to the study, suggesting existing hypoperfusion, did not benefit from optimization, whereas those without hypoperfusion at entry to the study did see reduced mortality.

- Rivers *et al.* [65] studied the effect of goal-directed therapy applied early in sepsis before organ failure was fully established. They found that patients went on to develop less-severe organ dysfunction and had a lower in-hospital mortality.

It would appear that where organ failure is already established, there is little to gain from pursuing supranormal values: increased cardiac output and oxygen delivery is more likely to benefit when used in a preventive way.

The perioperative role of beta-blockers

Beta-blockers have several properties, not all of which may be beneficial:

- reduction in blood pressure and heart rate;
- anti-arrhythmic;
- negative inotropism;
- Anti-renin/angiotensin;
- prolongation of coronary diastolic filling time;
- up-regulation of cardiac beta$_1$ receptors;
- anti-inflammatory effects (after prolonged use);
- inhibition of catecholamine-induced cardiac necrosis (apoptosis); and
- increased left ventricular volume (thus increasing wall stress and oxygen requirements).

Perioperative myocardial infarction probably involves two mechanisms. Half may be due to coronary plaque rupture, leading to thrombus formation and subsequent vessel occlusion. The rest may be due to surgical stress causing an increase in sympathetic tone. This raises myocardial oxygen demand, leading to a myocardial oxygen supply/demand mismatch that, when sustained, causes infarction. Several of the above properties of beta-blockers may be responsible for their putative beneficial effect perioperatively [66].

Meta-analyses of perioperative beta-blocker use offer conflicting evidence. It has been suggested [66] that the conflicting results from the many perioperative beta-blocker trials might relate to:

- failure to titrate beta-blocker dose to heart rate adequately;
- timing of beta-blocker therapy and onset/lag times for anti-inflammatory effects; or
- duration of beta-blocker action and rebound effects from shorter-acting agents.

Further studies to clarify best the choice of beta-blocker, the dose of agent and the timing and duration of treatment are needed.

A strategy for perioperative cardiovascular optimization

As we have seen, there is a large body of evidence to suggest that the use of perioperative cardiovascular optimization and also somewhat paradoxically the use of beta-blockers can improve postoperative outcome. Reported reductions in length of hospital and critical care stay associated with goal-directed fluid therapy suggest there are substantial cost savings to be made. The challenge is to identify:

- the patients who will benefit from cardiovascular fluid optimization and those who will benefit from the further addition of inotropes;
- the appropriate goals to direct optimization therapy; and
- the patients at risk from cardiac ischemia who might be put at risk by overstimulation by inotropes, but who may benefit from the protection of beta-blockade.

Identifying the patients who will benefit from cardiovascular optimization

- Shoemaker [7] and Lee [67] have defined useful criteria to identify high-risk patients (Table 5.1 and Table 5.2). Lee's revised cardiac risk index (RCRI) is further discussed in Chapter 3. We have seen that where perioperative risk is low, there is little benefit from optimization regimens. In fact, some studies have seen increased risk in optimized patients. In selecting patients who might benefit from optimization, the anesthetist has to balance the risks of the surgery, the patient's own physiological reserve limitation and potential for inadequate fluid filling against the possible detrimental effects of over-hydration, overstimulation with inotropes and the morbidity from invasive monitoring (Figure 5.1).

- The recent studies using intraoperative fluid optimization [45–53] using esophageal Doppler have not suggested morbidity from this technique, but considerable benefits. The principle of proper fluid filling is well established in anesthesia. It would seem a reasonable strategy, therefore, to use this technique (or other flow-directed techniques) for all patients undergoing major surgery and identified as high risk by the criteria of

Table 5.2 The Revised Cardiac Risk Index in major non-cardiac surgery of Lee *et al.*

Criteria	Number of criteria	Risk of major cardiac complication (%)	
		Derivation cohort	Validation cohort
(1) High-risk type of surgery	0	0.5	0.4
(2) History of ischemic heart disease	1	1.3	0.9
(3) History of congestive heart failure	2	4.0	7.0
(4) History of cerebrovascular disease	3 or more	9.0	11.0
(5) Preoperative treatment with insulin			
(6) Preoperative serum creatinine >200 mg l^{-1} (176.8 μmol^{-1})			

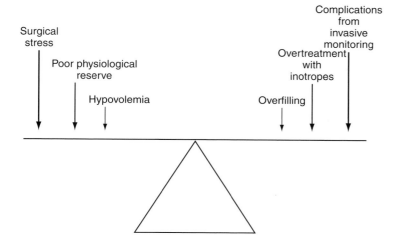

Figure 5.1 The balance of risks in perioperative optimization

Shoemaker or Lee. There are no studies comparing intraoperative goal-directed fluid therapy with the same treatment extending into the postoperative period. Given that there are studies showing benefit where goal-directed fluid optimization was commenced only in the postoperative period, it would seem reasonable to start fluid optimization intraoperatively and to continue, where practical, for 12–24 h, or even longer where fluid shifts related to surgery continue.

- The work of Older *et al.* [9, 10] has proved extremely effective to sensitively and specifically identify those patients at very high risk. Perhaps it is this group of patients with an anerobic threshold below $11\,\mathrm{ml\,min^{-1}\,kg^{-1}}$ who we should be considering for the additional use of inotropes. Others have suggested that patients with initial oxygen delivery of less than $450\,\mathrm{ml\,min^{-1}\,m^{-2}}$ should be targeted. A meta-analysis of perioperative goal-directed therapy has suggested that patients with a perioperative risk above 20% should be targeted [55].

The appropriate goals to direct optimization therapy

- Shoemaker [30] has suggested therapeutic goals to target therapy: the supranormal values described previously; a cardiac index of $4.5\,\mathrm{l\,min^{-1}\,m^{-2}}$, oxygen delivery of $600\,\mathrm{ml\,min^{-1}}$ $\mathrm{m^{-2}}$ and oxygen consumption of $170\,\mathrm{ml\,min^{-1}\,m^{-2}}$.

- It is a matter for judgement and experience on the part of the anesthetist to enhance cardiovascular function sufficiently to allow the demands of surgery to be met, whilst at the same time not overstressing the myocardium and precipitating ischemia or arrhythmia.

Patients at risk from cardiac ischemia

- We have seen that beta-blockers may be protective in a cohort of patients identified as high risk from untoward perioperative cardiac events. The strategy of beta-blockade and inotropic cardiovascular optimization would seem to be mutually exclusive.

- Use of beta-blockade, however, does not preclude the use of fluid optimization.

79

- We can identify patients as being at high risk from cardiac ischemia either from a history, by exercise testing, or by stress echocardiography. More specifically, the work of Lindenauer *et al.* [68] might suggest that it is important to select those with two or more criteria from the RCRI of Lee *et al.* [67] (Table 5.2). The American Heart Association–American College of Cardiology has also stratified cardiac risk and given guidance for perioperative beta-blockade (see Chapters 3 and 4).

- Where coronary revascularization is not indicated or cannot be achieved in a timely manner, these patients should receive flow-directed fluid therapy optimization but under the protection of beta-blockade and without inotropic support.

Further reading

Kern JW, Shoemaker WC. Meta-analysis of hemodynamic optimization in high-risk patients. *Crit Care Med* 2002; **30**: 1686–92.

Uusaro A, Russell JA. Could anti-inflammatory actions of

catecholamines explain the possible beneficial effects of supranormal oxygen delivery in critically ill surgical patients? *Intensive Care Med* 2000; **26**: 299–304.

References

1. Pearse RM, Harrison DA, James P, *et al.* Identification and characterisation of the high-risk surgical population in the United Kingdom. *Critical Care* 2006; **10**: R81.

2. National Confidential Enquiry into Perioperative Deaths (NCEPOD). *Then and now – the 2000 report of the National Confidential Enquiry into Perioperative Deaths*. London, NCEPOD; 2000.

3. Goldman L, Caldera D, Nussbaum S, *et al.* Multifactorial index of cardiac risk in non-cardiac surgical procedures. *New Engl J Med* 1977; **297**: 845–50.

4. Detsky AS, Abrams HB, Forbath N, *et al.* Cardiac assessment for patients undergoing non-cardiac surgery. A multifactorial clinical risk index. *Arch Int Med* 1986; **146**: 2131–4.

5. Boyd AD, Tremblay RE, Spencer FC, *et al.* Estimation of cardiac output soon after intracardiac surgery with cardio pulmonary bypass. *Ann Surg* 1959; **150**: 613–25.

6. Clowes GHA, Del Guercio LRM. Circulatory response to trauma of surgical operations. *Metabolism* 1960; **9**: 67–81.

7. Shoemaker WC, Czer LS. Evaluation of the biologic importance of various hemodynamic and oxygen transport variables: which variables should be monitored in postoperative shock? *Crit Care Med* 1979; 7: 424–31.

8. Reilly DF, McNeely MJ, Doerner D, *et al.* Self-reported exercise tolerance and the risk of serious perioperative complications. *Arch Intern Med* 1999; **159**: 2185–92.

9. Older P, Hall A. Clinical review: How to identify high-risk surgical patients. *Critical Care* 2004; **8**: 369–72.

10. Older P, Hall A, Hader R. Cardiopulmonary exercise testing as a screening test for perioperative management of major surgery in the elderly. *Chest* 1999; **116**: 355–62.

11. Charlson ME, Mackenzie CR, Gold JP, *et al.* Preoperative characteristics predicting intraoperative hypotension and hypertension among hypertensives and diabetics undergoing noncardiac surgery. *Ann Surg* 1990; **212**: 66–81.

12. Stone JG, Foex P, Sear JW, *et al.* Risk of myocardial ischaemia during anaesthesia in treated and untreated hypertensive patients. *Br J Anaesth* 1988; **61**: 675–9.

13. McFalls EO, Ward HB, Moritz TE, *et al.* Coronary artery revascularization before elective major vascular surgery. *N Engl J Med* 2004; **351**: 2795–804.

14. van den Berghe G, Wouters P, Weekers F, *et al.* Intensive insulin therapy in the

critically ill patients. *New Eng J Med* 2001; **345**: 1359–67.

15. Furnary AP, Gao G, Grunkemeier GL, *et al.* Continuous insulin infusion reduces mortality in patients with diabetes undergoing coronary artery bypass grafting. *J Thorac Cardiovasc Surg* 2003; **125**: 1007–21.

16. Gandhi GY, Nuttall GA, Abel MD, *et al.* Intensive intraoperative insulin therapy versus conventional glucose management during cardiac surgery: A randomized trial. *Ann Int Med* 2007; **146**: 233–43.

17. Groban L, Butterworth J. Perioperative management of chronic heart failure. *Anesth Analg* 2006; **103**: 557–75.

18. Grocott MP, Mythen MG, Gan TJ, *et al.* Perioperative fluid management and clinical outcomes in adults. *Anesth Analg* 2005; **100**: 1093–106.

19. Human albumin administration in critically ill patients: Systematic review of randomised controlled trials – Cochrane Injuries Group Albumin Reviewers. *BMJ* 1998; **317**: 235–40.

20. Soop M, Nygren J, Myrenfors P, *et al.* Preoperative oral carbohydrate treatment attenuates immediate postoperative insulin resistance. *Am J Physiol Endocrinol Metab* 2001; **280**: 576–83.

21. Melis GC, van Leeuwen PA, von Blomberg-van der Flier BM, *et al.* A carbohydrate-rich beverage prior to surgery prevents surgery-induced immunodepression: A randomized, controlled, clinical trial. *J Parenteral Enteral Nutr* 2006; **30**: 21–6.

22. Noblett SE, Watson DS, Huong H, *et al.* Preoperative oral carbohydrate loading in colorectal surgery: A randomized controlled trial. *Colorectal Dis* 2006; **8**: 563–9.

23. Rigg JR, Jamrozik K, Myles PS, *et al.* MASTER Anaesthesia Trial Study Group. Epidural anaesthesia and analgesia and outcome of major surgery: A randomized trial. *Lancet* 2002; **359**: 1276–82.

24. Liu S, Wu C. Effect of postoperative analgesia on major postoperative complications: A systematic update of the evidence. *Anesth Analg* 2007; **104**: 689–702.

25. MRC/BHF. Heart Protection Study of cholesterol lowering with simvastatin in 20,536 high-risk individuals: A randomized placebo-controlled trial. *Lancet* 2002; **360**: 7–22.

26. Noordzij PG, Poldermans D, Schouten O, *et al.* Beta-blockers and statins are individually associated with reduced mortality in patients undergoing noncardiac, nonvascular surgery. *Coron Artery Dis* 2007; **18**: 67–72.

27. Schouten O, Poldermans D, Visser L, *et al.* Fluvastatin and bisoprolol for the reduction of perioperative cardiac mortality and morbidity in high-risk patients undergoing non-cardiac surgery: rationale and design of the DECREASE-IV study. *Am Heart J* 2004; **148**: 1047–52.

28. Wallace AW, Galindez D, Salahieh A, *et al.* Effect of clonidine on cardiovascular morbidity and mortality after noncardiac surgery. *Anesthesiology* 2004; **101**: 284–93.

29. Shoemaker WC, Montgomery ES, Kaplan E, *et al.* Physiologic patterns in surviving and nonsurviving shock patients. Use of sequential cardiorespiratory variables in defining criteria for therapeutic goals and early warning of death. *Arch Surg* 1973; **106**: 630.

30. Shoemaker WC, Pierchala C, Chang P, *et al.* Prediction of outcome and severity of illness by analysis of the frequency distributions of cardiorespiratory variables. *Crit Care Med* 1977; **5**: 82.

31. Shoemaker WC, Appel PL, Waxman K, *et al.* Clinical trial of survivors' cardiorespiratory patterns as therapeutic goals in critically ill postoperative patients. *Crit Care Med* 1982; **10**: 398.

32. Schultz RJ, Whitfield GF, LaMura JJ, *et al.* The role of physiologic monitoring in patients with fractures of the hip. *J Trauma* 1985; **25**: 309–16.

33. Shoemaker WC, Appel PL, Kram HB, *et al.* Prospective trial of supranormal values of survivors as therapeutic goals in high-risk surgical patients. *Chest* 1988; **94**: 1176–86.

34. Berlauk JF, Abrams JH, Gilmour IJ, *et al.* Preoperative optimization of cardiovascular hemodynamics improves outcome in peripheral vascular surgery. A prospective, randomized clinical trial. *Ann Surg* 1991; **214**: 289–97.

35. Fleming A, Bishop M, Shoemaker W, *et al.* Prospective trial of supranormal values as goals of resuscitation in severe trauma. *Arch Surg* 1992; **127**: 1175–9.

36. Bishop MH, Shoemaker WC, Appel PL, *et al.* Prospective, randomized trial of survivor values of cardiac index, oxygen delivery, and oxygen consumption as resuscitation endpoints in severe trauma. *J Trauma* 1995; **38**: 780–7.

37. Boyd O, Grounds RM, Bennett ED. A randomized clinical trial of the effect of deliberate perioperative increase of oxygen delivery on mortality in high-risk surgical patients. *JAMA* 1993; **270**: 2699–707.

38. Ziegler DW, Wright JG, Choban PS, *et al.* A prospective randomized trial of preoperative "optimization" of cardiac function in patients undergoing elective peripheral vascular surgery. *Surgery* 1997; **122**: 584–92.

39. Valentine RJ, Duke ML, Inman MH, *et al.* Effectiveness of pulmonary artery catheters in aortic surgery: A randomized trial. *J Vasc Surg* 1998; **27**: 203–11.

40. Takala J, Meier-Hellmann A, Eddleston J, *et al.* Effect of dopexamine on outcome after major abdominal surgery: A prospective, randomized, controlled multicenter study. European Multicenter Study Group on Dopexamine in Major Abdominal Surgery. *Crit Care Med* 2000; **28**: 3417–23.

41. Wilson J, Woods I, Fawcett J, *et al.* Reducing the risk of major elective surgery: Randomised controlled trial of preoperative optimisation of oxygen delivery. *BMJ* 1999; **318**: 1099–103.

42. Byers RJ, Eddleston JM, Pearson RCRJ, *et al.* Dopexamine reduces the incidence of acute inflammation in the gut mucosa after abdominal surgery in high-risk patients. *Crit Care Med* 1999; **27**: 1787–93.

43. Snowden C, Roberts D. More than an abstract: "To optimise or not to optimise that is the question". *CPD Anaesth* 2000; **2**: 43–44.

44. Stone MD, Wilson RJ, Cross J, *et al.* Effect of adding dopexamine to intraoperative volume expansion in patients undergoing major elective abdominal surgery. *Br J Anaesth* 2003; **91**: 619–24.

45. Mythen MG, Webb AR. Perioperative plasma volume expansion reduces the incidence of gut mucosal hypoperfusion during cardiac surgery. *Arch Surg* 1995; **130**: 423–9.

46. Pölönen P, Ruokonen E, Hippeläinen M, *et al.* A prospective, randomized study of goal-oriented hemodynamic therapy in cardiac surgical patients. *Anesth Analg* 2000; **90**: 1052–59.

47. McKendry M, McGloin H, Saberi D, *et al.* Randomised controlled trial assessing the impact of a nurse delivered, flow monitored protocol for optimization of circulatory status after cardiac surgery. *Br Med J* 2004; **329**: 258.

48. Sinclair S, James S, Singer M. Intraoperative intravascular volume optimisation and length of hospital stay after repair of proximal femoral fracture: Randomised controlled trial. *BMJ* 1997; **315**: 909–12.

49. Venn R, Steele A, Richardson P, *et al.* Randomized controlled trial to investigate influence of the fluid challenge on duration of hospital stay and perioperative morbidity in patients with hip fractures. *Br J Anaesth* 2002; **88**: 65–71.

50. Conway DH, Mayall R, Abdul-Latif MS, *et al.* Randomised controlled trial investigating the influence of intravenous fluid titration using oesophageal Doppler monitoring during bowel surgery. *Anaesthesia* 2002; **57**: 845–9.

51. Gan TJ, Soppitt A, Maroof M, *et al.* Goal-directed intraoperative fluid administration reduces length of hospital stay after major surgery. *Anesthesiology* 2002; **97**: 820–6.

52. Wakeling HG, McFall MR, Jenkins CS, *et al.* Intraoperative oesophageal Doppler guided fluid management shortens postoperative hospital stay after major bowel surgery. *Br J Anaesth* 2005; **95**: 634–42.

53. Noblett SE, Snowden CP, Shenton BK, *et al.* Randomized clinical trial assessing the effect of Doppler-optimized fluid management on outcome after elective colorectal resection. *Br J Surg* 2006; **93**: 1069–76.

54. Pearse R, Dawson D, Fawcett J, *et al*. Early goal-directed therapy after major surgery reduces complications and duration of hospital stay. A randomised, controlled trial. *Crit Care* 2005; **9**: R687–93.

55. Kern JW, Shoemaker-William C. Meta-analysis of hemodynamic optimization in high-risk patients. *Crit Care Med* 2002; **30**: 1686–92.

56. Poeze M, Greve JW, Ramsay G. Meta-analysis of hemodynamic optimization: relationship to methodological quality. *Crit Care* 2005; **9**: R771–9.

57. Rubenfeld GD, McNamara-Aslin E, Rubinson L, *et al*. The pulmonary artery catheter, 1967–2007 rest in peace? *JAMA* 2007; **298**: 458–61.

58. Bundgaard-Nielsen M, Holte K, Secher NH, *et al*. Monitoring of peri-operative fluid administration by individualized goal-directed therapy. *Acta Anaesthesiol Scand* 2007; **51**: 331–40.

59. Edwards JD, Brown GC, Nightingale P, *et al*. Use of survivors' cardiorespiratory values as therapeutic goals in septic shock. *Crit Care Med* 1989; **17**: 1098–103.

60. Tuchschmidt J, Fried J, Astiz M, *et al*. Elevation of cardiac output and oxygen delivery improves outcome in septic shock. *Chest* 1992; **102**: 216–20.

61. Hayes MA, Yau EH, Timmins AC, *et al*. Response of critically ill patients to treatment aimed at achieving supranormal oxygen delivery and consumption. Relationship to outcome. *Chest* 1993; **103**: 886–95.

62. Yu M, Levy MM, Smith P, *et al*. Effect of maximizing oxygen delivery on morbidity and mortality rates in critically ill patients: A prospective, randomized, controlled study. *Crit Care Med* 1993; **21**: 830–8.

63. Gattinoni L, Brazzi L, Pelosi P, *et al*. A trial of goal-oriented hemodynamic therapy in critically ill patients. SvO2 Collaborative Group. *New Engl J Med* 1995; **333**: 1025–32.

64. Gutierrez G, Palizas F, Doglio G, *et al*. Gastric intramucosal pH as a therapeutic index of tissue oxygenation in critically ill patients. *Lancet* 1992; **339**: 195–9.

65. Rivers E, Nguyen B, Havstad S, *et al*. Early goal-directed therapy collaborative group: Early goal-directed therapy in the treatment of severe sepsis and septic shock. *New Engl J Med* 2001; **345**: 1368–77.

66. Schouten O, Bax JJ, Dunkelgrun M, *et al*. Pro: Beta-blockers are indicated for patients at risk for cardiac complications undergoing noncardiac surgery. *Anesth Analg* 2007; **104**: 8–10.

67. Lee TH, Marcantonio ER, Mangione CM, *et al*. Derivation and prospective validation of a simple index for prediction of cardiac risk of major noncardiac surgery. *Circulation* 1999; **100**: 1043–9.

68. Lindenauer PK, Pekow P, Wang K, *et al*. Perioperative beta-blocker therapy and mortality after major noncardiac surgery. *New Engl J Med* 2005; **353**: 349–61.

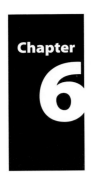

Chapter 6

Respiratory risk and complications

J. Granton

A great deal has been made of scoring systems and protocols for the assessment of risk surrounding perioperative cardiac complications [1]. Although effort has been made, the quantification of perioperative risk for respiratory complications has not met with the same acceptance. Perhaps the reason is related to difficulty in defining what a respiratory complication entails. Beyond just a definition, one must further decide what complications are clinically relevant. If atelectasis on postoperative day one is found on routine chest X-ray and the patient is discharged on schedule in good health, can we even call this a complication?

Despite the lack of consensus on what constitutes a respiratory complication, this does not diminish their impact on mortality or clinically relevant morbidity. The rates of complications have a wide variability depending on definitions of complications, type of surgeries and preoperative status of patient.

- In one prospective study of elective surgery, 11% of patients undergoing nonthoracic surgery with an expected admission greater than 24 h suffered a postoperative respiratory complication. However, this could encompass a wide variety of definitions, including atelectasis [2].

- In a study of patients with advanced chronic obstructive pulmonary disease (COPD) undergoing nonthoracic surgery, 37% had one or more postoperative pulmonary complications, the most common of which was prolonged ICU stay and refractory bronchospasm [3].

- In patients undergoing major noncardiac surgery, 1.5% can be shown to develop postoperative pneumonia [4].

- In elderly patients, pulmonary complications are more predictive of long-term mortality after surgery than cardiac complications [5].

One could cite studies that try to quantify the incidence of pulmonary complications, including pneumonia, prolonged mechanical ventilation, bronchospasm, atelectasis, pneumothorax, and even death. But for the practising anesthesiologist the question remains, "What are the chances that my patient is going to have a complication?" This is a very difficult question to answer. The variety of scoring systems available are difficult to apply due to the complexities of an individual patient. Thus we are left with trying to understand what puts an individual patient at risk by trying to extrapolate from studies that demonstrate what puts a population of patients in jeopardy for a perioperative complication. To do this, we must look at patient factors and surgical factors, and decide how best to improve our accuracy of prediction using preoperative investigation. However, once we decide that any given patient is at risk of a postoperative pulmonary complication, besides canceling the surgery, is there anything we can do to reduce risk?

Anesthesia for the High Risk Patient, ed. I. McConachie. Published by Cambridge University Press.
© Cambridge University Press 2009.

Who is at risk of perioperative respiratory complications?

Patient factors

1. Pre-existing respiratory disease
To a large extent respiratory disease is related to chronic obstructive pulmonary disease (COPD).

- The risk of perioperative bronchospasm, ventilation/perfusion mismatch, gas trapping and the respiratory depressant effects of inhalational agents are all more profound in patients with COPD [6].

- Obviously these risks are related to the severity of the disease and the definition of a complication with relative risks ranging from 2.7 to 4.7 for a perioperative respiratory incident [7].

- The American College of Physicians guidelines for risk assessment for patients undergoing noncardiac surgery indicate that COPD is the most commonly identified risk factor for the development of postoperative pulmonary complications [5].

It is not clear what additional risk asthma confers regarding perioperative respiratory complications. It would seem that most evidence indicates asthma is not routinely an independent predictor of respiratory complications [5]. However, frequency of complications may be elevated in older asthmatics, those with active symptoms, or recent flare up of symptoms [8]. Some studies do exist showing asthma to be predictive of respiratory complications in the postanesthetic care unit (PACU) [9, 10].

2. Smoking
Although not completely clear, smoking is a potential risk factor for the development of perioperative respiratory complications – even if the patient is not suffering from COPD as a result of smoking [7]. This is further discussed in Chapter 11.

3. Age
After COPD, the guidelines put forward by The American College of Physicians indicated that advanced age was the second most commonly identified risk factor for the development of perioperative respiratory complications.

- The odds ratio was 2.09 and 3.04 for patients aged 60–69 and 70–79, respectively, when compared to patients less than 60 years of age [5].

- However, there is a concern that the presence of co-existing disease may be a confounder in many studies, thus potentially negating age as an independent predictor [7].

4. Overall health
Generally, higher ASA classification (for example IV vs. III) is predictive of an increased risk of perioperative respiratory complications [5, 7, 11]. This holds true in particular for those with significant pre-existing respiratory disease [3]. Not surprisingly, patients with lower exercise tolerance have an increased incidence of perioperative pulmonary complications [7, 12].

5. Obesity

Interestingly, most studies have found no correlation between obesity and perioperative respiratory complications [5, 13, 14]. In ambulatory surgery, obesity did not increase the need for unanticipated hospital admission [15].

It should be remembered that obesity (BMI >30) and large neck circumference are associated with obstructive sleep apnea (OSA) [16]. These patients may be more difficult to intubate and may also experience problems in the recovery room with hypertension, low saturations and recurrent airway obstruction [17].

This is further discussed in Chapter 10.

6. Preoperative sputum production

A history of preoperative sputum production has been linked to an increased risk of postoperative respiratory complications [2].

Surgical factors

1. Duration of anesthetic

Generally the longer the duration of anesthesia (greater than 3 h), the greater the risk of postoperative respiratory complications [5, 7].

- In prospective studies of patients undergoing nonthoracic surgery, duration of anesthesia was found to be a risk factor for postoperative complications [2, 13].
- In a systemic review of the literature, Fisher *et al.* found that duration of anesthesia was found as an associated risk factor for respiratory complications in multiple studies [18].

Table 6.1 illustrates the effect of various patient and surgical risk factors on the odds ratio for developing postoperative respiratory complications.

Table 6.1 Patient and surgical risk factors and odds ratio for developing respiratory complications.

Risk factor	Odds ratio for developing a respiratory complication
Age > 60	2.09 (95% CI, 1.70–2.58)
COPD	1.79 (95% CI, 1.44–1.56)
Cigarette smoking	1.26 (95% CI, 1.10–1.56)
ASA greater than II	4.87 (95% CI, 3.34–7.10)
Duration of surgery of greater than 3 h	2.14 (95% CI, 1.33–3.46)
General anesthesia	1.83 (95% CI, 1.35–2.46)
Emergency surgery	2.21 (95% CI, 1.57–3.11)

Adapted from Qaseem A, Snow V, Fitterman N, *et al.* Risk assessment for and strategies to reduce perioperative pulmonary complications for patients undergoing noncardiothoracic surgery: A guideline from the American College of Physicians. *Ann Int Med* 2006; **144**: 575–80.

Table 6.2 Influence of surgical site on rates of postoperative pulmonary complications.

Surgical incision site	Range of % cases with complications*
Thoracic	10–40
Upper abdomen	13–33
Lower abdomen	0–16
Laparoscopic	0.3–0.4

*Range provided by nine studies with varying co-morbid states and complication definitions.
Adapted from Smetana GW. Preoperative pulmonary evaluation. *New Engl J Med* 1999; **340**: 937–44.

2. Nasogastric tube insertion

Surprisingly, nasogastric (NG) tube insertion has often been found to be an independent predictor of postoperative respiratory complications [18].

- In a prospective study of risk factors for postoperative pulmonary complications the most predictive was NG tube insertion with an odds ratio of 21.8! [18].
- It is not clear what mechanism is responsible for the risk associated with NG tube insertion.
- Some theories include: impaired cough, bacteria transfer from oral pharynx to the lungs, and diaphragmatic dysfunction [18].

3. Site of surgery

Incisions of the upper abdomen carry a greater risk of postoperative respiratory complications when compared to the lower abdomen [11], although this author believes that quantifying the amount of additional risk is difficult at best. Incisions involving the thorax are often quoted as having a greater risk. This is illustrated in Table 6.2.

4. Anesthetic technique

The evidence is not completely clear whether avoidance of a general anesthetic and the use of an alternate technique are protective in reducing the risk of pulmonary complications. Without a doubt, there are those who strongly believe that avoidance of general anesthesia in patients with preoperative respiratory dysfunction is of benefit.

- Two well-received reviews on risk factors for respiratory complications seem to add weight to the argument favoring avoidance of general anesthesia in this patient population [5, 7].
- In addition, the technique used for postoperative pain control may have an impact on postoperative respiratory complications [19, 20]. This will be discussed in greater detail later.

5. Emergency surgery

Multiple studies have indicated that emergency surgery can increase the risk of postoperative respiratory complications [5].

Preoperative investigations

Pulmonary function test (PFT)

Although it can be tempting to quote risks of pulmonary complications based on things such as forced vital capacity (FVC), in this author's experience too many patient and surgical factors are varying, and using PFTs as a means to predict outcome is far from an exact science. The patients' exercise capacity and overall health status are likely more important.

- Because the evidence is conflicting, support for a prohibitive spirometric value, below which surgery should be canceled, is not universal [5].
- In a well done prospective cohort study, McAlister *et al.* found that a forced expiratory volume in 1 s (FEV$_1$) that was less than 1 l was predictive of complications in patients undergoing elective nonthoracic surgery [13].
- In addition, the use of spirometry to improve bronchodilator therapy perioperatively makes good sense [7].

Special mention should be devoted to those patients undergoing lung resection surgery. A wide variety of tests are performed to predict perioperative pulmonary risk. Based on the planned resection, postoperative predicted spirometry values and diffusion capacity (DL$_{co}$) can be calculated [11]. Others have used measurement of exercise oxygen consumption (MVO$_2$) and the six-minute walk test as methods to assess viability of lung resection surgery. Regarding cardiac surgery, there is some evidence that poor spirometry results may be predictive of worse morbidity and mortality, although cut-off spirometric values cannot be stated [21].

Blood gases

Similar to PFTs, using preoperative blood gases to predict postoperative respiratory complications is difficult. Some have suggested that a pCO$_2$ greater than 45 is predictive of complications, but this is debatable [7].

Chest radiographs

For the most part, physicians can predict the likelihood of perioperative respiratory complications without the use of chest radiographs. In a meta-analysis of routine preoperative chest radiographs, in only 1.3% of the films were abnormalities unexpected, and in only 0.1% of cases did this result in a change in management [22]. Nothing can be stated as to whether this change in management resulted in improved outcomes.

Additional laboratory values

Interestingly, low serum albumin levels (less than 35 g l^{-1}) are predictive of perioperative risk [5]. A very large prospective cohort study of VA medical centers in the United States demonstrated that a serum albumin level less than 30 g l^{-1} was a powerful indicator of postoperative respiratory failure [23]. The same study also found that a blood urea nitrogen (BUN) greater than 10.7 mmol l^{-1} (30 g dl^{-1}) was predictive of respiratory complications.

Risk index

Due to the complexities of patient and surgical factors, it is tempting to use a risk index to help predict postoperative complications. Recently, authors involved in the National Veterans Administration Surgical Quality Improvement Program have produced and validated a multi-factor risk index for predicting postoperative pneumonia and respiratory failure (postoperative ventilation for greater than 48 h or reintubation) for noncardiac surgery [4, 23]. They assign a point value to specific patient and surgical factors and several investigative findings that were found to be predictive. These points are totaled, and this total allows the patients risk to be classified.

Can we do anything to reduce a patient's risk of perioperative respiratory complications?

Smoking cessation

Smoking is associated with a wide variety of co-morbid illnesses, in particular coronary artery disease and chronic lung disease. Current smoking is associated with increased incidence of postoperative respiratory complications [24]. However, controversy exists regarding the timing and effectiveness of smoking cessation as a method of perioperative respiratory complication reduction.

- Cigarette smoke can acutely reduce airway ciliary function and increase carbon monoxide levels.
- It may take weeks to months to find an objective improvement in respiratory function after smoking cessation.
- The best evidence would suggest that at least two months is required before smoking abstinence reduces the risk of pulmonary complications [25].
- Some have a concern that smoking cessation in the short term before an anesthetic may actually worsen cough and sputum production.
- One must also keep in mind smoking's effect on wound healing and cardiac events.
- What can be said is that longer durations of cessation appear to be more effective in reducing postoperative complications, but the exact duration required is difficult to quantify [26].

Anesthetic technique

As was stated previously, it would seem that duration of anesthesia can impact the risk of respiratory complications. However, what is far more controversial is the difference in risk between neuraxial combined with general anesthesia, neuraxial alone, and general anesthesia alone.

- In a widely cited meta-analysis including 9559 patients, Rodgers *et al.* found that there was a statistically significant reduction in mortality in those patients who received neuraxial blockade or neuraxial blockade combined with general anesthesia versus those who received general anesthesia alone.
- Looking at pulmonary complications, this study demonstrated a reduction in pneumonia (odds ratio 0.61, CI 0.48–0.76) and postoperative respiratory depression (odds ratio 0.41, CI 0.23–0.73) in patients receiving neuraxial blockade [27].
- It should be noted that this paper has met with its skeptics, who question the heterogeneous populations involved, as well as older anesthetic techniques and agents [5].

This author believes that the decision to offer neuraxial techniques should be made on an individual patient and surgery basis. Blanket statements that neuraxial techniques will offer a reduction in complications are not warranted.

89

The type of neuromuscular blockade used for general anesthesia has been shown to influence postoperative respiratory complications. The risk of prolonged blockade with a long-acting agent (pancuronium), may contribute to an increased incidence of respiratory complications postoperatively [5].

Pain control

It seems to make intuitive sense that adequate postoperative pain control should reduce respiratory complications in those incisions that are particularly painful (upper abdominal and thorax). For patients undergoing laparotomy or major thoracic surgery, a well-placed and functioning epidural provides superior pain relief when compared to intravenous narcotics [19, 20].

- In a randomized study of patients undergoing abdominal surgery, patients managed with an epidural for postoperative pain relief had a reduction in postoperative respiratory complications when compared to controls, although no difference in mortality was found [19].

- In a large Veterans study in the United States, the use of epidural anesthesia for post-operative pain control compared to systemic opiates found that for abdominal aortic surgery patient's epidurals significantly reduced major complications including intubation time and duration of intensive care unit stay [20].

Obviously the risks of epidural analgesia need to be taken into consideration also.

Postoperative lung expansion

A variety of techniques are available for postoperative lung expansion. This includes incentive spirometry, assisted cough, percussion and vibration, deep suctioning and ambulation. The use of postoperative incentive spirometry has been shown to reduce postoperative respiratory complications [28]. However, there is minimal evidence that one technique is superior to another [5]. The choice likely revolves around what the patient can cooperate with and the services available in an individual hospital.

The sleep apnea patient

Special mention is made here about the patient that suffers from obstructive sleep apnea (OSA). Care should be taken to avoid excessive use of sedation and narcotics in the perioperative period, as this may lead to an increased incidence of airway obstruction and desaturation [16]. If practical, most would agree that the preferable choice would be regional or neuraxial anesthesia. Regarding the choice for postoperative pain control, a technique or regime that avoids extensive reliance on narcotics would seem prudent. Thus multimodal analgesia and/or regional nerve blockade would serve these patients well. Finally, the decision to perform surgery on an outpatient basis is controversial. Practice guidelines put forth by the American Society of Anesthesiologists in 2006 attempted to reach a consensus regarding outpatient surgery. It would seem that minor procedures not involving the airway are reasonable for outpatient bookings. However, there was a lack of agreement amongst many experts on surgery requiring a general anesthetic [29]. Clinical judgment is required in coming to any decision on discharge home. Considerations should include: severity of the sleep apnea, need for analgesia, support at home, and stability of saturation prior to discharge.

Further reading

Rock P, Passannante A. Preoperative assessment: Pulmonary. *Anesthesiol Clin North Am* 2004; **22**: 77–91.

Watson CB. Respiratory complications associated with anesthesia. *Anesthesiol Clin North Am* 2002; **20**: 513–37.

References

1. Fleisher LA. Risk of anesthesia. In: Miller DL, ed. *Miller's Anesthesia*, 6th edn. Philadelphia, PA: Elsevier, Churchill Livingstone. 2005; 908.

2. Mitchell CK, Smoger SH, Pfeifer MP, *et al.* Multivariate analysis of factors associated with postoperative pulmonary complications following general elective surgery. *Arch Surg* 1998; **33**: 194–8.

3. Wong DH, Weber EC, Schell MJ, *et al.* Factors associated with postoperative pulmonary complications in patients with severe chronic obstructive pulmonary disease. *Anesth Analg* 1995; **80**: 276–84.

4. Arozullah AM, Khuri SF, Henderson WG, *et al.* Development and validation of a multifactorial risk index for predicting postoperative pneumonia after major noncardiac surgery. *Ann Int Med* 2001; **135**: 847–57.

5. Qaseem A, Snow V, Fitterman N, *et al.* Risk assessment for and strategies to reduce perioperative pulmonary complications for patients undergoing noncardiothoracic surgery: A guideline from the American College of Physicians. *Ann Int Med* 2006; **144**: 575–80.

6. Seigne PW, Philip PM, Simon C. Anesthetic considerations for patients with severe emphysematous lung disease. *Int Anesthesiol Clin* 2000; **38**: 1–23.

7. Smetana GW. Preoperative pulmonary evaluation. *New Engl J Med* 1999; **340**: 937–44.

8. Warner DO, Warner MA, Barnes RD, *et al.* Perioperative respiratory complications in patients with asthma. *Anesthesiology* 1996; **85**: 460–7.

9. Shnaider I, Chung F. Outcomes in day surgery. *Curr Opin Anesthesiol* 2006; **19**: 622–9.

10. Chung F, Mezei G, Tong D. Pre-existing medical conditions as predictors of adverse events in day-case surgery. *Br J Anaesthesia* 1999; **83**: 262–70.

11. Ferguson MK. Preoperative assessment of pulmonary risk. *Chest* 1999; **115**: 58S–63S.

12. Williams-Russo P, Charlson ME, MacKenzie CR, *et al.* Predicting postoperative pulmonary complications: Is it a real problem? *Arch Int Med* 1992; **152**: 1209–13.

13. McAlister FA, Bertsch K, Man J, *et al.* Incidence of and risk factors for pulmonary complications after nonthoracic surgery. *Am J Resp Crit Care Med* 2005; **171**: 514–17.

14. Eichenberger A, Proietti S, Wicky S, *et al.* Morbid obesity and postoperative pulmonary atelectasis: An underestimated problem. *Anesth Analg* 2002; **95**: 1788–92.

15. Servin F. Ambulatory anesthesia for the obese patient. *Curr Opin Anesthesiol* 2006; **19**: 597–9.

16. Den Herder C, Schmeck, JDJK, Appelboom DJK, *et al.* Risks of general anaesthesia in people with obstructive sleep apnoea. *Br Med J* 2004; **329**: 955–9.

17. Bryson GL, Chung F, Finegan BA, *et al.* Patient selection in ambulatory anesthesia – an evidence-based review: Part I. *Can J Anesthes* 2004; **51**: 768–81.

18. Fisher BW, Majumdar SR, McAlister FA. Predicting pulmonary complications after nonthoracic surgery: A systemic review of blinded studies. *Am J Med* 2002; **112**: 219–25.

19. Rigg JR, Jamrozik K, Myles PS, *et al.* Epidural anaesthesia and analgesia and outcome of major surgery: A randomized trial. *Lancet* 2002; **359**: 1276–82.

20. Park WY, Thompson JS, Lee KK. Effect of epidural anesthesia and analgesia on perioperative outcome: A randomized, controlled Veterans Affairs cooperative study. *Ann Surg* 2001; **234**: 569–71.

21. Hirose H, Gill IS, Kavuru M, *et al.* Pulmonary function parameters and outcomes after cardiac surgery. *Chest* 2006; **130**:4, 124S.

22. Archer C, Levy AR, McGregor M. Value of routine preoperative chest X-rays: A meta-analysis. *Can J Anesthes* 1993; **40**: 1022–7.

23. Arozullah AM, Daley J, Henderson WG, *et al.* Multifactorial risk index for predicting postoperative respiratory failure in men after major noncardiac surgery. *Ann Surg* **2000**; **232**: 242–53.

24. Bluman LG, Mosca L, Newman N, *et al.* Preoperative smoking habits and postoperative pulmonary complications. *Chest* 1998; **113**: 883–9.

25. Warner DO. How surgical patients quit smoking: Why, when and how. *Anesth Analg* 2005; **101**: 481–7.

26. Theadom A, Cropley M. Effects of preoperative smoking cessation on the incidence of intraoperative and postoperative complications in adult smokers: A systemic review. *Tobacco Control* 2006; **15**: 352–8.

27. Rodgers A, Walker N, Schug S, *et al.* Reduction of postoperative mortality and morbidity with epidural or spinal anaesthesia: Results from overview of randomized trials. *Br Med J* 2000; **321**: 1–12.

28. Fleisher LA, Roizen MF. Anesthesia implications of concurrent disease. In: Miller DL, ed. *Miller's Anesthesia*, 6th edn. Philadelphia, PA: Elsevier, Churchill Livingstone. 2005; 1086.

29. American Society of Anesthesiologists Task Force on Perioperative Management of Patients with Obstructive Sleep Apnea. Practice guidelines for the perioperative management of patients with obstructive sleep apnea. *Anesthesiology* 2006; **104**: 1081–93.

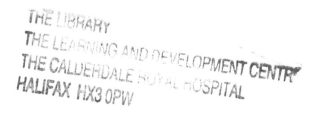

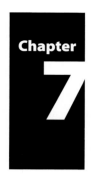

Chapter 7

Analgesia for the high-risk patient

C. Clarke and P. Morley-Forster

Introduction

Ancient texts refer to the struggles of Greek physicians to relieve pain. Within the practice of modern day anesthesia, the tools at our disposal have increased greatly in number and complexity, but challenges remain.

- The patient who is at high risk either because of extensive surgery or poor physiological reserve requires effective pain relief to avoid morbidity and even mortality.
- At the same time, there are more potential limitations to certain drugs and regional techniques in the elderly, or those with systemic illness.
- Multiple factors must be weighed by the Acute Pain Service (APS) in formulating an individual management plan.
- There are some exciting analgesic strategies being developed for high-risk patients such as peripheral opioid agonists, long-acting depot local anesthetics, magnetic neuromodulation, and technology to detect postsurgical nerve injury earlier.

This chapter serves as a guide to evidence-based considerations and practices in the perioperative pain management of high-risk patients.

The Acute Pain Service (APS)

A well-organized, multi-disciplinary APS is essential to ensure optimal pain management is achieved in "high-risk" patients.

- The multi-disciplinary approach to perioperative pain management was first described by Ready *et al.* in 1988 [1].
- Gould *et al.* demonstrated prospectively that the introduction of an acute pain service to the surgical wards improved pain levels as assessed by Visual Analog Scales [2].
- A recent review of the literature concluded that not only does an APS improve pain scores and patient satisfaction, but it also significantly reduces cost, nausea and patient morbidity [3]

The APS team at most centers now consists of at least one dedicated nurse and an anesthesia consultant. A pharmacist and/or a physiotherapist may complement the team.

Pathophysiology of acute pain

The classic nociceptive system responsible for the transmission of pain sensations is well-understood.

Anesthesia for the High Risk Patient, ed. I. McConachie. Published by Cambridge University Press.
© Cambridge University Press 2009.

- Peripheral Aδ and C fibers sense the noxious stimuli of a pressure, cutting, thermal or chemical nature and transmit them via an action potential in the axon to the dorsal horn of the spinal cord.
- At the dorsal horn, these signals are then relayed to the ascending spinothalamic tract. The dorsal horn is more than a simple relay point: it acts as a signal modulator, enhancing or inhibiting signals from the periphery [4].
- From the thalamus, the signal is transferred to the somato-sensory cortex, which is responsible for the localized perception of pain and activating either a withdrawal or nonmovement response.

Clinical pain differs from the nociceptive model seen in the laboratory of the neurophysiologist. In order to appreciate the need for multi-modal pain management in the perioperative period, one must understand the contributions of peripheral and central sensitization to the pain experience.

- Trauma releases inflammatory mediators from tissues, mast cells, macrophages and lymphocytes.
- Vasodilatation and increased capillary permeability augments the inflammatory response.
- The "sensitizing soup" of mediators promotes the depolarization of sympathetic and sensory nerve fibers. A stimulus which is normally perceived as nonpainful, such as pressure, becomes painful. The excitation threshold of peripheral nociceptors is lowered, causing stimuli to initiate a stronger pain response than occurs in the nonsensitized state [5].
- Central sensitization is the phenomenon of enhanced perception of peripheral stimuli via facilitated transmission at spinal cord synapses [6]. This amplified pain response after surgery appears to be mediated by up-regulation of prostaglandins and interleukins in the central nervous system [7]. The neurotransmitter, glutamate, plays a crucial role in sensitization at the dorsal horn by binding to the N-methyl-D-aspartate (NMDA) receptor and facilitating sodium conductance intracellularly [8].
- The involvement of NMDA receptors, prostaglandins and calcium-permeable AMPA (α-amino-3-hydroxy-5-methyl-4-isoxazoleproprionic acid) receptors in the development of central sensitization explain why ketamine, nonsteroidal anti-inflammatory drugs (NSAIDs) and gabapentin/pregabalin are important pharmacologic agents in treatment and prevention of postsurgical pain [9].
- Early identification and treatment of neuropathic pain, due to peripheral or central nervous system dysfunction, is important. Neuropathic pain is often described as "burning" or "shooting" and may be elicited by touch or pressure on the affected area. It is poorly responsive to opioids; anticonvulsant therapy is more effective.

Pain assessment

Due to cultural, social or emotional influences, patients demonstrate broad variation in their reactions to pain, necessitating individualized assessment. Although it is important to understand the patient suffering component that may be added to the pain sensation, this section will focus on effective tools for evaluating pain *intensity*.

- When assessing postoperative pain, it is important to differentiate between surgical incision pain and pre-existing pain from other causes. Use of a pre-admission pain diagram may be helpful for this reason.

- The pre-admission consultation should identify high-risk patients and establish a pain management plan before the day of surgery, and determine whether inpatient, or ICU, admission will be required.

- The most practical tool for assessment of pain at the bedside is the Numerical Rating Scale (NRS). The patient is asked to rate their pain from 0 to 10; 0 represents no pain and 10 represents the worst imaginable pain. This scale consistently gives the most reproducible scores and is easy to apply [10].

- The faces pain scale is a variation of the NRS containing a series of facial expressions ranging from happy to sad. Patients are asked to rate their pain to choose the face they feel is most representative of their own pain. This will yield a score which depends on the number of faces the patient has to choose from. This scale has been shown to be effective in patients with cognitive impairment, particularly in the ICU setting [11].

- The Visual Analog Scale is a 10 cm line bordered by the phrase "no pain" and "worst imaginable pain". The patient is asked to place a mark on the line to demonstrate the intensity of their pain. This mark is then measured, in mm, from 0 giving a pain score from 0 to 100. This pain scale has been demonstrated to give the most statistically robust data for research trials, but can demonstrate user variability as great as 20%, with patients scoring different pain values without stating any difference in their perceived pain. This yields false results that may be determined as clinically significant [10].

The key points in choosing a pain assessment tool are that it is quick and easy to use, used regularly, repeated soon after any intervention, and applied both at rest and on movement. It is important to provide an intervention if the pain score is over halfway up the scale. From a clinical perspective, patients should be comfortably able to take a deep breath and cough. Changes in the *type* or *intensity* of the pain being experienced by the patient should be noted, as this may indicate either failure of the analgesic technique, e.g. an epidural catheter falling out or becoming disconnected, or possibly deterioration in the patient's condition such as compartment syndrome.

Site of surgery/trauma

In the overall assessment of analgesia requirements for the high-risk patient, the site of surgery must be considered in conjunction with the patient's medical condition.

Chest wall

Patients having chest surgery can experience severe postoperative pain that significantly alters chest wall mechanics, making the patient vulnerable to atelectasis, ventilation/perfusion mismatching, hypoxemia and infection [12]. Although many techniques for postthoracotomy analgesia are discussed in the literature, there is no doubt that pain control in this surgical population is best attained by a thoracic epidural. Other commonly used techniques are intravenous opioids by patient-controlled analgesia with NSAIDs, intercostal nerve blocks, and paravertebral nerve blocks as adjuncts.

Upper/lower abdomen

A significant proportion of patients in this category will present as emergency cases with the possibility of concomitant sepsis, dehydration, electrolyte imbalance and other physiological deficits. Upper abdominal surgery adversely affects postoperative pulmonary function. Does effective analgesia avoid this development? A systematic review of the literature supports the ability of epidural analgesia to reduce perioperative pulmonary complications in the high-risk patient following abdominal surgery [13]. The majority of lower abdominal or pelvic surgery cases are elective (e.g. gynecologic) and tend to cope very well with patient-controlled analgesia (PCA) or traditional opioid dosing.

Peripheral sites

The main concern in those with peripheral limb surgery is impairment of mobility since this predisposes the patient to thromboembolic phenomenon as well as atelectasis [14]. The analgesic objectives should be to promote early mobilization. A multi-modal analgesic regime with consideration of regional anesthesia, where appropriate, is optimal.

Pain in more than one location

This is a common problem following major trauma. Although an epidural may be indicated to treat pain from chest trauma, or a laparotomy, it will not provide effective analgesia for concomitant limb fractures. One strategy is to use local anesthetic only in the epidural infusion and allow the patient to use a standard PCA to treat the pain not managed by the epidural. This strategy can also be used when epidural analgesia is inadequate due to a missed segment, or when low epidural placement misses the top end of a surgical wound.

Major considerations of pain management for co-existing disease

Coronary artery disease

- Approximately 50% of surgical patients have one or more cardiac risk factors [15].
- Uncontrolled pain can initiate a sympathetic response, causing an increase in arterial pressure, heart rate, and myocardial contractility.
- In addition, this response may trigger hypercoagulability and vasospasm [16].
- All the above can contribute to altering myocardial supply and demand ratios resulting in ischemia or infarction.
- Therefore, it is important to recognize patients with coronary arterial disease and manage them effectively.

The use of thoracic epidurals has been well-studied in cardiac disease. In addition to decreasing the negative physiologic responses to pain, data suggest that thoracic epidurals may foster a physiologic environment that is favorable for myocardial perfusion. Thoracic epidurals seem to increase oxygen supply by increasing the diameter of coronary arteries while maintaining perfusion pressure [17]. This technique increases myocardial blood supply despite sympathetic stimulation [18].

There is still scant evidence in the literature to support the concept that optimal pain control will decrease the incidence of perioperative cardiac events. However, one clinical trial in patients undergoing revascularization demonstrated that superior pain control reduced the frequency and severity of ischemic events [19].

It is important to note that ketamine at high doses may negatively affect the myocardium prone to ischemia. Previous studies have demonstrated that ketamine decreases catecholamine re-uptake, causing an increased sympathomimetic tone, and increases myocardial contractility at induction doses. No studies have examined the effect of ketamine on myocardial ischemia in the low doses used for pain management.

Patients with fixed cardiac output

In patients with severe aortic stenosis, severe mitral valve stenosis or hypertrophic obstructive cardiomyopathy, it may be necessary to obtain echocardiography before proceeding with any neuraxial analgesia. Decreased venous return from the pharmacologic sympathectomy may cause profound hypotension.

Respiratory

Chronic obstructive pulmonary disease, and reactive airways disease, are both highly prevalent in the surgical population.

- A large meta-analysis of several studies was conducted in 1998 looking at various analgesic strategies to reduce postoperative respiratory complications.

- The studies reviewed looked at epidural opioid, epidural local anesthetic, epidural opioid with local anesthetic, thoracic versus lumbar insertion, intercostal nerve blocks, wound infiltration with local anesthetic and intrapleural local anesthetic. Outcomes assessed were clinically significant atelectasis, respiratory infection and any pulmonary complication (e.g. hypoxia, need for ventilatory support).

- They determined that patients undergoing abdominal and thoracic surgery had the greatest benefit from epidural analgesia with local anesthetic. Patients who received local anesthetic epidurals had higher PaO_2, and a lower incidence of atelectasis, pulmonary infections and overall pulmonary complications [20].

This analgesic strategy should be considered when anesthetizing patients with COPD or asthma for thoracic procedures.

Despite studies demonstrating the efficacy of epidural analgesia in reducing perioperative pulmonary complications, there has been concern raised that it may actually be detrimental to the patient with obstructive pulmonary disease.

- Insertion of a high thoracic epidural block has been shown to initially reduce vital capacity and forced expiratory volume by 8–10%, primarily as a result of the decreased function of intercostal muscles [21].

- However, abdominal and thoracic surgery patients may have postoperative reductions in vital capacity and forced expiratory volume by as much as 60% due to diaphragmatic dysfunction.

- The small initial loss of lung volumes with epidural insertion is compensated by its later protective effects [22].

97

- The theoretical concern of an increase in airway reactivity in sympathectomized patients does not appear to be borne out in reality, since evidence shows that epidural analgesia causes up to a 20% reduction in airway reactivity. This phenomenon appears to be explained mainly by the fact that intravenous local anesthetics block neurally mediated airway constriction [22].

Ketamine has several benefits in the respiratory-compromised patient.

- Firstly, ketamine has been demonstrated to cause an increase in spontaneous respiratory rate.
- Secondly, it has been shown to have bronchodilatory effects.

These two qualities, in addition to its pain-relieving and opioid-sparing benefits, make it an excellent analgesic to consider in the patient with obstructive pulmonary disease.

The patient with reactive airway disease or nasal polyps may be more likely to manifest hypersensitivity to aspirin and other NSAIDs even if they do not have a documented sensitivity.

Sleep apnea

Sleep apnea can be categorized as central or obstructive.

- Central sleep apnea generally occurs as a function of neurologic or neuromuscular disorders.
- Obstructive sleep apnea is attributed to anatomical obstruction of the airway from fatty tissue infiltration and a decrease of protective muscle tone.

Many analgesics contribute to sedation and muscle relaxation, which exacerbate both types of sleep apnea syndromes.

- Opioids contribute to obstruction in sleep apnea by preferential depression of upper airway muscle activity similar to the effect of sleep. It appears that both dose and route of administration are important for alteration of upper airway muscle function [23]. A recent study concluded that there is a dose-dependent relationship between opioids and obstructed/ataxic breathing. However, the clinical relevance of these findings has yet to be established [24].
- Ketamine may develop a role in pain management for the patient with sleep apnea. Its intense analgesic properties at sub-anesthetic doses, and the fact that it is relatively devoid of respiratory depressant activity, provide theoretical support for its postoperative use in the sleep apneic patient, although there are no clinical trials confirming its efficacy.

Hepatic disease

Liver disease accounts for a significant proportion of hospitalized patients.

- The most important consideration with liver disease is that the duration and effect of analgesics can be significantly affected; furthermore, pharmacodynamics and pharmacokinetics are altered depending on the degree of organ dysfunction.
- In addition, patients with liver failure, particularly those with hepatic encephalopathy, are much more sensitive to the sedative effects of opioid analgesics.
- Finally, when planning the analgesic technique, one must be aware of the coagulation status of the patient. Although, in general, a neuraxial technique may offer the best pain relief, in some individuals the risk of an epidural hematoma may be too high.

The liver is the major site for biotransformation of essentially all opioids, with the exception of remifentanil, which is metabolized by ester hydrolysis in the plasma. Even in hepatic failure, remifentanil pharmacokinetics do not appear to change significantly [25]. If one chooses to administer opioids, it is important to titrate the dose specifically to the patient's level of pain, and vital signs. Initial dosing should not occur on a standard scheduled regime until the duration of drug effect in that individual is determined.

Administration of codeine to patients with hepatic dysfunction is a poor choice. Codeine relies for its efficacy upon hepatic biotransformation into morphine. Thus, if metabolism of codeine is seriously impaired, the expected analgesic action will not occur.

The use of acetaminophen in patients with liver disease has been controversial in the past. However, a recent systematic review concluded that *acetaminophen is safe to use in patients with chronic liver disease*. Although the elimination of acetaminophen in hepatic dysfunction occurs more slowly than in patients without liver disease, repeated administration of the drug does not result in accumulation. Hepatotoxicity seems to be confined to those who misuse acetaminophen, intentionally or accidentally. The use of therapeutically recommended doses does not appear to increase hepatotoxicity in patients with chronic liver disease [26].

The literature carries conflicting reports as to whether or not NSAIDs contribute to acute hepatic toxicity or worsens chronic hepatic insufficiency. NSAIDs should be avoided in patients who are already taking potentially hepatotoxic drugs, or have autoimmune disease [27]. Patients with severe liver disease are also predisposed to gastrointestinal bleeds and hepato-renal syndrome, which could be further exacerbated by the use of NSAIDs. In summary, the use of NSAIDs in patients with liver disease should be undertaken only after a careful analysis of the risk–benefit ratio.

Renal disease

In selecting the analgesic regime of choice in this patient population, it is important to consider which drugs possess active metabolites which are renally excreted or which possess a prolonged renal clearance themselves.

- The literature supports alfentanil, sufentanil, remifentanil, fentanyl, ketamine, and acetaminophen as being the safest for use in renal impairment, as no specific change in dosing appears to be required [28].

- In the presence of renal disease, one should not use NSAIDs, since they have the potential to cause renal failure or worsen existing renal disease. This vulnerability is particularly enhanced during the use of angiotensin-converting enzyme inhibitors, diuretics and beta-blockers, all commonly used in the surgical population [29].

Meperidine, morphine and NSAIDs have the potential for serious adverse sequelae in renal insufficiency. The active metabolite of meperidine, normeperidine, accumulates in renal insufficiency causing central nervous system excitatory symptoms of anxiety, agitation, hyperreflexia, myoclonus, tremors, and seizures. These effects have been seen in patients with renal failure since normeperidine, which is excreted by the kidneys, accumulates in renal insufficiency. Meperidine is clearly contraindicated in patients in renal failure.

The active metabolite of morphine, morphine-6-glucuronide, is excreted renally and is approximately 10 times as potent as morphine. In renal insufficiency it has the ability to accumulate and cause significant respiratory depression. Another opioid such as hydromorphone or fentanyl is preferable.

In summary, one should avoid meperidine, morphine and all NSAIDs in patients with renal disease. All other analgesics should have their doses adjusted according to the estimated renal clearance remaining.

Sepsis

Patients with sepsis are at risk of developing multi-organ dysfunction or failure. The goal of analgesia in the septic patient is to decrease the perception of pain while avoiding suppression or deterioration of the cardiovascular, respiratory, hepatic, or renal systems. Despite the proven benefits of neuraxial techniques in other classes of high-risk patients, this option is relatively contraindicated in sepsis due to the risk of CNS infection and the risk of coagulation defects, either from decreased production of coagulation factors secondary to hepatic failure or from disseminated intravascular consumption of platelets and clotting factors. All systems must be assessed carefully before implementing an analgesic strategy.

Obesity

Obese patients display a higher incidence of diabetes, renal failure, respiratory failure, hypertension, and coronary artery disease, all of which can influence considerations of an analgesic strategy.

- Changes in tissue distribution produced by obesity can markedly affect the apparent volume of distribution of the anesthetic drugs. For example, the loading dose of lipophilic opioids should be based on total body weight, but the maintenance doses should be reduced because of the higher sensitivity of the obese patient to the depressant effects of these agents [30].

- There are other changes induced by obesity that can affect the pharmacokinetic profile of anesthetic drugs, such as the absolute increase in total blood volume and cardiac output (CO) and alterations in plasma protein binding [31].

- Changes related to obesity can induce severe glomerular injury, leading to chronic renal disease [32]. In these cases, the estimation of creatinine clearance from standard formulae is inaccurate, and the dosing of renally excreted drugs must be adjusted according to the measured creatinine clearance [33].

- Although fatty infiltration of the liver is often seen in obese patients, hepatic metabolization of drugs is often preserved or even enhanced [31].

In summary, the obese patient is at risk of co-morbid disease and has pharmacokinetic and pharmacodynamic changes that reduce their ability to handle analgesic drugs.

Elderly

Pain in the elderly is often underdiagnosed and undertreated due to its myriad presentations. Inadequate pain management in the elderly can exacerbate emotional distress and depression, delirium, anxiety, sleep disturbances, and delay mobilization. Compounding these concerns is that fact that they are subject to polypharmacy, and a high prevalence of co-morbidities.

The elderly patient demonstrates age-related reduction in organ function affecting pharmacokinetics and pharmacodynamics.

- Drugs display increased potency and prolonged duration of effect due to a reduced volume of distribution, decreased clearance and reduction in protein binding [34].

- Patient controlled analgesia (PCA) appears to be the analgesic modality of choice in this patient population, as it allows for individual tailoring of dosing to the patient. When compared with intramuscular narcotic administration, PCA has demonstrated superiority in that there is a lower incidence of confusion and pulmonary complications [35].

Specific modalities

Multi-modal analgesia

Multi-modal analgesia implies the use of two or more analgesic agents used in combination to affect different targets in the pain pathway.

- A multi-modal approach has been shown to produce better pain relief, to reduce the total amount of analgesics required, and to lower side effects. In addition to opioids, many other compounds have been added to the multi-modal regimen including acetaminophen, NSAIDs, ketamine, local anesthetics, clonidine, anti-convulsants and atypical anti-psychotics.
- Although there exist small studies to support the use of the individual adjuncts mentioned above, the most significant results have been demonstrated with ketamine and NSAIDs.
- In large meta-analyses, these two have demonstrated opioid-sparing and a reduction in overall pain scores [13].

Intravenous patient controlled analgesia (PCA)

The principle of PCA is that the patient self-titrates an opioid, most commonly morphine, in small doses, generally 1–2 mg, using a patient request button. Each time a dose is administered the system "locks out" for a set period, during which time the request button is ineffective, a feature integral to patient safety. Subsequent requests, after each lockout, will result in further doses.

- This method is excellent for maintaining analgesia once achieved.
- Pre-loading of the patient via the IV or IM routes is mandatory to the success of the technique, as using the button alone can take hours to achieve a steady serum level of analgesic drug.
- The patient must have the mental and physical capabilities to understand the concept and to press the button.
- PCA has been demonstrated to yield greater patient satisfaction and to lower pain scores while showing a higher rate of opioid consumption when compared to traditional staff-administered dosing [36].
- As well as recognizing that individuals vary widely in their metabolism of opioids and serum levels required for analgesia, this technique offers the potential for increased analgesia during periods where pain intensity is increased due to therapeutic interventions, e.g. physiotherapy, dressing changes, etc.

Epidural analgesia (EA) and patient-controlled epidural analgesia (PCEA)

The pros and cons of EA are much debated.

- When comparing EA of all types with PCA analgesia, superior postoperative analgesia is demonstrated with the epidural technique [37].

- A recent meta-analysis has concluded that adding EA to a conventional anesthetic for thoracic and abdominal surgery results in a number of benefits including reduced time to extubation, need for re-intubation, ICU stay, pain scores, and opioid consumption [38].
- A Cochrane review further extols the benefits of EA, stating that after abdominal aortic surgery, epidural local anesthetics decrease overall cardiac complications, myocardial infarctions, and gastric and renal complications when compared to systemic opioid analgesia [39].
- However, with the exception of this small high-risk subset of the surgical population, EA has failed to demonstrate a significant reduction in postoperative mortality [40].

Epidural opioids are effective when used in conjunction with a local anesthetic.

- This synergism reduces the required dose and side effects associated with either the local anesthetic or opioid alone.
- Infusion regimes vary, but usually incorporate mixtures of bupivacaine at a concentration of 0.0625–0.15% with a lipid-soluble opioid (not morphine) such as Diamorphine (maximum 40 mcg ml^{-1}) or Fentanyl (maximum 5 mcg ml^{-1}).
- These mixtures are infused at rates of up to 14 ml per hour depending upon the site of insertion.
- Insertion of the epidural at an appropriate segmental level is important, as spread of drugs within the epidural space is limited.
- In practice, hypotension due to autonomic blockade by the local anesthetic is a far bigger problem than respiratory depression, although lowering the dose of the opioid may be wise if respiratory depression is a significant patient risk factor.

There are always situations where epidural analgesia is impossible or should be used with care. These include:

- patient refusal (absolute contraindication);
- infection at the site of insertion (absolute contraindication);
- anticoagulation (consider reversal if for elective surgery);
- fixed cardiac output states, e.g. aortic stenosis, hypertrophic obstructive cardiomyopathy. Epidural blockade may precipitate profound cardiovascular collapse in these patients (use with care including full hemodynamic monitoring and ICU monitoring).

PCEA is a modification of epidural analgesia. Similar opioid/local anesthetic mixtures tend to be used but with a lower background infusion rate.

- The main difference is that the patient is able to self-administer extra doses of the mixture to supplement analgesia if required. PCEA allows greater flexibility of dose and better patient response to increases in pain intensity, such as during physiotherapy.
- A typical setting for PCEA would be 6 ml background infusion of bupivacaine 0.125% with morphine 50 μg ml^{-1} with 5 ml bolus permitted every 15 min.

If an epidural is contraindicated, other types of blocks might warrant consideration:

- intrapleural or paravertebral infusions are useful for unilateral incisions such as open cholecystectomy. A left intrapleural block has been advocated for the treatment of pancreatitis pain;

- an infusion of local anesthetic directly into the wound via a catheter sited during wound closure can contribute significantly to postoperative analgesia and is of value alongside standard PCA opioids.

Continuous peripheral nerve blocks

Continuous peripheral nerve blocks by infusion of local anesthetic through an indwelling catheter have been demonstrated to yield reduced pain scores and lower side effects compared to PCA or IM opioid regimes [41].

- Some single-shot blocks of the brachial plexus have a prolonged action often extending into the first or even second postoperative day, and are well worth considering particularly in patients where avoidance of opioids is desirable.
- However, a recent meta-analysis has failed to demonstrate any reduction in morbidity and mortality with the use of peripheral nerve analgesia compared to traditional techniques [13].

Specific medications

Opioids

The body of knowledge surrounding opioid medication is vast and beyond the scope of this chapter. It is well known that all opioids may produce the same general side effects including respiratory depression, urinary retention, cough suppression, nausea, rigidity, pruritis and sedation-related hypotension. However, this section will highlight distinct points to consider regarding specific opioids in the management of high-risk patients.

Morphine

Morphine has the potential for histamine release. In human studies, 10% of patients receiving morphine had increased levels of plasma histamine; these levels have been directly correlated with hypotension. One should avoid large bolus doses of morphine in the hemodynamically unstable patient. As mentioned previously, morphine should not be administered in renal failure due to accumulation of the morphine-6-glucuronide metabolite.

Hydromorphone

Hydromorphone has a lower incidence of histamine release compared to morphine. It is a fast-acting opioid with 5–8 times the potency of morphine. The most beneficial quality of hydromorphone is that its metabolites are inactive.

Oxycodone

Oxydone (in combination with acetaminophen) is the most commonly prescribed opioid in the United States [42]. Controlled studies demonstrating its efficacy have been performed in postoperative pain, cancer pain, osteoarthritis-related pain, postherpetic neuralgia and diabetic neuropathy.

Codeine

Patients in hepatic failure may be unable to convert codeine to morphine, resulting in diminished analgesia from codeine.

Meperidine

The most important consideration with meperidine is the possibility of the accumulation of the excitatory metabolite, normeperidine. Normeperidine has a long half-life of up to 40 h. Thus, patients with renal impairment or those that have been receiving the drug over several days are at increased risk of seizures or agitation.

Fentanyl and analogs

Fentanyl and its analogs sufentanil and alfentanil have minimally active metabolites. They do not cause histamine release or direct myocardial depression. Fentanyl, in particular, has been demonstrated to be safe for use in PCA. Studies have demonstrated that fentanyl and morphine PCA have the same safety, side effect and patient satisfaction profile [43].

Tramadol

Tramadol is a recent addition to North American markets. It is often referred to as an atypical opioid since it is only a weak mu-opioid agonist and exerts its primary action as a serotonin and noradrenaline reuptake inhibitor.

- Tramadol, at equianalgesic doses, appears to have a lower side effect profile than the other opioids. This includes a smaller effect on bowel motility, and less respiratory depression [44, 45].
- It has been available in several European countries since the 1970s, where it has been used intravenously in trauma, labor, myocardial emergencies, intraoperatively and postoperatively [46]. However, the majority of support for tramadol revolves around oral dosing in post-operative pain.

Acetaminophen/paracetamol

Acetaminophen has been shown to be a useful adjunct to opioids in the management of postoperative pain. The analgesic effect occurs centrally by activating descending serotonergic pathways [47]. It is important to note that intravenous paracetamol has been used to provide rapid and effective postoperative pain control in European countries for over 20 years. As mentioned previously, therapeutic dosing does not exacerbate existing hepatic disease.

Nonsteroidal anti-inflammatory drugs (NSAIDS)

Nonsteroidal anti-inflammatory medications have been shown in many clinical trials to possess opioid-sparing capabilities using a variety of postoperative pain models. Whether or not this contributes to a significant clinical difference in patient outcome remains open for debate.

- NSAIDs produce analgesia by inhibiting cyclooxygenase (COX), an enzyme that converts arachidonic acid into thromboxane and prostaglandins, important messengers in the inflammatory pathway.

- Nonselective NSAIDs inhibit both COX-1 and COX-2 enzymes and selective NSAIDs inhibit only COX-2.

- The anti-inflammatory properties are derived from COX-2 inhibition whereas the adverse gastrointestinal and renal events are derived from COX-1 inhibition. The major side effects of nonselective NSAIDs include platelet inhibition, inhibition of renal function, and erosion of gastric mucosa.

- The chance of worsening renal failure appears significant for patients with renal disease, or on ACE inhibitors, as well as those patients that are volume-depleted [29].

- The selective COX-2 inhibitors, although they do not have as high an incidence of gastrointestinal (GI) complications or platelet inhibition, do have their own side effects including adverse renal and cardiac events.

- The most important consideration when using COX-2 inhibitors is that *prolonged use* may predispose patients to an increased risk of thrombotic cardiovascular events [48]. Several COX-2 inhibitors have been withdrawn from the market due to concerns over cardiovascular side effects.

Ketamine

Ketamine is a noncompetitive antagonist of the *N*-methyl-D-Aspartate (NMDA) receptor that induces significant sedation and analgesia. Intraoperative sub-anesthetic doses have been demonstrated to possess opioid-sparing properties in addition to the ability to prevent central and peripheral sensitization from surgical interventions [49].

Gabapentin and pregabalin

Both act via modulation of the α_2-δ subunit of voltage-gated calcium channels. Binding to the α_2-δ subunit results in attenuation of calcium flux into the neuron, which in turn inhibits the release of various pain-inducing neurotransmitters. Although they function at the same receptor, pregabalin achieves its efficacy at lower doses than gabapentin, and thus seems to have a lower side effect profile.

- Gabapentin and pregabalin have both been shown to be effective adjuncts to perioperative analgesia, providing reductions in pain scores, opioid consumption and opioid-related side effects [50].

- Furthermore, there is a possibility that the perioperative use of gabapentin may prevent the development of chronic pain related to surgery [51].

Lidocaine

Intraoperative intravenous lidocaine infusions for the reduction of postoperative pain and opioid-sparing have been mentioned in the literature since the 1960s. However, until recently, intravenous lidocaine had been primarily utilized for the treatment of chronic pain.

- The perioperative use of lidocaine has again been featured in the literature demonstrating opioid-sparing, decreased pain scores and shortened hospital stays [52].

- The mechanism of action is postulated to be a combination of anti-inflammatory effects and antagonism of the NMDA receptor [53, 54].

- Larger randomized control trials must be carried out in order to establish this as a truly effective option.

Outcome studies

- A recent systematic review of the postoperative analgesia literature concluded that "there is insufficient evidence to confirm or deny the ability of postoperative analgesia techniques to affect postoperative mortality or morbidity". The authors attribute this to underpowering of previous clinical trials, and call for more large-scale outcome studies, since significant adverse events like pulmonary embolus and myocardial infarction are relatively rare [13, 55].

- However, White and Kehlet [55] argue that the major benefits of good analgesia lie in shortening recovery and hospital discharge times and in promoting early ambulation.

- Such benefits would be more apparent if multi-modal analgesia were incorporated along with minimally invasive surgery, and other aspects of fast-track recovery care.

Further reading

Joshi G, ed. Current concepts in postoperative pain management. *Anesthesiol Clin N Am* 2005; **23**: 1–234.

References

1. Ready LB, Oden R, Chadwick MD, *et al.* Development of an anesthesiology-based post-operative pain management service. *Anaesthesiology* 1988; **68**: 100–06.

2. Gould TH, Crosby DL, Harmer M, *et al.* Policy for controlling pain after surgery: Effect of sequential changes in management. *BMJ* 1992; **305**: 1187–93.

3. Werner M, Soholm L, Rotboll-Nielsen P, *et al.* Does an acute pain service improve postoperative outcome? *Anesth Analg* 2002; **95**: 1361–72.

4. Willis WD, Westlund KN. Neuroanatomy of the pain system and of the pathways that modulate pain. *J Clin Neurophysiol* 1997; **14**: 2–31.

5. Woolf CJ, Ma Q. Nociceptors – noxious stimulus detectors. *Neuron* 2007; **55**: 353–64.

6. Woolf CJ, Salter MW. Neuronal plasticity: Increasing the gain in pain. *Science* 2000; **288**: 1765–8.

7. Buvanendran A, Kroin JS, Berger RA, *et al.* Upregulation of prostaglandin E2 and interleukins in the central nervous system and peripheral tissue during and after

surgery in humans. *Anesthesiology* 2006; **104**: 403–10.

8. Neugebauer V, Lucke T, Schailble HG. N-methyl-D-aspartate (NMDA) and non-NMDA antagonists block the hyperexcitability of dorsal horn neurons during development of acute arthritis in rat's knee joints. *J Neurophysiol* 1993; **70**: 1365–77.

9. Buvanendran A, Kroin JS. Useful adjuvants for postoperative pain management. *Best Pract Res Clin Anaesthesiol* 2007; **21**: 31–49.

10. Williamson A, Hoggart B. Pain: A review of three commonly used pain rating scales. *Iss Clin Nursing* 2005; **14**: 798–804.

11. Terai T, Yukioka H, Asada A. Pain evaluation in the intensive care unit: Observer-reported faces scale compared with self-reported visual analog scale. *Reg Anesth Pain Med* 1998; **23**: 147–51.

12. Richardson J, Sabanathan S, Shah R. Post-thoracotomy spirometric lung function: The effect of analgesia. *J Cardiovasc Surg* 199; **40**: 445–56.

13. Liu SS, Wu CL. Effect of post-operative analgesia on major

post-operative complications: A systematic update of the evidence. *Anesth Analg* 2007; **104**: 689–702.

14. Lewis KS, Whipple JK, Michael KA, *et al.* Effect of analgesic treatment on the physiologic consequences of pain. *Am J Hosp Pharm* 1994; **15**: 1539–54.

15. Devereaux PJ, Goldman L, Cook DJ, *et al.* Perioperative cardiac events in patients undergoing non-cardiac surgery: A review of the magnitude of the problem, the pathophysiology of events and methods to estimate and communicate risk. *CMAJ* 2005; **173**: 727–34.

16. Warltier DC, Pagel PS, Kersten JR. Approaches to the prevention of perioperative myocardial ischemia. *Anesthesiology* 2000; **92**: 253.

17. Meissner A, Rolf N, Van Aken H. Thoracic epidurals and the patient with heart disease: Benefits, risks and controversies. *Anesth Analg* 1997; **85**: 517–28.

18. Nygard E, Kofoed KF, Freiberg J, *et al.* Effects of high thoracic epidural analgesia on myocardial blood flow in patients with ischemic heart disease. *Circulation* 2005; **111**: 2165–70.

19. Mangano DT, Siliciano D, Hollenberg M, *et al.* Postoperative myocardial ischemia: Therapeutic trials using intensive analgesia following surgery. *Anesthesiology* 1992; **76**: 342–53.

20. Ballantyne JC, Carr DB, deFerranti S, *et al.* The comparative effects of postoperative analgesic therapies on pulmonary outcome: Cumulative meta-analyses of randomized controlled trials. *Anesth Analg* 1998; **86**: 598–612.

21. Groeben H, Schwalen A, Irsfeld S, *et al.* High thoracic epidural anesthesia does not alter airway resistance and attenuates the response to an inhalational provocation test in patients with bronchial hyperreactivity. *Anesthesiology* 1994; **81**: 868–74.

22. Groeben H. Epidural anesthesia and pulmonary function. *J Anesthesia* 2006; **20**: 290–9.

23. Catley DM, Thornton C, Jordan C, *et al.* Pronounced, episodic oxygen desaturation in the postoperative period: Its association with

ventilatory pattern and analgesic regimen. *Anesthesiology* 1985; **63**: 20–8.

24. Walker JM, Farney RJ, Rhondeau SM, *et al.* Chronic opioid use is a risk factor for the development of central sleep apnea and ataxic breathing. *J Clin Sleep Med* 2007; **3**: 455–61.

25. Dershwitz M, Hoke JF, Rosow CE, *et al.* Pharmacokinetics and pharmacodynamics of remifentanil in volunteer subjects with severe liver disease. *Anesthesiology* 1996; **84**: 812–20.

26. Benson GD, Koff RS, Tolman KG. The therapeutic use of acetaminophen in patients with liver disease. *Am J Ther* 2005; **12**: 133–41.

27. O'Connor N, Dargan PI, Jones AL. Hepatocellular damage from non-steroidal anti-inflammatory drugs. *Quat J Med* 2003; **96**: 787–91.

28. Murphy EJ. Acute pain management pharmacology for the patient with concurrent renal or hepatic disease. *Anaesthesia Inten Care* 2005; **33**: 311–22.

29. Whelton A. Nephrotoxicity of nonsteroidal anti-inflammatory drugs: Physiologic foundations and implications. *Am J Med* 1999; **106**: 13S–24S.

30. Casati, A, Putzu M. Anesthesia in the obese patient: Pharmacokinetic considerations. *J Clin Anesth* 2005; **17**: 134–45.

31. Adams JP, Murphy PG. Obesity in anaesthesia and intensive care. *Br J Anaesthesiol* 2000; **85**: 91–108.

32. Henegar JR, Bigler SA, Henegar LK, *et al.* Functional and structural changes in the kidney in the early stages of obesity. *J Am Soc Nephrol* 2001; **12**: 1211–7.

33. Snider RD, Kruse JA, Bander JJ, *et al.* Accuracy of estimated creatinine clearance in obese patients with stable renal function in the intensive care unit. *Pharmacotherapy* 1995; **15**: 747–53.

34. Owen JA, Sitar DS, Berger L, *et al.* Age-related morphine kinetics. *Clin Pharmacol Therapeut* 1983; **34**: 364–8.

35. Egbert AM, Parks LH, Short LM, *et al.* Randomized trial of postoperative patient-controlled analgesia vs.

intramuscular narcotics in frail elderly men. *Arch Int Med* 1990; **150**: 1897–903.

36. Hudcova J, McNicol E, Quah C, *et al.* Patient controlled opioid analgesia versus conventional opioid analgesia for postoperative pain. *Cochrane Database Syst Rev* 2006 Oct **18**; (4): CD003348.

37. Wu C, Cohen S, Richman J, *et al.* Efficacy of postoperative patient-controlled and continuous infusion epidural analgesia versus intravenous patient-controlled analgesia with opioids: A meta-analysis. *Anesthesiology* 2005; **103**: 1079–88.

38. Guay J. The benefits of adding epidural analgesia to general anesthesia: A metaanalysis. *J Anesthesia* 2006; **20**: 335–40.

39. Nishimori M, Ballantyne JC, Low JH. Epidural pain relief versus systemic opioid-based pain relief for abdominal aortic surgery. *Cochrane Database Syst Rev* 2006 Jul **19**; 3: CD005059.

40. Bonnet F, Marret E. Postoperative pain management and outcome after surgery. *Best Pract Res Clin Anaesthesiol* 2007; **21**: 99–107.

41. Richman JM, Liu SS, Courpas G, *et al.* Does continuous peripheral nerve block provide superior pain control to opioids? *Anesth Analg* 2006; **102**: 248–57.

42. Coluzzi F, Mattia C. Oxycodone. Pharmacological profile and clinical data in chronic pain management. *Minerva Anestesiol* 2005; 7: 451–60.

43. Woodhouse A, Hobbes AF, Mather LE, *et al.* A comparison of morphine, pethidine and fentanyl in the postsurgical patient-controlled analgesia environment. *Pain* 1996; **64**: 115–21.

44. Wilder-Smith CH, Bettiga A. The analgesic tramadol has minimal effect on gastrointestinal motor function. *Br J Clin Pharmacol* 1997; **43**: 71–5.

45. Tarrkila P, Tuominen M, Lindgren L, *et al.* Comparison of respiratory effects of

tramadol and pethidine. *Eur J Anaesthesiol* 1998; **15**: 64–8.

46. Radbruch L, Grond S, Lehmann KA. A risk benefit assessment of tramadol in the management of pain. *Drug Saf* 1996; **15**: 8–29.

47. Graham GG, Scott KF. Mechanism of action of paracetamol. *Am J Therape* 2005; **12**: 46–55.

48. Iezzi A, Ferri C, Mezzetti A, *et al.* COX-2 friend or foe? *Curr Pharmacol Des* 2007; **13**: 1715–21.

49. DeKock MF, Lavand'homme PM. The clinical role of NMDA receptor antagonists for the treatment of postoperative pain. *Best Pract Res Clin Anaesthesiol* 2007; **21**: 85–98.

50. Tiippana EM, Hamunen K, Kontinen VK. Do surgical patients benefit from perioperative gabapentin/pregabalin? A systematic review of efficacy and safety. *Anesth Analg* 2007; **104**: 1545–56.

51. Fassoulaki A, Stramatakis E, Petropoulos G, *et al.* Gabapentin attenuates late but not acute pain after abdominal hysterectomy. *Eur J Anesthesiol* 2006; **23**: 136–41.

52. Omote K. Intravenous lidocaine to treat postoperative pain management: Novel strategy with a long-established drug. *Anesthesiology* 2007; **106**: 5–6.

53. Hollmann MW, Durieux ME. Local anaesthetics and the inflammatory response: A new therapeutic indication? *Anesthesiology* 2000; **93**: 858–75.

54. Sugimoto M, Uchida I, Mashimo T. Local anaesthetics have different mechanisms and sites of action at the recombinant N-methyl-D-aspartate (NMDA) receptors. *Br J Pharmacol* 2003; **138**: 876–82.

55. White PF, Kehlet H. Post-operative pain management and patient outcome: Time to return to work! *Anesth Analg* 2007; **104**: 487–9.

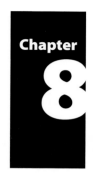

Regional anesthesia for the high-risk patient

S. Dhir

This chapter will discuss both regional analgesia and anesthesia techniques for the high-risk patient.

- Regional anesthesia (RA) is used as an alternative or additive to general anesthesia (GA) for various surgical procedures.
- It is increasing in popularity and the technology and clinical understanding of regional blocks has evolved greatly over the past few decades.
- The objective of this chapter is to describe the indications, limitations and practical aspects of regional techniques in high-risk patients, based on current evidence.

Central neuraxial blocks

- Epidural anesthesia and analgesia provides superior analgesia and segment-dependent sympatholysis in high-risk orthopedic patients [1].
- Extended spinal anesthesia using a micro-catheter as a primary method of anesthesia for colorectal surgery in high-risk patients in whom GA would have been associated with higher morbidity and mortality has also been used with success [2].
- RA alone (spinal or epidural) is an attractive and safe option for abdominal surgery in selected high-risk patients with severe pulmonary impairment [3].
- Neuraxial anesthesia may also reduce oxygen consumption due to a reduction in cardiac work (motor block), increased peripheral and splanchnic blood flow (sympathetic block), and a quiescent physiological state.

Epidural analgesia is the RA technique most often used in the ICU. It may not always improve mortality, but eases management and improves patient comfort in the ICU in patients with chest trauma, thoracic and abdominal surgeries, major orthopedic surgery, acute pancreatitis, paralytic ileus, cardiac surgery, and intractable angina pain [4].

With central neuraxial techniques, things to consider are:

- consent;
- sedation: safety of insertion in sedated patients is questionable. However, practices differ from region to region;
- positioning and confirmation of space: loss of resistance to air/saline, acoustic devices;
- drugs used;
- neurological assessment;

Anesthesia for the High Risk Patient, ed. I. McConachie. Published by Cambridge University Press.
© Cambridge University Press 2009.

- hemodynamics, e.g. bradycardia and hypotension;
- sepsis; and
- coagulation status: although there is no compelling evidence that there is increased risk of bleeding with developing coagulopathy or therapeutic anticoagulation, the benefits should be weighed against this risk.

Studies of central neuraxial versus general anesthesia suggest that modern neuraxial techniques may carry a lower risk for postoperative cardiac complications, but this finding remains controversial. Neuraxial anesthesia helps control pain, and may reduce pulmonary and thrombotic complications even if it may not lower cardiac risks [5]. However, there have been several randomized controlled trials (RCT) suggesting otherwise.

Peripheral nerve blocks for upper limb

These blocks provide sufficient good quality analgesia for shoulder and upper limb surgery in high-risk patients.

Points of consideration with specific upper limb blocks are as follows.

Interscalene block (ISB)

- The chance of spinal cord injury related to ISB or intrathecal drug injection can be minimized with the use of combination of ultrasound (US) with peripheral nerve stimulator (PNS) and lesser medial needle direction [6].
- Phrenic nerve blockade results in loss of hemidiaphragmatic function. This could be a serious consideration in patients with respiratory disease.
- Proximity of catheter to tracheostomy (if present).
- Patient positioning problems if C-spine injury.

Supraclavicular blocks

- Probably less popular now due to risk of pneumothorax.

Infraclavicular block

- High success rate with good analgesia for most arm, elbow and hand surgery.
- Very small risk of pneumothorax.
- Easy catheter fixation and maintenance.

Axillary block

- Catheter techniques are unreliable.
- Does not reliably provide full anesthesia for mid-arm/elbow surgery.
- Higher chance of incomplete blocks due to septae in the tissues preventing full spread of anesthetic.

Peripheral nerve blocks for lower limb

These blocks provide good analgesia for the management of acute pain from lower limb fractures in the interim period while awaiting surgical fixation.

The total dose of local anesthetic (LA) may need adjustment based on other blocks done concomitantly, drug interactions, disease states, etc.

Particular concerns with specific lower limb blocks are as follows.

Lumbar plexus block
- No analgesia to anterior aspect of lower limb.
- Possibility of epidural/spinal spread, renal injury, peritoneal injection, IV injection.
- Not suitable in anticoagulated patients.
- Positioning of patient may need small doses of IV analgesics.
- Difficult block to learn.
- Deep block – cannot use US guidance.

Femoral nerve block
- Incomplete block for knee surgery.

Saphenous nerve block
- Purely sensory nerve so PNS use is ineffective in localizing nerve.

Sciatic nerve block
- Low success rate with anterior approach.
- Patient positioning may be difficult following trauma.

Intravenous regional analgesia (IVRA)
- IVRA is simple, reliable, easy to administer and cost-effective.
- Prilocaine and lidocaine are used commonly, although some countries no longer have access to prilocaine.
- Various adjuvants like opioids, NSAIDs, tramadol, clonidine and muscle relaxants have been studied with variable effects to improve block efficacy, decrease tourniquet pain, and prolong duration of postdeflation analgesia.
- A successful block needs exsanguination of the limb, which may be uncomfortable in trauma patients.
- Unplanned deflation can result in LA toxicity.
- Not a suitable technique for prolonged and repeated procedures.
- Lower limb IVRA is not commonly used.

Nerve localization techniques
Nerve stimulators
- Traditional method.
- Inexpensive and easy to train personnel.
- May be painful in patients with trauma.

Ultrasound guidance

- Probably a superior method of nerve localization where nerves, needle path and LA spread can be seen.
- Not possible to see and differentiate deeper structures with present technology.
- Adequate training and equipment needed.
- Equipment is relatively expensive.

Additives to local anesthetics

Epinephrine

- Vaso-constriction of perineural vessels → decreased LA uptake → prolongs duration of LA action and reduced blood levels of drug, i.e. reduced toxicity.
- Intravascular injection marker due to resultant tachycardia.
- May accentuate injury in nerves with disrupted neural blood flow.

Clonidine

- May increase duration of LA in single-shot blocks.
- No apparent benefit in continuous peripheral nerve blocks.
- Significantly prolongs spinal anesthesia.
- Side effects include hypotension, bradycardia, and sedation.

Ketamine

- Blocks sodium and potassium currents in peripheral nerves.
- Central antinociception through NMDA receptors.

Opioids

- Uncertain clinical effects in peripheral nerve blocks.
- Pruritis, urinary retention, sedation when used in central neuraxial blocks.

NSAIDs

- Effects may depend on presence of inflammation at site.
- May attenuate hyperalgesic state caused by prostaglandin-induced afferent nerve sensitization.
- May improve postoperative analgesia and prolong tourniquet tolerance in IVRA.

Verapamil

- No significant advantage over epinephrine if expected duration is < 3.5 h.

Hyaluronidase

- Does not hasten block onset, reduce incidence of failed block, or affect LA blood concentration.
- Shortens block duration.

Indications for the use of regional anesthesia in high-risk patients

Cardiac surgery

- Thoracic epidural analgesia may be very beneficial in a selected population of cardiac surgery patients. The risks may be acceptable if strict protocols are followed with appropriate neurological monitoring.
- Unstable angina – increased coronary perfusion has been shown in many studies.
- Heart surgery while on or off cardiopulmonary bypass in very high-risk heart patients in whom there is unacceptable operative risk with GA (considered controversial).
- Careful patient selection and procedure is crucial, including screening of preoperative drug use and an initial normal coagulation profile. Attempts at placement should be limited. The catheter is best placed the day prior to surgery. Catheters should be removed when coagulation status is normal.
- Much of the debate on the value of epidural analgesia following cardiac surgery through a median sternotomy centers around whether the risks of hematoma formation are worth the benefits of improved analgesia [7]. On critical review of the literature, enhanced postoperative analgesia appears to be the only clear benefit, as neuraxial techniques have no other clinically important effect on outcome [8].

Carotid surgery

- Regional anesthesia may be the anesthetic technique of choice when carotid endarterectomy is performed in high-risk patients [9]. This is further discussed in Chapter 17.

The elderly patient

- Continuous regional techniques have been used to provide effective analgesia with lower pain scores and better physiotherapy for the perioperative management of high-risk elderly patients undergoing major abdominal, vascular, or orthopedic surgery [10].
- Isolated orthopedic injuries in high-risk geriatric patients managed by RA have a lower risk of thromboembolism. With the use of minimal sedation, mental status and respiratory function is preserved.

Neonates and infants

Spinal anesthesia has been shown to provide a viable alternative to GA in high-risk infants undergoing appropriate procedures by providing stable hemodynamics and respiratory variables, rapid recovery, and discharge time [11].

Obstetrics

- RA techniques play an important role in pregnant patients as they do not interfere with maternal hemodynamic stability and fetal well-being. Many peripheral injuries can be managed entirely with RA with minimal effects on the mother and fetus.

- The biggest risk of spinal anesthesia during pregnancy is hypotension secondary to sympathetic nerve blockade that may reduce uterine blood flow and perfusion to the fetus. Fluid (predominantly crystalloid) prehydration is a common ritual despite its lack of efficacy [12]. Use of sympathomimetic drugs rather than fluids to treat or prevent associated hypotension is recommended. The use of ephedrine has been associated with lower uterine artery pH and phenylephrine has become more popular due to the realization that it does not have a detrimental effect on placental perfusion. However, it is noted to have a short duration of action and may produce maternal bradycardia. The combination of both drugs at reduced dosage is now recommended [13].
- When compared to other drugs used in anesthesia and analgesia, epidural LA seems to have the least impact on neonatal neurobehavior.

Obesity

Delayed recovery from GA and postoperative hypoxemia can be avoided if a regional technique is adopted for ambulatory surgery in obese patients. However, these patients are more likely to have a failed block [14].

Additional effects of regional techniques

Stress response and regional techniques

- RA blocks efferent autonomic neuronal pathways to adrenal medulla, liver, etc., and blocks afferent input from operative site to CNS and hypothalamic–pituitary axis.
- RA better preserves immune function.
- Reduced IL-6 and other cytokine responses.
- Smaller increases in cortisol, catecholamines and other stress hormonal changes.
- Reduction of stress and catabolic response with regional techniques provides enhanced recovery and dynamic pain control [15].
- However, one has to keep in mind that the attenuated inflammatory response in the immuno-compromised patient may diminish the clinical signs and symptoms associated with infection [16].

Mortality and morbidity

- There is a global reduction in postoperative complications such as deep vein thrombosis (DVT), pulmonary embolism (PE), pneumonia, cardiac events [17].
- There is a clear reduction in mortality in older studies, but no statistical difference has been seen in recent studies. This may be explained partially by the widespread modern use of thromboprophylaxis that was absent in older studies. Lower odds ratio of death at 7 and 30 days but no difference in overall major morbidity [18] has been observed.

Coagulation and DVT

There is a hypercoagulable state after surgery due to:

- potentiation of stress response;

- endothelial damage with tissue factor activation; and
- synergy with inflammatory responses.

This may result in vaso-occlusive and thrombotic events, e.g. DVT, PE, graft failure.

The use of regional anesthesia in high-DVT-risk surgery is thought to reduce this risk in comparison with general anesthesia. The sympathetic block leads to vasodilatation of the limbs and increased blood flow, resulting in less stasis both intra- and postoperatively, with reduced blood cell adhesion to damaged vessel walls. RA also reduces platelet aggregation, lowers mean arterial pressure, and alters coagulation and fibrinolytic responses to further prevent clotting (whereas general anesthesia is thought to completely inhibit fibrinolytic function) [19].

Vascular graft function [20]

- GA results in reduced blood flow in deep veins with increased risk for graft occlusion.
- Sympatholysis due to RA improves regional blood flow and microcirculation.
- RA promotes fibrinolytic activity:
  - ↓ postoperative rise in plasminogen activator inhibitor-1.
  - ↓ postoperative rise in platelet aggregation.
  - Rapid return of antithrombin III levels to normal.
  - Systemic LA absorption impairs platelet aggregation.
- Benefits may be seen only if RA is continued postoperatively.
- In addition to the above benefits, patients undergoing major vascular procedures may have a lower cardiac morbidity with epidural analgesia or anesthesia; however, there is not much effect on mortality/morbidity in peripheral vascular surgery [21]. Postoperative thoracic epidural analgesia has been shown to reduce postoperative myocardial infarction by as much as 40% [22]. This is important because many high-risk patients cannot tolerate beta-adrenergic blockers, which also reduce postoperative myocardial infarction.

Gastrointestinal

Effects of regional anesthesia and analgesia on the GI tract are due to:

- LAs block afferent and efferent limbs of nociceptive arc (parasympathetic innervation by vagus is intact);
- systemic absorption of LA improves bowel motility (direct excitatory effect in GI smooth muscle);
- reduction of opioid use;
- blockade of inhibitory spinal reflex arc; and
- pharmacological sympathectomy increases GI blood flow resulting in improved colonic motility.

There is good evidence that regional anesthetic techniques with the avoidance of general anesthesia (particularly opioid-based analgesia) are associated with reduced incidence of postoperative GI dysfunction. It has also been demonstrated that ileus during intra-abdominal surgery is shorter if epidural is used with LA without the addition of epidural opioids [23].

Excessive fluid loading in an attempt to correct epidural-induced hypotension may have a potential effect on anastomotic integrity by compromising microcirculation. Vasoparesis rather than absolute hypovolemia is usually the cause of hypotension, and therefore it is illogical to treat it with fluids alone, especially in high-risk patients where GI tract perfusion may be critical [24].

Pulmonary

- Postoperative epidural with LA and/or opioids is known to reduce pulmonary morbidity and decrease atelectasis [25].
- The use of regional anesthetic techniques in high-risk patients undergoing noncardiac surgery has been shown to decrease the incidence of postoperative pulmonary complications [26].

Blood loss

- It has been shown that there is significant positive correlation between morphine consumption and blood loss in providing good quality pain relief.
- Sympathectomy can lead to vasodilatation, pooling and decrease of preload.
- This collectively reduces blood loss and has been demonstrated in cesarean section, hysterectomy, prostatectomy, and hip arthroplasty.

Joint mobility

Early mobilization after major orthopedic surgery plays a vital role in successful functional rehabilitation, as postoperative pain often reduces or even prevents effective physiotherapy. There is enough evidence that improved joint mobility most likely resulting from potent analgesia provided by the nerve block [27, 28] helps in early functional recovery and achieves therapy goals with less narcotic consumption.

Other morbidity [29]

- Postoperative sleep disturbance – the anesthesia-related causes are thought to be pain, volatile agents, stress responses, and use of opioids. RA is known to reduce postoperative sleep disturbances by influencing all of these.
- Cognitive changes are discussed in the chapter on the elderly patient.
- Fatigue – this depends on surgical stress, and the causes are thought to be opioid use, postoperative sleep disturbances and inflammatory/endocrine response. RA improves fatigue, facilitating early mobilization and return to normal activities.

Complications

The majority of complications associated with RA are temporary and nondisabling. Less serious complications are common, while ones that are life-threatening are, fortunately, rare.

Peripheral nerve injury

- Potential exists with all blocks: incidence < 0.02–0.4%.
- May present as residual weakness, hypoesthesia, permanent paresis.

- Causes: needle/catheter-induced mechanical trauma, perineural edema, local anesthetic neurotoxicity, use of epinephrine (accentuates disruption of neural blood flow), and use of peripheral nerve stimulator at low currents [30]. Permanent injuries have been reported when blocks have been performed under deep sedation/general anesthesia.

Vascular injury

- Minor, inconsequential vessel puncture is common but may be reduced by US techniques.
- Transient vascular insufficiency due to vasospasm may occur after vascular puncture. It may lead to axonal loss, neural deficits and medial brachial fascial compartment syndrome [31].

Pneumothorax

More common with interscalene, supraclavicular and intercostals blocks.

Horner's syndrome following brachial plexus block

Cervical sympathetic block (Horner's syndrome) is possible due to the close proximity of the cervical sympathetic chain with the brachial plexus.

Meta-analysis and outcomes

- Numerous clinical trials have been published examining the efficacy of RA for the treatment of perioperative pain compared to systemic opioids.
- There have been many meta-analyses of RCTs and analyses comparing various analgesic techniques. While some find that RA techniques are associated with significantly decreased perioperative morbidity, mortality [32], superior postoperative analgesia [33], decrease in opioid-related side effects [34] and improved patient satisfaction [35], others find no difference [36].

Systemic effects and complications

- Positive systemic effects include: analgesia, bronchodilatation, neuroprotection, anti-inflammatory, anti-arrhythmic and anti-thrombotic actions.
- Negative effects: dose-dependent toxicity (neuro, cardiac, CNS), myotoxicity, and inhibition of wound healing.

Costs

- Increased direct costs: equipment, pumps for continuous blocks, and time to perform blocks. Some institutions staff specific "block room" with associated costs.
- Reduced indirect costs (although often difficult to identify) due to potential:
  - reduction in length of stay and superior pain control;
  - reduction in mortality, pulmonary/cardiac/other morbidity, graft failure;
  - early achievement of discharge criteria;
  - facilitation of early ambulation and enteral nutrition.

Conclusions

- RA using peripheral regional and central neuraxial blocks can play an important role in a multi-modal approach to pain management in high-risk patients.
- Morbidity may be improved by avoiding high doses of systemic opioids (and thereby reducing withdrawal, delirium and mental changes), and reducing GI dysfunction, fatigue, and sleep disturbances.
- Advantages also include, in selected high-risk patients, reducing the risks associated with general anesthesia.
- Indications must be carefully chosen, taking into consideration the anatomical variations and coagulation status. Practical aspects like physician experience and availability of equipment must also be considered.

Further reading

Gulur P, Nishimori M, Ballantyne JC. Regional anaesthesia versus general anaesthesia, morbidity and mortality. *Anaesthesia* 2008; **63**: 250–8.

Parker MJ, Handoll HH, Griffiths R. Anaesthesia for hip fracture surgery in adults. *Cochrane Database Syst Rev* 2004; **4**: CD000521.

Sites BD, Spence BC, Gallagher J, *et al.* Regional anesthesia meets ultrasound: A specialty in transition. *Acta Anaesthesiol Scand* 2008; **52**: 456–66.

References

1. Adams HA, Saatweber P, Schmitz CS, *et al.* Postoperative pain management in orthopaedic patients: No difference in pain scores but improved stress control by epidural anaesthesia. *Eur J Anaesth* 2002; **19**: 658–65.

2. Kumar CM, Corbett WA, Wilson RG. Spinal anaesthesia with a micro-catheter in high-risk patients undergoing colorectal cancer and other major abdominal surgery. *Surg Oncol* 2008; **17**: 73–9.

3. Savas JF, Litwack R, Davis K, *et al.* Regional anesthesia as an alternative to general anesthesia for abdominal surgery in patients with severe pulmonary impairment. *Am J Surg* 2004; **188**: 603–05.

4. Schulz-Stubner S, Boezaart A, Hata S. Regional analgesia in the critically ill. *Crit Care Med* 2005; **33**: 1400–1407.

5. Auerback A, Goldman L. Assessing and reducing the cardiac risk of noncardiac surgery. *Circulation* 2006; **113**: 1361–76.

6. Meier G, Bauereis C, Maurer H, *et al.* Interscalene plexus block. Anatomic requirements – Anaesthesiologic and operative aspects. *Anaesthesist* 2001; **50**: 333–41.

7. Castellano JM, Durbin CG. Epidural analgesia and cardiac surgery: Worth the risk? *Chest* 2000; **117**: 305–07.

8. Chaney MA. Intrathecal and epidural anesthesia and analgesia for cardiac surgery. *Anesth Analg* 2006; **102**: 45–64.

9. Stoner MC, Abbott WM, Wong DR, *et al.* Defining the high risk patient for carotid endarterectomy: An analysis of the prospective national surgical quality improvement program database. *J Vasc Surg* 2006; **43**: 285–95.

10. Michaloudis D, Petrou A, Bakos P, *et al.* Continuous spinal anaesthesia/analgesia for the perioperative management of high-risk patients. *Eur J Anaesth* 2000; **17**: 239–47.

11. Katznelson K, Mishaly D, Hegesh T, *et al.* Spinal anesthesia for diagnostic cardiac catheterization in high-risk infants. *Ped Anesth* 2005; **15**: 50–3.

12. Khaw KS, Ngan Kee WD, Wy Lee S. Hypotension during spinal anaesthesia for caesarean section: Implications, detection prevention and treatment. *Fetal Maternal Med Rev* 2006; **17**: 157–83.

13. Macarthur A, Riley ET. Obstetric anesthesia controversies: Vasopressor choice for postspinal hypotension during cesarean delivery. *Int Anesth Clin* 2007; **45**: 115–32.

14. Servin F. Ambulatory anesthesia for the obese patient. *Curr Opin Anaesth* 2006; **19**: 597–9.

15. Kehlet H, Dahl JB. Anaesthesia, surgery and challenges in postoperative recovery. *Lancet* 2003; **362**: 1921–8.

16. Horlocker TT, Wedel DJ. Regional anesthesia in the immunocompromised patient. *Reg Anesth Pain Med* 2006; **31**: 334–45.

17. Rodgers A, Walker N, Schug S, *et al.* Reduction of postoperative mortality and morbidity with epidural or spinal anaesthesia: Results from overview of randomized trials. *BMJ* 2000; **321**: 1493.

18. Wu CL, Hurley RW, Anderson GF, *et al.* Effect of postoperative epidural analgesia on morbidity and mortality following surgery in medicare patients. *Reg Anesth Pain Med* 2004; **29**: 525–33.

19. Edmunds MJR, Crichton JH, Runciman WB, *et al.* Evidence-based risk factors for postoperative deep vein thrombosis. *ANZ J Surg* 2004; **74**: 1082–97.

20. Breen P. General anesthesia vs. regional anesthesia. *Int Anesth Clin* 2002; **40**: 61–72.

21. Bode RH Jr, Lewis KP, Zarich SW, *et al.* Cardiac outcomes after peripheral vascular surgery: Comparison of general and regional anesthesia. *Anesthesiology* 1996; **84**: 3–13.

22. Beattie WS, Badner NH, Choi P. Epidural analgesia reduces postoperative myocardial infarction: A meta-analysis. *Anesth Analg* 2001; **93**: 853–8.

23. Mythen MG. Postoperative gastrointestinal tract dysfunction. *Anesth Analg* 2005; **100**: 196–204.

24. Low J, Johnston N, Morris C. Epidural analgesia – first do no harm. *Anaesthesia* 2008; **63**: 1–3.

25. Ballantyne JC, Carr DB, de Ferranti S, *et al.* Comparative effects of postoperative analgesic therapies on pulmonary outcome: Cumulative meta-analyses of randomized controlled trials. *Anesth Analg* 1998; **86**: 598–612.

26. Stevens R, Fleisher LA. Strategies in the high-risk cardiac patient undergoing non-cardiac surgery. *Best Pract Res Clin Anaesthesiol* 2004; **18**: 549–63.

27. Capdevila X, Barthelet Y, Biboulet P, *et al.* Effects of perioperative analgesic technique on the surgical outcome and duration of rehabilitation after major knee surgery. *Anesthesiology* 1999; **91**: 8–15.

28. Ilfeld BM, Wright TW, Enneking KF, *et al.* Joint range of motion after total shoulder arthroplasty with and without a continuous interscalene block: A retrospective case controlled study. *Reg Anesth Pain Med* 2005; **30**: 429–33.

29. Nielson K, Tucker MS, Steele S. Outcomes after regional anesthesia. *Int Anesthesiol Clin* 2005; **43**: 91–110.

30. Benumof JL. Permanent loss of cervical spinal cord function associated with interscalene block performed under general anesthesia. *Anesthesiology* 2000; **93**: 1541–4.

31. Tsao BE, Wilbourn AJ. Infraclavicular brachial plexus injury following axillary regional block. *Muscle Nerve* 2004; **30**: 44–8.

32. Rodgers A, Walker N, Schug S, *et al.* Reduction of postoperative mortality and morbidity with epidural or spinal anaesthesia: Results from overview of randomized trials. *BMJ* 2000; **321**: 1493.

33. Wu C, Cohen S, Richman J, *et al.* Efficacy of postoperative patient controlled and continuous infusion epidural analgesia versus intravenous patient controlled analgesia with opioids: A meta-analysis. *Anesthesiology* 2005; **103**: 1079–88.

34. Richman JM, Liu SS, Courpas G, *et al.* Does continuous peripheral nerve block provide superior pain control to opioids? A meta-analysis. *Anesth Analg* 2006; **102**: 248–57.

35. White PF, Issioui T, Skrivanek GD, *et al.* The use of a continuous popliteal sciatic nerve block after surgery involving the foot and ankle: Does it improve the quality of recovery? *Anesth Analg* 2003; **97**: 1303–9.

36. Peyton PJ, Myles PS, Silbert BS, *et al.* Perioperative epidural analgesia and outcomes after major abdominal surgery in high-risk patients. *Anesth Analg* 2003; **96**: 548–54.

chapter 9

Anemia, coagulopathy and blood transfusion

I. McConachie

Anemia and blood transfusion are relatively common in high-risk surgical and critically ill patients. In recent years, blood transfusion in these patients has been increasingly questioned. In addition, the necessary collection, processing, testing and storage infrastructure makes blood transfusion expensive and it should be our duty to use this scarce resource prudently.

Oxygen transport

Whole body oxygen delivery (DO_2) is determined by the product of cardiac output (CO in $l\,min^{-1}$) and arterial blood oxygen content (CaO_2 in $mg\,dl^{-1}$):

$$DO_2 = CO \times CaO_2$$

CaO_2 is determined primarily by the hemoglobin concentration (Hb in $g\,dl^{-1}$) and the degree of Hb oxygen saturation (HbO_2/Hb or SaO_2, as a fraction), so that

$$CaO_2 = (Hb \times SaO_2 \times K) + (pO_2 \times 0.003)$$

where K is Huffners constant (1.34) – the O_2-carrying capacity of 1 g Hb, and pO_2 is arterial oxygen tension in mmHg.

It can easily be seen that a fall in Hb may have a profound effect on global DO_2 unless compensatory mechanisms occur. It is on this premise that red blood cells are often transfused, that is, to augment DO_2 at a time when the increased cellular oxygen demands of major surgery or critical illness put a strain on already stressed cardiorespiratory systems so that such demands may be met.

- Experimental work suggests an optimal DO_2 at an Hb and hematocrit (Hct) of $10\,g\,dl^{-1}$ (or $100\,g\,l^{-1}$) and 30%, respectively, above which the rheological properties of blood cause a reduction in flow and hence a decreased DO_2 overall.
- A fall in CaO_2, e.g. due to a fall in Hb, results in an increase in erythropoetin (EPO) production within minutes. This EPO response appears to be blunted in the critically ill.
- The stimulus to EPO production is a drop in CaO_2 and so is brought about by both hypoxia and anemia.

Physiological response to anemia

In the normovolemic patient, a rapid drop in Hb brings about certain compensatory changes [1]:

- *Hemodynamic* – the decrease in plasma viscosity improves peripheral blood flow and thus enhances venous return to the right atrium. An immediate increase in stroke volume follows, by the Starling principle, in response to hemodilution and is nonsympathetically

---

Anesthesia for the High Risk Patient, ed. I. McConachie. Published by Cambridge University Press.
© Cambridge University Press 2009.

mediated. The reduced viscosity also reduces afterload, which may be an important mechanism in maintaining cardiac output in the impaired ventricle. Further increases in cardiac output are mediated through aortic chemoreceptors inducing sympathetically mediated increases in contractility (and so stroke volume), venomotor tone (and thus venous return) and heart rate.

- *Microcirculatory* – secondary to the increased cardiac output is an increased organ capillary blood flow and capillary recruitment. Both of these factors are dependent upon the degree of anemia and the individual organ concerned.

- *Oxyhemoglobin dissociation curve (ODC)* – a rightward shift in the ODC is seen, which increases the O_2 unloading by hemoglobin for a given blood pO_2. This is clearly advantageous in increasing cellular O_2 extraction. The primary reason for this is the increased red cell 2,3-diphosphoglycerate synthesis seen during anemia. Local temperature and pH cause a rightward shift in the curve, but their effect is thought to be less significant than that of 2,3-DPG.

Note: These are the responses to anemia. When anemia is due to acute blood losses the physiological responses to hypovolemia will also be triggered. In general, anemia is better tolerated than hypovolemia. A significant, acute fall in circulating blood volume, unless replaced or compensated for, is associated with progressive reductions in organ blood flow and function.

Anemia and the heart

Major surgery, critical illness, and anemia all place stress on the myocardium to increase cardiac output and hence global DO_2. To do so, myocardial DO_2 must increase to meet its own increased O_2 demand (MVO_2). As normal myocardial O_2 extraction runs at between 75% and 80%, any increase in MVO_2 shall be met primarily by an increase in coronary flow; that is, MVO_2 is "flow-restricted". In the presence of coronary artery disease, fixed coronary stenoses may prevent any increase in myocardial flow, thus limiting myocardial DO_2. Thus, during anemia the increased MVO_2 brought about by the demands of an increased cardiac output cannot be met, coronary blood flow is preferentially diverted to the subepicardial layers, and subendocardial ischemia or infarction ensue.

Effect of transfusion on oxygen transport

It has been assumed that an increase in global DO_2 (for example by red cell transfusion) would result in an increase in oxygen consumption (VO_2) in critical illness.

- However, Dietrich *et al.* [2] studied the increase of DO_2 by red cell transfusion in nonsurgical intensive care patients. After volume resuscitation, patients were transfused if their Hb was less than 10 g dl^{-1}. They showed neither an increase in VO_2 nor a decrease in blood lactate levels in any patient, and concluded that the shock state of this patient group was not improved by red cell transfusion.

- In postcardiac surgery patients, the oxygen transport responses to transfusion vary. Even in anemic patients there is no consistent VO_2 response to transfusion [3].

Thus, increasing DO_2 by red cell transfusion may not be of significant benefit in terms of increased oxygen uptake in the cells, but exposes the patient to the possible harmful effects of blood transfusion.

However, it must also be acknowledged that with significant, ongoing blood loss, at some point, blood transfusion *will* be required in addition to maintenance of blood volume and cardiac output. Progressive anemia will eventually reduce DO_2 below its critical level (the point below which further falls in DO_2 cannot be compensated for by increased oxygen extraction by the tissues with inevitable tissue hypoxia).

Role of anemia in morbidity and mortality

A possible effect of anemia on morbidity and mortality is the risks of associated blood transfusion. In addition, it has sometimes proved difficult to distinguish between any adverse influences on outcome of the anemia itself, the cause of the anemia, and possible adverse effects on outcome from treatment of the anemia – chiefly allogenic blood transfusion.

- Carson *et al.* [4] found no increased mortality in 8787 surgical patients down to Hb of $8\,g\,dl^{-1}$, amongst whom the presence of cardiac disease had no bearing on outcome.
- In a study of vascular surgery patients, Hb levels of $9\,g\,dl^{-1}$ were tolerated without adverse clinical outcome [5]. Patients did not compensate for anemia by increased myocardial work, but by increasing O_2 extraction in the peripheral tissues.

However:

- a recent, large study of over 5000 cardiac surgery patients [6] showed that $Hb < 11\,g\,dl^{-1}$ is associated with increased adverse effects especially in those patients with other comorbidities;
- another large, recent, retrospective study in elderly surgical patients found increased 30 day mortality in even mild anemia [7].

Transfusion seems to be commonly triggered by a certain Hb or hematocrit level without any evidence of impaired oxygenation of the tissues. A Hb of $10\,g\,dl^{-1}$ has been traditionally accepted as the level at which Hb should be maintained. In truth, there is little objective evidence to support this approach, and it seems as if this number has been chosen for little more than the fact that this is a nice round number!

However, evidence already outlined above may support a more liberal "trigger" for transfusion in those patients with cardiac disease.

Harmful effects of blood transfusion

Wrong blood

Sadly "wrong blood to patient" errors still occur – and are potentially lethal. Analysis of incident reports has revealed multiple errors of identification, often beginning when blood was collected from the blood bank [8]. The use of hospital protocols including systems for validation of patient identification by more than one person is vital.

Old blood

There may be several problems arising from the transfusion of old blood in critically ill or high-risk patients, although their exact clinical significance is still debated.

- Stored blood has reduced levels of 2,3-DPG, causing a leftward shift in the oxyhemoglobin dissociation curve and a reduced unloading of O_2 from hemoglobin.
- The reduced membrane deformability of red cells, brought about through their storage, is thought to impede their passage through the narrow confines of a capillary bed,

with potential implications for ischemic organs and tissues. The high hematocrit of packed red cells will increase blood viscosity and further threaten perfusion of such areas.

- A small retrospective study of patients with severe sepsis found that the age of the stored transfused RBC was directly associated with mortality [9].

- While some studies have found no evidence of increased morbidity in cardiac surgery patients when old blood is transfused [10], the most recent (and largest) study has clearly found an association between length of storage and morbidity and also short- and long-term survival [11].

- From a trauma unit database, multi-variate analysis has identified that the mean age of blood transfused, number of units older than 14 days, and number of units older than 21 days are independent risk factors for the development of organ failures [12]. They suggest that fresh blood may be more appropriate for the initial resuscitation of trauma patients requiring transfusion.

- Stored blood undergoes progressive losses, mainly of factors V and VIII. Platelets are rapidly lost such that after 48 h there are negligible amounts of functional platelets remaining in solution.

Hemolytic reactions

An estimated 1 in 250 000 transfusions result in an overt hemolytic reaction, most commonly secondary to minor red blood cell (RBC) antigens. This is almost certainly an underestimate due to underreporting and failure to recognize such a reaction during either surgery or the course of a critical illness at a time when the signs (hypotension, tachycardia, disseminated intravascular coagulation (DIC), pyrexia) can be attributed to a more common pathology.

Transfusion-related acute lung injury (TRALI)

Acute lung injury following blood transfusion is thought to result from the activation of recipient neutrophils by donor antibodies and donor RBC-derived membrane lipids. Such neutrophil activation increases endothelial permeability with extravasation of inflammatory mediators and fluid. The resultant clinical picture is indistinguishable from ARDS.

- In the perioperative or critically ill patient there are often other factors that could explain why a patient should develop ARDS, and so the incidence of TRALI is probably underestimated.

- It is possible that the use of leucodepleted blood may reduce the incidence of TRALI.

Increase in cytokines?

- Laboratory studies have shown that RBC transfusion activates neutrophils causing a release of inflammatory cytokines [13].

- Intraoperative transfusion in cardiac surgery patients increases the inflammatory response [14]. During storage, the leucocytes lose their membrane integrity and release substances such as bactericidal permeability increasing (BPI) protein into the plasma. BPI was found in all units of packed red blood cells tested at concentrations up to 15 times preoperative plasma levels in patients.

- However, the issues are complex. For example, one study [15] has found a greater increase in cytokine concentration after autologous blood transfusion than after allogeneic blood transfusion. The lower response in the latter may result from transfusion-induced suppression of cellular immunity.

Transmission of infection by blood transfusion

- Direct transmission of infection via contaminated blood is small but still possible.
- *HIV*. This risk is associated with the donation of blood during the immunologically silent "window period" of infection prior to the host antibody response. The current risk is estimated to be extremely low.
- *Hepatitis B*. The risk of transfusion-associated hepatitis B has fallen dramatically since routine surface antigen testing (1975) and is expected to fall further as the use of the hepatitis B vaccine becomes increasingly widespread. The current risk is between 1 in 30 000 and 1 in 250 000 unit transfusions and accounts for about 10% of all posttransfusion hepatitis [16].
- Transfusion is becoming an increasingly rare cause of hepatitis C infection, possibly as a result of HIV high-risk donation exclusion but with a high associated morbidity.
- Transmission of other viruses such as Parvovirus and West Nile Fever have been reported in the literature, but are rare.
- Bacterial contamination of stored blood is related to the length of storage, but is associated with a high mortality. Transmission rates of other quoted transfusion-associated nonviral infections such as *Plasmodium* and *Trypanosoma cruzi* are vanishingly small.
- The potential for transmission by blood products of protein containing prion particles such as those responsible for human variant Creutzfeldt Jacob Disease (vCJD) represents an unknown risk. There has been one case of blood donation from someone carrying the vCJD prion resulting in the later death from vCJD of both the donor and the recipient. The UK Government has recently banned the donation of blood by anyone who has received a blood transfusion since 1980 (to limit donation to those who received transfusion prior to the assumed introduction of the Bovine Spongiform Encephalopathy prion into the UK food chain). A screening test for the vCJD prion in blood donors is also being developed. Additional attempts to minimize transmission of vCJD by blood products include the purchasing of plasma products from the USA and the universal leucodepletion of blood components (at a cost of £85 million per year).

Immunosuppressive effects of blood transfusion

The immunosuppressive effects of allogeneic blood transfusion are well established [17]. The clinical relevance primarily revolves around two areas of concern.

Postoperative infection

The effects of blood transfusion-induced immunosuppression have been thought to increase the risk of postoperative infection including wound infections. Many studies have suggested such an increased infection rate in patients undergoing colorectal, orthopedic, gynecological, trauma and coronary artery bypass graft surgery. Much of the evidence is retrospective, and the results of prospective trials do not demonstrate an increased risk despite several observational trials that suggested increased risk [18].

Cancer recurrence

Observational data exist to support the concept of increased tumor recurrence in patients who have received perioperative transfusion whilst undergoing potentially curative surgery for colorectal, breast, lung, sarcoma, hepatic and head and neck cancers. Subsequent prospective trials, however, have been unable to demonstrate negative consequences [18].

Vamvakas [19] has disputed much of the evidence for infection and tumor recurrence, stating that most is retrospective and that analysis of prospective, randomized, controlled trials show very little difference between those transfused and those not transfused. He suggests that differences are due to retrospective trial design and that immunosuppression may occur secondary to the variables that lead to the transfusion, and not as a result of the transfusion itself.

Leucodepleted blood transfusion

The evidence from randomized, controlled trials of infection and recurrence rates comparing allogeneic with either leucodepleted or autologous blood are, as yet, inconclusive.

- Leucodepletion reduces the levels of BPI and other substances in stored blood [20].
- The use of leucoreduced blood was associated with a decrease in the postoperative length of stay in a study of cardiac surgery patients [21].
- Canada has recently introduced a universal leucoreduction programme. A retrospective "before and after" study of hip fracture patients, cardiac surgery patients and surgical and trauma admissions to ICU has shown reduced inhospital mortality rates but no decrease in serious nosocomial infections [22]. The frequency of posttransfusion fever and antibiotic use also decreased significantly following leucoreduction.

The widespread adoption of leucodepleted blood has rendered much of the above debate academic.

Transfusion and outcome

Current recommendations with regard to transfusion practice apply to the broadest spectrum of pathology and pathology severity. Often no mention is made of the critically ill or high-risk surgical patient in whom metabolic demands and cardiorespiratory physiology are altered in the extreme. Many studies examining transfusion and mortality potentially are exposed to confounding influences relating to the patient's comorbidities or other treatment effects.

- The most significant study on this issue has been the TRICC (Transfusion Requirements in Critical Care) study [23]. This Canadian multi-center, prospective, randomized study compared a restrictive with a liberal transfusion strategy in 838 general ICU patients. Those in the restrictive strategy group were transfused at an Hb $< 7\,\mathrm{g\,dl^{-1}}$ with packed red cells to maintain their Hb at $7–9\,\mathrm{g\,dl^{-1}}$. Those in the liberal strategy group were transfused with packed red cells at an Hb $< 10\,\mathrm{g\,dl^{-1}}$ to maintain their Hb at $10–12\,\mathrm{g\,dl^{-1}}$. In those patients with an APACHE score less than 20 and in patients aged less than 55 years, the 30-day survival and overall hospital mortality was significantly better in those randomized to the restrictive transfusion strategy. Amongst patients with cardiac disease, the 30-day mortality was reduced, but not significantly so, if allocated to the restrictive strategy. This groundbreaking trial – the first large, prospective study of blood transfusion strategy on outcome in ICU – also showed a significant decrease in organ dysfunction and cardiac complications in the restrictive strategy group.

- A similar negative effect of transfusion on outcome was demonstrated in patients having coronary artery bypass surgery [24]. They also demonstrated a significantly increased risk of left ventricular dysfunction and mortality in the high and medium Hct groups compared to the low Hct group. The authors proposed that increased blood viscosity may require increased myocardial work while reducing coronary flow.
- In a study from a major US trauma center, blood transfusion seems to be an independent predictor of mortality, need for ICU admission, and ICU and hospital length of stay (even after controlling for severity of shock and injury) [25].

As a final word, recommendations by the ASA Task Force on Blood Component Therapy [26] state that transfusion is:

- rarely required above an Hb of $10\,\mathrm{g\,dl}^{-1}$; and
- almost always indicated when Hb is less than $6\,\mathrm{g\,dl}^{-1}$.

Reducing the need for blood transfusion

A major trend in recent years has been a greater reluctance to expose patients to the problems associated with allogeneic blood transfusion. This in part reflects greater understanding of these problems, but also a realization that the beneficial effects of transfusion are less apparent in many groups of patients. Thus, one should be able to justify the use of blood products at all times and, for each patient, question whether the benefits of transfusion are worth the risks – recognizing that the days of routine transfusion of blood for mild degrees of anemia should be gone.

Requirement for allogeneic blood transfusion can be reduced by:

- accepting the appropriateness of a restrictive transfusion strategy for most patients;
- increasing the use perioperatively of predonation and other forms of autologous blood transfusion; and
- preventing or reducing blood or red cell loss.

Prevention of blood loss

A detailed account of perioperative methods of reducing surgical blood loss lies outside the scope of this text, but these include:

- hypotensive anesthetic techniques;
- improved surgical techniques including minimally invasive surgery;
- appropriate attention to patient positioning, CO_2 tension and venous drainage;
- use of tourniquets and infiltration of vasoconstrictors;
- use of antifibrinolytic and other drugs to reduce bleeding (see below);
- surgery under spinal or epidural anesthesia as opposed to general anesthesia;
- in addition, the loss of *red blood cells* may be reduced by the use of hemodilution techniques and the use of cell saver strategies; and

- erythropoietin (EPO) therapy. EPO therapy is expensive and the benefits are, so far, controversial. Studies have shown conflicting effects on the need for allogeneic blood in different types of surgery. However, if it reduces red cell transfusion requirements and avoids the harmful effects of transfusion, it may well be a highly cost-effective therapy for the critically ill patient.

Society of Cardiovascular Anaesthetists guidelines [27] recently produced suggest that *all* possible modalities that can be utilized to reduce the need for allogeneic blood transfusion should be employed for all cardiac surgery patients, e.g. routine use of pharmacological adjuncts already discussed. This included the use of aprotinin, but this has been overtaken by the recent events surrounding this drug (see below). This aggressive approach to reduce the need for blood transfusion in cardiac surgery has been challenged [28], pointing out that at least some of these modalities may have greater risks associated with their use compared to the proven risks of allogeneic blood transfusion.

Blood substitutes

All intravenous infusions of asanguinous fluids can be considered to be "blood substitutes". However, in this context we mean oxygen-carrying red cell substitute fluids.

Interest continues in the use of such blood substitutes to reduce the need for allogeneic blood transfusion. In general, there may be toxicity relating to the cell debris contained within preparations of hemoglobin – chiefly, renal toxicity. Another source of concern in early studies of free hemoglobin in solution was a marked vasopressor effect, probably related to scavenging of the endogenous vasodilator, nitric oxide. This in itself may be harmful for trauma patients in the field if it encourages further bleeding.

There are several main areas of research.

- Diasprin cross-linked hemoglobin (DCLB). Recent multi-center trials show some effect in limiting the transfusion of allogeneic blood. However, two large multi-center trials have now been terminated early owing to safety concerns. Interest in this product thus seems to have waned.

- Polymerized human hemoglobin. Seems to be free of significant side effects and early reports regarding efficacy are encouraging.

- Bovine hemoglobin. This has been used successfully in surgery associated with major blood loss, but there are concerns related to increased blood pressure and production of antibodies. Nevertheless, a commercial product has been approved for use in South Africa.

- Human recombinant hemoglobin. Likely to be expensive, but may prove useful in the future.

- Perfluorocarbons carry increased oxygen in solution, but have a requirement for a high FiO_2. Early trials suggest a reduction in the requirement for transfusion of allogeneic blood.

Massive transfusion

Massive blood transfusion (MBT) in the high-risk surgical patient can occur in most surgical subspecialities, but is especially common in trauma, vascular, obstetric and oncology surgery. Morbidity and mortality remain high, but this reflects the underlying pathology as much if not more than the harmful effects of the blood products themselves.

Various definitions of MBT have been proposed:

- one or more blood volumes is lost in a 24 h period;
- replacement of 50% of the blood volume within 3 h;
- transfusion of more than 20 units of red cells.

The different clinical situations represented above may carry different clinical implications, e. g. rapid loss versus slower, sustained loss with different hemodynamic effects.

The main problems associated with MBT include the following.

- Inability to "keep up" with volume loss with resultant hemodynamic instability and shock.
- Hemodilution with eventual fall in DO_2 below critical oxygen delivery if replacement with only clear fluids.
- Acidosis – Multi-factorial, but includes acidosis from shock and hypothermia. Administration of sodium bicarbonate should only be guided by blood gas measurements.
- Hypothermia. MBT contributes significantly to perioperative hypothermia especially if products are given straight from refrigeration units. The adverse effects of perioperative hypothermia are discussed fully in Chapter 14.
- Citrate toxicity is a theoretical problem, but unlikely to be a clinical problem unless liver disease reduces citrate metabolism.
- Hyperkalemia is common (stored blood contains approximately 20 mmol K) and is exacerbated by acidosis.
- Hypocalcemia is also a theoretical problem (partly from citrate), but most authors no longer recommend administration of calcium in all but the most extreme situations. Measurement of ionized calcium is recommended prior to replacement.
- Reduced levels of 2,3-DPG in stored blood reduces oxygen release from Hb at the tissues, but is probably not as big a clinical problem as many people believe (or no one would survive replacement of their blood volume with stored blood).
- Coagulopathy results from dilution with crystalloids and colloids, acidosis and hypothermia [29] and the reduced clotting factors and platelets found in stored blood (see above). Coagulation problems are not usually severe until 1–2 blood volumes have been replaced in the patient. Release of tissue factors into the circulation (especially in trauma patients), cell fragments and mediators from stored blood may cause disseminated intravascular coagulation (DIC) with consumption of clotting factors.

Management of MBT

Hospitals should have local guidelines in place which, ideally, should be tested in hospital-wide drills. Full discussion of the management of MBT and, in particular, prevention and treatment of coagulopathies is beyond the scope of this text, but the following is a summary of some of the principles recommended by the UK Blood Transfusion services [30].

- Restore circulating volume and tissue oxygenation as initial priority.
- Contact key personnel in the OR and laboratories. Laboratories need to be kept informed so as to provide good service, especially as many areas have centralized storage of blood components. Hematologists provide invaluable advice for interpretation of investigations and management of MBT.

- Control bleeding by surgical efforts and/or correcting coagulation abnormalities.
- Request appropriate laboratory investigations. However, the dynamics of the situation change rapidly, and components may have to be given before test results (often already out of date) are available. Frequent testing is encouraged to discourage indiscriminate use of clotting factors.
- Request suitable red cells products. O-negative blood is rarely essential, but most laboratories can supply group-specific blood very quickly (with ongoing cross-match checks while the blood is being delivered). Whole blood is ideal but not often available.
- If possible, blood warmers and/or a rapid infusion device should be used. Rapid infusion devices are useful due to the speed at which blood may be pumped into the patient but, more crucially, they are able to adequately warm blood even at very high flow rates. This has been shown to limit the eventual total blood requirement by maintaining body temperature and preventing acidosis and coagulopathy [31].
- Employ cell-saver technology if available and if the wound is not heavily contaminated.
- Request platelets (e.g. 1 unit 10 kg weight), fresh frozen plasma (FFP) (e.g. $10-15\,\mathrm{ml\,kg^{-1}}$) and cryoprecipitate (e.g. 6 unit pool) according to local guidelines. The use of Factor VIIa is controversial and will be discussed below.
- Suspect DIC if clotting factor correction does not result in clinical improvement.

Coagulation and coagulopathy

This is a simplified account of the classic coagulation cascade.

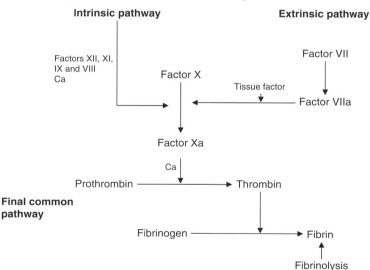

However, recently [32] it has been recognized that:

- coagulation is regulated by processes at the cell surfaces;
- the most important initiating event in blood clot formation is the formation of the tissue factor or TF/factor VIIa complex;

- this complex of factor VIIa and TF activates factor X;
- the small amount of thrombin generated activates platelets with subsequent amplification of thrombin production leading to clot formation;
- circulating protease inhibitors limit coagulation to specific cell surfaces and prevent widespread, harmful clotting; and
- this process of thrombin release and formation of a stable clot is necessary for effective wound healing.

Management of surgical bleeding

- First and foremost, bleeding from damaged blood vessels requires surgical control. Occasionally with trauma patients, and less commonly with vascular surgery patients, conventional surgical techniques are ineffective and "damage control surgery" is recommended to prevent the lethal triad of coagulopathy, acidosis and hypothermia and prevent the development of irreversible shock. Damage control surgery [33] involves packing the abdomen, not closing the abdomen, ventilating the patient in ICU and correcting coagulation defects, hypothermia and acidosis. The patient undergoes definitive surgery when stable. This approach reduces the side effects of massive transfusion and saves the lives of trauma patients.
    All other "nonsurgical" bleeding can be termed microvascular bleeding.
- Microvascular bleeding due to clotting factor deficiency is less common than surgical bleeding and hypothermia and rarely occurs in surgery under 1 h and with transfusion of less than 10 units of blood. Prothrombin, factor V and factor VII levels are critically reduced if losses exceed approximately twice the blood volume.
- Clotting factor replacement with fresh frozen plasma is recommended by the ASA [26]:
    - microvascular bleeding in the presence of PT/PTT > 1.5 × normal;
    - microvascular bleeding in patients transfused with more than 1 blood volume without PT/PTT measurement;
    - dose should be calculated to achieve at least 30% factor concentration.
- Platelet deficiency is probably more common than deficiency of clotting factors. After replacement of 1 blood volume probably only 30–40% of platelets remain. Platelet replacement has also been recommended by ASA guidelines [26]:
    - microvascular bleeding with platelet count < 50;
    - microvascular bleeding with 50 < platelet count < 100 and risk of more significant bleeding;
    - microvascular bleeding with known platelet dysfunction.
- Cryoprecipitate replacement for fibrinogen deficiency is also covered by the ASA [26] guidelines:
    - microvascular bleeding with fibrinogen concentration < 80–100 mg dl^{-1} (or when fibrinogen measurement is not available).
- Factor VII replacement is controversial, and is discussed further below.

Factor VII in surgical bleeding

Recombinant factor VII was developed as replacement therapy for hemophilia and has also been used for patients with antibodies to other factors. The rationale for the use of factor VII in uncontrolled surgical bleeding is based on the cellular based coagulation model described above.

- At *pharmacological* doses, recombinant factor VIIa binds to the surface of locally activated platelets, resulting in a massive "thrombin burst".
- The requirement for locally activated platelets limits unwanted clot formation away from the site of injury.
- Recombinant Factor VIIa also reduces fibrinolysis of the resultant clot.

There is a growing body of literature (but few randomized, prospective trials) suggesting that recombinant Factor VIIa may have some role [34] in treating massive or uncontrolled hemorrhage resulting from many different etiologies:

- thrombocytopenia and platelet function defects;
- liver failure;
- anticoagulant overdose;
- factor deficiency (VII, IX);
- postcerebral hemorrhage;
- postpartum hemorrhage;
- trauma. Hemorrhage is a major factor in mortality in trauma patients;
- surgical bleeding. Reports have appeared chiefly for liver surgery, neurosurgery, cardiac surgery, orthopedic and prostatic surgery.

However, there are concerns over safety, efficacy and costs as a result of increasing nonapproved use. Dosage is also not well established, but a common dose in hemophiliacs is 40–80 mcg kg^{-1}. Recombinant factor VIIa has a short half-life, so may have to be repeated after 2 h. Monitoring is problematic, and the best available monitor may be a clinical reduction in bleeding!

The main safety concern relates to unwanted thrombosis, which has been reported in various settings [35].

European consensus guidelines have been produced [36] and graded according to conventional principles from A to E based on strength of evidence ("A" being strongest evidence). In summary, they suggest:

Recommended in:

- blunt trauma (grade B);
- may be beneficial in postpartum hemorrhage (grade E);
- uncontrolled bleeding in surgical patients (grade E);
- bleeding following cardiac surgery (grade D).

Not recommended in:

- penetrating trauma (grade B);
- prophylactically in elective surgery (grade A) or liver surgery (grade B);
- bleeding episodes in patients with Child–Pugh A cirrhosis (grade B). Efficacy of rFVIIa was considered uncertain in bleeding episodes in patients with Child–Pugh B and C cirrhosis (grade C).

The use of recombinant factor VIIa should not replace conventional therapies and strategies for control of hemorrhage, and should be used only after discussion with a hematologist. Indeed, the majority of institutions will limit its availability solely to occasions when its use has been authorized by a hematologist!

Pharmacological adjuncts to coagulation

Many drugs have been used with varying success in an attempt to aid hemostasis without causing unwanted thrombosis or other side effects. Recombinant factor VIIa has already been discussed. Other agents include:

- *Aprotinin.* Aprotinin has been widely used, especially in cardiac and liver surgery. Aprotinin is an inhibitor of serum proteases including plasmin and kallikrein, thus reducing fibrinolysis. The resultant lesser accumulation of fibrin degradation products (FDPs) also improves platelet function. (FDPs inhibit platelet aggregation and inhibit fibrin crosslinking.)

  In cardiac surgery, a meta-analysis confirmed the effectiveness of aprotinin in reducing blood loss and requirement for allogeneic blood transfusion [37]. Aprotinin has also been used in liver surgery, especially transplantation, but with less evidence of efficacy [38].

  However, a more recent study has shown that aprotinin increases the incidence of renal dysfunction and cardiac and cerebral complications following CABG surgery [39]. In a follow up study, the same group subsequently reported a long-term increase in mortality in patients given aprotinin [40]. At the time of writing, aprotinin has been withdrawn by its manufacturers worldwide awaiting results from further trials.

- *Tranexamic acid.* Tranexamic acid (TXA) blocks conversion of plasminogen to plasmin and prevents plasmin from breaking down fibrin. The reduced plasmin results in less fibrinolysis, and also reduces the formation of FDPs which have anticoagulant properties as discussed above. TXA has also been found to be effective in reducing blood loss and the requirement for allogeneic blood transfusion in cardiac surgery, and is recommended over aprotinin by some due to reduced costs, no allergic potential and no adverse renal effects. TXA has also been shown to be effective in orthopedic surgery with high potential for bleeding [41].

Note: Both aprotinin and TXA inhibit clot breakdown, i.e. relatively normal clotting ability is required to produce clot in the first place.

- *Desmopressin.* Desmopressin or 1-deamino-8-D-arginine vasopressin (DDAVP) is a synthetic analog of vasopressin with prolonged antidiuretic effects but without any vasoconstrictor effects. Desmopressin causes release of von Willebrand factor (vWf) (and acts as a protein carrier for, and increases levels of, factor VIII) and improves coagulation in the most common form of von Willebrand's disease, mild forms of hemophilia and other platelet disorders, e.g. uremia. DDAVP also improves platelet adhesiveness. DDAVP ($0.3\,mg\,kg^{-1}$) produces rapid rises in vWf but may need to be repeated. Use of DDAVP is controversial, but some papers have shown reduced blood loss and requirement for blood products, especially in those patients taking aspirin. Others have not [42].

- *Fibrin sealant.* Fibrin sealants and other topically applied substances show some promise in controlling surgical bleeding [43], but, depending on their source, some may have the potential for undesirable immune effects.

Further reading

Monk TG, Goodnough LT. Issues in transfusion medicine. *Anesthesiol Clin N Am* 2005; **23**: 241–396.

Supplement on Perioperative Anaemia. *Br J Anaesthesia* 1998; **81**: 1–82.

References

1. Hebert PC, Hu L, Biro G. Review of physiological response to anaemia. *Can Med Assoc J* 1997; **156** (Suppl 11): S27–40.

2. Dietrich KA, Conrad SA, Hebert CA, *et al.* Cardiovascular and metabolic response to red blood cell transfusion in critically ill volume-resuscitated nonsurgical patients. *Crit Care Med* 1990; **18**: 940–5.

3. Casutt M, Seifert B, Pasch T, *et al.* Factors influencing the individual effects of blood transfusions on oxygen delivery and oxygen consumption. *Crit Care Med* 1999; **27**: 2194–200.

4. Carson JL, Duff A, Berlin J, *et al.* Perioperative blood transfusion and postoperative mortality. *JAMA* 1998; **279**: 199–205.

5. Bush RL, Pevec WC, Holcroft JW. A prospective, randomized trial limiting perioperative red blood cell transfusions in vascular patients. *Am J Surg* 1997; **174**: 143–8.

6. Kulier A, Levin J, Moser R, *et al.* Impact of preoperative anemia on outcome in patients undergoing coronary artery bypass graft surgery. *Circulation* 2007; **116**: 471–9.

7. Wu WC, Schifftner TL, Henderson WG, *et al.* Preoperative hematocrit levels and postoperative outcomes in older patients undergoing noncardiac surgery. *JAMA* 2007; **297**: 2481–8.

8. Williamson LM, Lowe S, Love EM, *et al.* Serious hazards of transfusion (SHOT) initiative: Analysis of the first two annual reports. *BMJ* 1999; **319**: 16–9.

9. Purdy FR, Tweeddale MG, Merrick PM. Association of mortality with age of blood transfused in septic ICU patients. *Can J Anaesth* 1997; **44**: 1256–61.

10. Vamvakas EC, Carven JH. Length of storage of transfused red cells and postoperative morbidity in patients undergoing coronary artery bypass graft surgery. *Transfusion* 2000; **40**: 101–9.

11. Koch CG, Li L, Sessler DI, *et al.* Duration of red-cell storage and complications after cardiac surgery. *N Engl J Med* 2008; **358**: 1229–39.

12. Zallen G, Offner PJ, Moore EE, *et al.* Age of transfused blood is an independent risk factor for postinjury multiple organ failure. *Am J Surg* 1999; **178**: 570–2.

13. Zallen G, Moore EE, Ciesla DJ, *et al.* Stored red blood cells selectively activate human neutrophils to release IL-8 and secretory PLA2. *Shock* 2000; **13**: 29–33.

14. Fransen E, Maessen J, Dentener M, *et al.* Impact of blood transfusions on inflammatory mediator release in patients undergoing cardiac surgery. *Chest* 1999; **116**: 1233–9.

15. Avall A, Hyllner M, Bengtson JP, *et al.* Postoperative inflammatory response after autologous and allogeneic blood transfusion. *Anesthesiology* 1997; **87**: 511–6.

16. Schreiber GB, Busch MP, Kleinman SH. The risk of transfusion-transmitted viral infections. *N Engl J Med* 1996; **334**: 1685–9.

17. Landers DF, Hill GE, Wong KC, *et al.* Blood transfusion-induced immunomodulation. *Anesth Analg* 1996; **82**: 187–204.

18. Vamvakas EC, Blajchman MA. Deleterious clinical effects of transfusion-associated immunomodulation: Fact or fiction? *Blood* 2001; **97**: 1180–95.

19. Vamvakas EC. Transfusion-associated cancer recurrence and postoperative infection: Meta-analysis of randomised, controlled clinical trials. *Transfusion* 1996; **36**: 175–86.

20. Fransen EJ, Rombout-Sestrienkova E, van Pampus EC, *et al.* Prestorage leucocyte reduction of red cell components prevents release of bactericidal permeability increasing protein and defensins. *Vox Sang* 2002; **83**: 119–24.

21. Fung MK, Rao N, Rice J, et al. Leukoreduction in the setting of open heart surgery: A prospective cohort-controlled study. *Transfusion* 2004; **44**: 30–5.

22. Hebert PC, Fergusson D, Blajchman MA, et al. Clinical outcomes following institution of the Canadian universal leukoreduction program for red blood cell transfusions. *JAMA* 2003; **289**: 1941–9.

23. Hebert PC, Wells G, Blajchman MA, et al. A multicentre, randomised, controlled clinical trial of transfusion requirements in critical care. *N Engl J Med* 1999; **340**: 409–17.

24. Speiss BD, Ley C, Body SC, et al. Haematocrit value on intensive care unit entry influences the frequency of Q-wave myocardial infarction after coronary artery bypass grafting. *J Thorac Cardiovasc Surg* 1998; **116**: 460–7.

25. Malone DL, Dunne J, Tracy JK, et al. Blood transfusion, independent of shock severity, is associated with worse outcome in trauma. *J Trauma* 2003; **4**: 898–905.

26. Practice guidelines for perioperative blood transfusion and adjuvant therapies: an updated report by the American Society of Anesthesiologists Task Force on Perioperative Blood Transfusion and Adjuvant Therapies. *Anesthesiology* 2006; **105**: 198–208.

27. Spiess BD, Shore-Lesserson L, Stafford-Smith M, et al. Perioperative blood transfusion and blood conservation in cardiac surgery: The Society of Thoracic Surgeons and The Society of Cardiovascular Anesthesiologists clinical practice guideline. *Ann Thorac Surg* 2007; **83** (5 Suppl): S27–86.

28. Karkouti K, McCluskey SA. Perioperative blood conservation – The experts, the elephants, the clinicians, and the gauntlet. *Can J Anaesth* 2007; **54**: 861–7.

29. Ferrara A, MacArthur JD, Wright HK, et al. Hypothermia and acidosis worsen coagulopathy in the patient requiring massive transfusion. *Am J Surg* 1990; **160**: 515–18.

30. Stainsby D, MacLennan S, Thomas D, et al. Guidelines on the management of massive blood loss. *Br J Haematol* 2006; **135**: 634–41.

31. Dunham CM, Belzberg H, Lyles R, et al. The rapid infusion system: A superior method for the resuscitation of hypovolemic trauma patients. *Resuscitation* 1991; **21**: 207–27.

32. Hoffman M, Monroe DM. Coagulation 2006: A modern view of hemostasis. *Hematol Oncol Clin North Am* 2007; **21**: 1–11.

33. Hirshberg A, Mattox KL. "Damage control" in trauma surgery. *Br J Surg* 1993; **80**: 1501–2.

34. Welsby IJ, Monroe DM, Lawson JH, et al. Recombinant activated factor VII and the anaesthetist. *Anaesthesia* 2005; **60**: 1203–12.

35. Goodnough LT, Shander AS. Recombinant factor VIIa: Safety and efficacy. *Curr Opin Hematol* 2007; **14**: 504–9.

36. Vincent JL, Rossaint R, Riou B, et al. Recommendations on the use of recombinant activated factor VII as an adjunctive treatment for massive bleeding – A European perspective. *Crit Care* 2006; **10**: R120.

37. Laupacis A, Fergusson D. Drugs to minimize perioperative blood loss in cardiac surgery: Meta-analyses using perioperative blood transfusion as the outcome. The International Study of Peri-operative Transfusion (ISPOT) Investigators. *Anesth Analg* 1997; **85**: 1258–67.

38. Lentschener C, Roche K, Ozier Y. A review of aprotinin in orthotopic liver transplantation: Can its harmful effects offset its beneficial effects? *Anesth Analg* 2005; **100**: 1248–55.

39. Mangano DT, Tudor IC, Dietzel C. The risk associated with aprotinin in cardiac surgery. *N Engl J Med* 2006; **354**: 353–65.

40. Mangano DT, Miao Y, Vuylsteke A, et al. Mortality associated with aprotinin during 5 years following coronary artery bypass graft surgery. *JAMA* 2007; **297**: 471–9.

41. Zufferey P, Merquiol F, Laporte S, et al. Do antifibrinolytics reduce allogeneic blood transfusion in orthopedic surgery? *Anesthesiology* 2006; **105**: 1034–46.

42. Pleym H, Stenseth R, Wahba A, et al. Prophylactic treatment with desmopressin does not reduce postoperative bleeding after coronary surgery in patients treated with aspirin before surgery. *Anesth Analg* 2004; **98**: 578–84.

43. Schwartz M, Madariaga J, Hirose R, et al. Comparison of a new fibrin sealant with standard topical hemostatic agents. *Arch Surg* 2004; **139**: 1148–54.

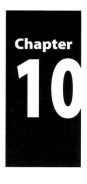

Chapter 10

The obese or malnourished patient

S. Balasubramanian and P. S. Hegde

Malnutrition includes both overnutrition and undernutrition. Overnutrition is called "obesity" (*obesus*, Latin "fattened by eating"), while undernutrition is more commonly referred to as "malnutrition". In clinical practice, both these variants pose a formidable challenge to the anesthetist.

Assessment of nutritional status

Malnutrition is very common in hospital patients.

- Common sense clinical examination will be helpful, e.g. history of weight loss and food intake, measured versus usual weight, specific features, e.g. of vitamin deficiencies and signs of muscle weakness and atrophy. Measured height and weight should be compared to standard tables.
- Anthropometric measurements, e.g. triceps skin fold thickness and mid-arm muscle circumference may be useful, but are operator-dependent to some degree and may not be reproducible.
- Albumin as an index of visceral protein mass is useful in pure malnutrition. However, in high-risk or critically ill patients, influences of decreased synthesis due to liver disturbances and loss due to capillary leak confuse the picture.
- Serum transferrin has been suggested as a better index of body proteins as it has a longer circulating half-life and is not an acute-phase protein.
- Lymphocyte count and skin tests for common allergens (an index of immune competence which is depressed in malnutrition) are useful in pure malnutrition but, again, are less useful in high-risk or critically ill patients.
- Of experimental interest at present are accurate measurements from bioelectrical impedance, which quantitatively measures lean body mass.

In summary, there are no simple tests appropriate for assessing acute malnutrition in critical or high-risk patients. Clinical impression and serial estimations of weight compared to premorbid weight are probably as useful as more complex tests [1].

Obesity (overnutrition)

Obesity is complex and multi-factorial, and is defined as a condition of excessive fat accumulation in adipose tissue to the extent that health may be impaired [2]. It occurs when the net energy intake exceeds the net energy expenditure.

Anesthesia for the High Risk Patient, ed. I. McConachie. Published by Cambridge University Press.
© Cambridge University Press 2009.

Epidemiology

- Globally there are as many overnourished as undernourished persons.
- In developed countries such as the UK, half the population is either overweight or obese, while in developing countries such as China, 15% of the population is overweight.
- The Health Survey for England predicts that more than 12 million adults and 1 million children will be obese by 2010 if no action is taken.
- The USA has the highest rate of obesity in the developed world.

Etiology

- Genetic and environmental factors.
- Ethnic influences – Asian immigrants to the UK have more central distribution of fat than native Caucasians. In the USA, African and Mexican Americans have a higher risk of obesity than white Americans.
- Diet and lifestyle – unhealthy eating habits, sedentary lifestyle and lack of exercise.
- Socioeconomic factors – in developed countries, obesity is more common amongst the lower socioeconomic class; however, in developing countries, it is associated with affluence [3].
- Behavioral – psychiatric/emotional disorders.
- Diseases – diabetes mellitus, hypothyroidism, Cushing's disease, hypothalamic lesions.
- Drugs – hormones (steroids, insulin, progestogens), antidepressants (amitriptyline, imipramine), antihypertensives (clonidine, prazosin, propranolol), valproic acid, phenothiazines, lithium.

Classification

Body Mass Index (BMI) = weight (kg)/height^2 (m^2)
Visceral obesity = waist > 102 cm (M) or > 88 cm (F)

Classification of overweight and obesity by BMI, waist circumference, and associated disease risk* [4]

	BMI** (kg m^{-2})	Risk relative to normal weight and waist circumference	
		Men < 102 cm Women < 88 cm	Men > 102 cm Women > 88 cm
Underweight	18.5	Not increased	Not increased
Normal	18.5–24.9	Not increased	Increased
Overweight	25.0–29.9	Increased	High
Obesity (Class I)	30.0–34.9	High	Very high
Obesity (Class II)	35.0–39.9	Very high	Extremely high
Extreme obesity (Class III)	>40.0	Extremely high	Extremely high

* Disease risk for type 2 diabetes, hypertension, and cardiovascular disease.
** Limitations: heavily muscled individuals will be classed as overweight. Elderly patients with decreased lean body mass and relatively increased body fat may have normal BMI.

Clinical implications

Patients with obesity are different by physical, physiological, psychological, and co-existing pathological factors. They also have altered pharmacokinetics.

Outcome

- In ICU, studies have shown conflicting results as to whether obesity increases mortality, but length of stay is prolonged.

- Similarly, in cardiac surgery patients, obesity is associated with more postoperative complications and longer hospitalization, but not with an increased early or long-term mortality [5].

- In obese general surgical patients there are increased technical problems with surgery, increased complications and, often, increased length of stay, but studies differ in their prediction of the effects of obesity on mortality.

Airway

Difficulties in airway management in obese patients arise from limitations in neck movement (especially when BMI >40) and excessive adiposity in front of neck, submental area and chest. Additionally they may have retropalatal redundant pharyngeal tissue narrowing the airway [6]. Obstructive sleep apnea (5%) may co-exist.

Respiratory system

Obese patients produce excessive carbon dioxide (VCO_2) and have increased oxygen consumption (VO_2). This is related to an increased effort and work of breathing of up to 70% [7]. The excessive chest wall adiposity results in atelectasis. The reduced functional residual capacity may be below the closing capacity. Morbidly obese patients can have alveolar closures even when upright. Such patients rapidly desaturate and may need intubation in a semi-reclining position. Splinting of the diaphragm due to pressure from abdominal contents in supine and Trendelenberg positions can cause ventilation perfusion mismatch [8]. The co-existing pathologies include increased incidence of asthma, pulmonary hypertension and obesity hypoventilation syndrome (8%).

Cardiovascular system

The circulatory volume and consequently the stroke volume are increased. The increased cardiac output reduces the ability for further increases if need arises. Patients may show a normal left ventricular function with diminished compliance. In extreme cases, ventricular dysfunction can become significant with associated pulmonary hypertension. Comorbidities include hypertension (mild to moderate 50–60%, severe 5–10%), atherosclerosis, coronary artery disease, cerebrovascular injury, and deep vein thrombosis (DVT) risk.

Gastrointestinal system

Fasting obese patients often have a gastric pH < 2.5 along with increased residual gastric volume. Co-existing gastroesophageal reflux and hiatus hernia can predispose to pulmonary aspiration. Hyperlipidemia and fatty liver have been associated.

Others

- Endocrinal – diabetes mellitus, insulin resistance, hypothyroidism.
- Musculoskeletal – arthritis.
- Metabolic – gout.
- Psychological – depression, anxiety, low self-esteem, social problems.

Pharmacokinetics

Ideal Body Weight (IBW) = Height (cm) – x
   ($x = 100$ for adult males and 105 for adult females)

- The bioavailability of oral drugs is unaffected in obese patients. Intramuscular route is unpredictable.
- Obese patients have increased circulating volume, hence water-soluble drugs have more volume of distribution (Vd). The Vd for fat-soluble drugs is significantly increased.
- Clearance (Cl) and termination of drugs remain similar to lean patients.
- The loading dose of a drug is calculated based on Vd and infusion rates are calculated based on Cl. Loading dose of drugs with distribution restricted to lean tissues only are calculated based on IBW. Drugs which are equally distributed to lean and fat tissues should have loading dose calculations based on actual body weight (ABW).
- If Cl of the drug increases with obesity, then the infusion rate is calculated based on ABW. Drugs whose Cl remains unaffected or decreased by obesity should have calculation of infusion rates based on IBW.
- Propofol – Vd and Cl are increased and hence the dosage should be based on ABW and not IBW.
- Thiopentone – induction dose should be increased. The duration of action is prolonged due to longer elimination half-life.
- Midazolam – the Vd increases but not Cl, hence a single dose should be based on ABW, while infusion is based on IBW.
- Inhalation agents show no difference in minimum alveolar concentration (MAC) and equilibrium is rapidly reached.
- Succinylcholine has increased dose requirements due to higher levels of pseudocholinesterase in obesity [9].
- Nondepolarizing muscle relaxants (NDMR) – dose should be based on IBW except for pancuronium, which requires higher dose, and atracurium, whose duration of action is unaffected. Minimal data are available on mivacurium, but dose may need to be increased relative to IBW.
- Opiates must be titrated to effect judiciously. Morphine is based on IBW. Alfentanil (reduced Cl and prolonged half-life) and remifentanil should be given on the basis of IBW. Fentanyl is given on the basis of ABW [10].

The above-mentioned are broad guidelines. There is interpatient variability in response, hence case-by-case clinical assessment and titration of dose to effect remains central to the delivery of a safe anesthetic.

Anesthetic considerations

Apart from general surgery, obese patients can present for restrictive/malabsorptive bariatric surgery. An intragastric balloon sited via endoscopy under sedation in patients with BMI > 60 facilitates weight loss, enabling them to undergo more definitive procedure safely. Open abdominal procedures are increasingly being replaced by endoscopic and laparoscopic procedures. Patients are encouraged to lose weight prior to elective procedures by changing dietary habits and exercising.

Preoperative phase

- Obese patients are best assessed in a lying down position as this highlights physiological limitations and positioning problems.

- Preoperative investigation is directed by the history and examination findings of the patient and the nature of the proposed surgery. It may include full blood count (to exclude polycythemia), chest X-ray, supine and upright blood gases and overnight oximetry [11]. Spirometry as a preassessment screening tool does not make any difference in predicting postoperative pulmonary complications [12].

- Preoperative nasal continuous positive airway pressure (CPAP) and bilevel-positive airway pressure (BIPAP) will benefit patients with obstructive sleep apnea [13].

- A preoperative discussion about the need for extubation when fully awake and in a sitting position may minimize patient anxiety and improve cooperation during recovery.

- Standard precautions such as preoperative fasting, H_2 inhibitors, metoclopramide, and nonparticulate antacids are given to avoid aspiration injury.

- Morbidly obese patients often have difficulties lying flat. A wide electric tilting bed is useful since narrow trolleys cause cramping of the head and shoulders, compromising airway management.

Positioning

The anesthetist

- Standing at the head end, on a little platform if needed, looking down the airway. This minimizes undue strain while attempting to safely bag, mask and secure the patient's airway, particularly when the patient is semi-reclined.

The patient

- Proper support ("ramping") with the head neutral or slightly flexed.

- Head and neck positioning of patient to align the oral, laryngeal and pharyngeal axes. Alignment can be guided by being able to draw an imaginary horizontal line between tragus and sternum.

- Use of shorter handles and polio laryngoscope blade will optimize the chances of successful laryngoscopy. The efficacy of cricoid pressure in obese patients has been questioned [14]. In extreme cases, awake fiberoptic intubation of the trachea is indicated.

- Special arm boards are used for proper positioning. Padded support along the whole length of the arms, with joints in slight flexion, will avoid the risk of brachial plexus, nerve compression and joint injuries. Nerves may also be vulnerable due to vitamin deficiencies secondary to inappropriate dieting [15].

- Lumbar spine extension may be a problem due to buttocks fulcruming the legs. Flexion of the hips by supporting the knees will minimize strain on lumbar spine.

Monitoring

- Breath sounds are distant and $ETCO_2$ is very important. Endotracheal tubes tend to move in obese patients especially undergoing laparoscopic surgery [16]. A visual confirmation using a fiberoptic scope may well be indicated.
- Pulse oximetry to monitor oxygenation is similar to the lean patient.
- Noninvasive blood pressure (NIBP) monitoring of the upper arm is a problem because of the girth and the conical shape of the upper arm. NIBP in the forearm is usually simple and reliable, but may show slightly wider pulse pressure.
- Invasive blood pressure and blood gas monitoring using an arterial line are not always indicated, but are useful in prolonged cases. They carry their own risks and challenges.
- Central venous pressure monitoring is used only if clinically indicated. Ultrasound guidance will minimize failure and avoidable risks. Intravenous cannulation may be a problem due to excessive subcutaneous tissue and might warrant central access.
- Monitoring neuromuscular function in the presence of NDMRs is important. Complete reversal is mandatory prior to attempting extubation.

Intraoperative phase

Low oxygen saturations, high $ETCO_2$ and high airway pressures are not uncommon. An initial high concentration of inspired oxygen followed by pulse oximetry/blood gas-guided titration is recommended. Ventilation and oxygenation can be improved by:

- positive end expiratory pressure (PEEP);
- reverse Trendelenberg position to offload the abdomen;
- discussion with the surgeon regarding abdominal packing;
- offloading the pressure by manually or mechanically lifting the abdominal pannus [17];
- barotrauma is possible; consider "pressure" rather than "volume" controlled ventilation. Maintaining minute ventilation by increasing the respiratory rate while limiting the tidal volume may minimise barotrauma;
- risk of aspiration during extubation can be reduced by extubating the obese patient while fully awake and in the sitting position. This facilitates increased tidal volumes as the abdominal contents gravitate away from the diaphragm.

Postoperative phase

- Patients with preoperative hypoxia, those undergoing thoracic or upper abdominal surgery, and those with significant co-morbidity should be nursed in high-care areas in the immediate postoperative period. Supplemental oxygen remains valuable.
- Good pain relief is necessary to avoid postoperative complications, ideally using regional techniques. Nonopioid analgesics have a role in balanced analgesia. Opiates require

careful titration, since overdosage can cause postoperative respiratory depression, while poor pain control can lead to difficulty in chest expansion with resultant atelectasis and respiratory infection. Reduced mobility can cause DVT.

- Nursing in a semi-reclined position helps to unload the diaphragm and improve ventilation and oxygenation.
- Low molecular weight heparin, stockings, and sequential compression devices as prophylaxis against DVT are important. Physiotherapy and early ambulation is helpful.
- The risk of wound infection is high. Meticulous attention to pressure points is essential.

Regional anesthesia/analgesia

- Excessive somnolence and airway obstruction is a risk with opioid analgesia. Regional blockade is a useful option and significantly reduces the risks, although it is technically challenging.
- Standard epidural needles can often be used, since the majority of obese patients have an epidural space less than 8 cm deep [18]. Obese patients have fatty infiltration of epidural space and increased blood volume secondary to increased abdominal pressure. This reduces the potential epidural space, leading to unpredictable spread of local anesthetic solution. Local anesthetic requirements for epidural and spinal are reduced up to 20–25% of normal in the morbidly obese.
- Successful ultrasound-guided nerve blocks in obese patients have been reported [19].

Rhabdomyolysis

This is a well known, potentially fatal complication of bariatric surgery, in particular during prolonged procedures in a large immobile patient [20]. Gluteal muscle necrosis due to pressure from the operating room table can lead to rhabdomyolysis and compartment syndrome. Consequent renal failure may be fatal.

Preventive measures include:

- suitable intraoperative padding,
- meticulous positioning, and
- limiting the duration of the operation.

Routine serial creatine phosphokinase (CPK) measurements with aggressive hydration and diuresis is advised if CPK rises above $5000 \, IU \, l^{-1}$ [21].

The obese obstetric patient

- Increased risk of hypertension, pre-eclampsia, diabetes and exacerbation of asthma.
- Higher incidence of difficult labor/instrumental delivery; increased risk to the fetus.
- Increased risk of failed intubation and aspiration.
- Longer cesarean sections. Complications include wound infection, dehiscence, chest infection and DVT.
- Hypoxemia due to supine position is worsened by intercostal muscle weakness because of the spinal anesthetic.

141

- Precipitous drop in venous return due to aortocaval compression and PEEP during general anesthetic is possible.
- Early siting of an epidural for labor analgesia, under more controlled conditions, gives the option of epidural top-up during an emergency. It has the added advantage of reducing DVT risk. Although not the norm, cesarean section is possible under local anesthetic infiltration. General anesthesia is best avoided whenever possible. The incidence of failed intubation is higher in obese parturients. In anticipated difficult intubation, a rapid sequence induction may be unsafe and an awake fiberoptic intubation must be considered.

Malnutrition (undernutrition)

Malnutrition is defined as "the cellular imbalance between supply of nutrients and energy and the body's demand for them to ensure growth, maintenance, and specific functions". Underweight adults have a BMI < 20 while a BMI < 17 indicates protein energy malnutrition (PEM). It is a marker of poor outcome after surgery.

Epidemiology

Undernutrition is seen in 10–40% of patients admitted to the hospital [22]. In a perioperative context, about 40–60% of patients presenting for major abdominal surgeries are malnourished [23]. The elderly population [24] and the long-term hospitalized patients [25] often remain undiagnosed. In high-risk or critically ill patients, the catabolic process exacerbates and magnifies the patient's nutritional deficiencies.

Etiology and classification

- Primary malnutrition is caused by inadequate dietary intake. More common in the elderly and in developing countries.
- Secondary malnutrition can result from reduced absorption (gastrointestinal diseases) or increased nutritional requirements (sepsis, burns, growth). More common in the developed countries.

Starvation in children

In children, PEM can manifest as kwashiorkor, marasmus or marasmic kwashiorkor.

- Kwashiorkor (edematous PEM) – kwashiorkor results when the diet predominantly has nonprotein calories from starch or sugar and is deficient in total protein and essential amino acids. The abdomen is protruded due to edematous intestine and fatty infiltration of the liver. They often have muscle wasting.
- Marasmus (nonedematous PEM) – marasmus results when there is severe inadequacy of energy and nutrients causing total exhaustion. Unlike kwashiorkor, the abdomen is flat. Intermediate forms are termed marasmic-kwashiorkor.

Adult starvation

Adult patients can withstand up to 40% of weight loss below their ideal body mass, but death is almost certain when BMI < 13.

Obese starvation

Obese persons sometimes go on an unsupervised starvation as a way of dieting with resultant electrolyte, vitamin and mineral deficiencies.

Eating disorders (anorexia nervosa and bulimia nervosa)

Anorexia nervosa is a psychiatric diagnosis characterized by BMI < 17.5, self-induced weight loss and obsessive fear of gaining weight. In bulimia nervosa, weight may be normal because of alternating binge eating with intentional purging resulting in malnutrition.

Micronutrient (vitamins and minerals) disorders

Description of individual nutrient deficiency is beyond the scope of this chapter. Deficiencies in iron, iodine and vitamins A and D are prevalent. Fat-soluble vitamins (A, D, E and K) are stored in significant quantities and their deficiency may not surface clinically for months. Water-soluble vitamins (except B_{12}), on the other hand, have minimal storage and deficiency can manifest in weeks.

Screening for malnutrition

All doctors have a responsibility to identify and manage patients at risk of malnutrition [26]. The Malnutrition Universal Screening Tool (MUST) [27] is a reliable and valid tool for determining the presence of malnutrition. It identifies malnutrition risk by incorporating:

- weight loss in the previous 3–6 months,
- current weight (BMI), and
- predicted future weight.

More detailed assessments are carried out after the patients at risk are identified. Some tools for nutritional assessment are included in an appendix at the end of this chapter.

Nutrition support should be considered in people at risk of malnutrition. The National Institute of Health and Clinical Excellence (NICE) [28] guideline in the UK recommends that nutritional support should be considered in people who are malnourished, as defined by:

- BMI < 18.5,
- unintentional weight loss greater than 10% within the last 3–6 months,
- BMI < 20 and unintentional weight loss greater than 5% within the last 3–6 months.

Clinical implications

Malnourished patients are different by physical, physiological, psychological, and co-existing pathological factors. They also have altered pharmacokinetics.

Outcome

- Low BMI (but not high BMI) is an independent risk factor for increased mortality in ICU [29].
- Outcome is worse in cardiac surgery patients with low BMI [4].

- Cancer patients with low BMI have a worse prognosis (30) – perhaps because they are less able to tolerate chemotherapy.
- Preoperative weight loss is a predictor of poor outcome following colonic surgery [31].

Respiratory system
- Starvation has the effect of decreasing lung elasticity, resulting in decreased pulmonary compliance.
- Respiratory rate may be low.
- In extreme eating disorders, self-induced vomiting can lead to aspiration pneumonia and spontaneous pneumothoraces.
- Malnourished patients have poor cough efforts and hence are more prone for respiratory infections.

Cardiovascular system
- Malnourished patients have a low metabolic rate with resultant hypotension and bradycardia.
- Arrhythmias are common. Electrocardiographic changes include atrioventricular block, prolonged QT, ST depression and T-wave inversion.
- Decreased myocardial and left ventricular function has been demonstrated.

Others
- Gastrointestinal: esophageal strictures, gastric dilatation, hyperamylasemia and fatty liver.
- Renal – reduced glomerular filtration rate, proteinuria, raised blood urea nitrogen and concentrated urine.
- Metabolic – electrolyte imbalances including hypomagnesemia. Hypocalcemia due to vitamin D deficiency.
- Hematological – anemia, leucopenia and thrombocytopenia.
- Decrease in immune function.
- Musculoskeletal – generalized myalgia, osteoporosis, muscle dysfunction is common [32].
- Neurological – alterations in autonomic nervous system, decreased pain sensitivity, neuropathies and generalized weakness.
- Skin – decreased skin turgor and dry mucus membranes predispose to poor wound healing.
- In ICU patients, impaired weaning off ventilatory support.

Pharmacokinetics
- Metabolic pathways are deranged with reductions in albumin and plasma cholinesterase.
- Fat-soluble drug redistribution and excretion is altered along with fluid and electrolyte imbalance, as is the neuromuscular junctional activity and sensitivity to narcotics.
- Hypoalbuminemia results in increased nonprotein-bound active form of the drugs in plasma and results in enhanced potency of many drugs.
- The low metabolic rate can delay drug breakdown and elimination. Consequently, the dose of most anesthetic drugs needs reduction on a weight-for-weight basis and should be carefully titrated against response.

Anesthetic considerations

Preoperative phase

- Preoperative nutritional status has a significant impact on surgical outcome. Nonurgent surgery should be deferred in favor of improving nutritional status. It is recommended that a patient with serum albumin level of 34 g dl^{-1} or less and total lymphocyte count less than 1200 cells μl^{-1} should not be considered for elective major surgeries until nutritional problems are corrected with the appropriate intervention.

- Beware of overzealous correction of the nutritional deficiency in a severely malnourished patient since it carries the risk of "refeeding syndrome" [33]. Refeeding syndrome is characterized by severe electrolyte and fluid shifts associated with metabolic abnormalities in malnourished patients undergoing rapid refeeding by any route [34]. Nutrient and calorie supplementation can provoke undesirable transcellular shifts of electrolytes, with notable risk of hypophosphatemia. The syndrome can present with heart failure, respiratory failure, and derangement of hepatic and renal function, neuropsychiatric events, coma and death.

- The World Health Organization [35] recommends a slow and progressive three-phase refeeding protocol (for enteral and parenteral feeds) to ensure adequate time for normal physiology to be restored, namely:
  - acute resuscitation phase,
  - stabilizing phase,
  - rapid catch-up growth or weight gain phase.

- History and examination findings dictate the preoperative investigations. A full blood count, urea and electrolytes, liver function tests, glucose, calcium, phosphorus, and magnesium level measurements should be carried out before surgery. ECG is useful.

Intraoperative phase

- Loss of subcutaneous fat (compounded by anemia and hypotension) increases susceptibility to pressure necrosis and nerve palsies, necessitating meticulous positioning and padding of pressure points.

- Hypothermia is common and rectal temperatures may fall below 36.3°C preoperatively. Active warming measures are necessary.

- Cardiovascular changes are a major concern, especially in patients with pre-existing hemodynamic compromise. In view of peripheral vasoconstriction, invasive monitoring may be indicated for major surgery.

- Electrolyte abnormalities and neuromuscular comorbidity can alter the sensitivity of the patient to muscle relaxants. NMDR dosages should be carefully titrated, guided by the neuromuscular monitoring.

- Low body fat and hypoalbuminemia alter pharmacokinetics. Doses of most drugs are reduced.

Postoperative phase

- Complications are higher in patients with albumin levels below 34 g dl^{-1}.

- Higher incidence of infections and delayed healing [36].

- Early intervention to correct hypoglycemia, which can be profound [37] due to depleting hepatic glucogen reserves as well as gluconeogenic substrates, is important. Normally in the presence of low serum glucose levels ketone bodies are efficiently oxidized by the brain. However, in the malnourished, marked depletion of fat stores impairs ketogenesis and can cause central nervous system damage.

Appendix

Nutritional metrics

Subjective Global Assessments and Nutritional Risk Index nutrition tests have shown to be predictive for malnutrition and postoperative complications in patients undergoing major abdominal surgery [23].

Subjective Global Assessment (SGA) [38]

A clinical score performed by a trained physician using a standard proforma including food intake and complaints such as vomiting, diarrhea and loss of weight helps classification into three categories: A – well nourished, B – moderately malnourished, C – severely malnourished.

Nutritional Risk Index (NRI) [39]

A simple equation that uses serum albumin and recent weight loss.

$$NRI = (1.489 \times \text{serum albumin g l}^{-1}) + 41.7 \times (\text{present weight/usual weight})$$

NRI > 100 = not malnourished
NRI 97.5–100 = mild malnourishment
NRI 83.5–< 97.5 = moderate malnourishment
NRI < 83.5 = severe malnourishment

Triceps skin-fold thickness (TSF)

Subcutaneous fat is measured with a skin calliper on the posterior upper arm between the acromian process and olecranon process. TSF: 4–8 mm = borderline fat stores; TSF: <3 mm = severe depletion.

Mid-arm circumference (MAC)

Tape is measured midway between the acromian and olecranon process of the non-dominant arm. (MAC < 15 cm in adult = severe muscle mass depletion.)

Mid-arm muscle circumference (MAMC) [40]

MAMC is calculated to estimate muscle mass and lean tissue stores as :

$$MAMC \text{ (cm)} = MAC \text{ (cm)} - (TSF \text{ (mm)} \times 0.3142)$$

Further reading

Choban PS, Flancbaum L. The impact of obesity on surgical outcomes: A review. *J Am Coll Surg* 1997; **185**: 593–603.

Sattar N, Lean M, eds. ABC of obesity. London, BMJ Blackwell, 2007.

Mora RJ. Malnutrition: Organic and functional consequences. *World J Surg* 1999; **23**: 530–5.

References

1. Baker JP, Detsky AS, Wesson DE. Nutritional assessment: A comparison of clinical judgment and objective measurement. *N Engl J Med* 1982; **306**: 969–72.

2. Garrow JS. *Obesity and Related Diseases*. London, Churchill Livingstone, 1988.

3. Sobal J, Stunkard A. Socioeconomic status of obesity: A review of the literature. *Psychol Bull* 1989; **105**: 206–75.

4. Han TS, Sattar N, Lean M. Assessment of obesity and its clinical implications. *BMJ* 2006; **333**: 695–8.

5. Perrotta S, Nilsson F, Brandrup-Wognsen G, *et al.* Body mass index and outcome after coronary artery bypass surgery. *J Cardiovasc Surg* 2007; **48**: 239–45.

6. Brodsky JB, Lemmens HJ, Brock-Utne JG, *et al.* Morbid obesity and tracheal intubation. *Anaesth Analg* 2002; **94**: 732–6.

7. Koenig SM. Pulmonary complications of obesity. *Am J Med Sci* 2001; **321**: 249–79.

8. Brown BR, ed. Anaesthesia and the obese patient. *Contemporary Anaesthesia Practise Series*. Philadelphia, FA Davis, 1982.

9. Bently JB, Borel JD, Vaughan RW, *et al.* Weight, pseudocholinesterase activity and succinylcholine requirement. *Anesthesiology* 1982; **57**: 48–9.

10. Bently JB, Borel JD, Gillespie TJ. Fentanyl pharmacokinetics in obese and non-obese patients. *Anesthesiology* 1981; **55**: A177.

11. Adams JP, Murphy PG. Obesity in anaesthesia and intensive care. *Br J Anaesth* 2000; **85**: 91–108.

12. Crapo RO, Kelly TM, Elliott CG, *et al.* Spirometry as a preoperative screening test in morbidly obese patients. *Surgery* 1986; **99**: 763–8.

13. Shafer H, Ewing S, Hasper E, *et al.* Failure of CPAP therapy in obstructive sleep apnoea syndrome: Predictive factors and treatment with bi-level positive airway pressure. *Resp Med* 1998; **92**: 208–15.

14. Brimacombe JR, Berry AM. Cricoid pressure. *Can J Anaesth* 1997; **44**: 414–17.

15. Sawyer RJ, Richmond MN, Hickey JD, *et al.* Peripheral nerve injuries associated with anaesthesia. *Anaesthesia* 2000; **55**: 980–91.

16. Ezri T, Hazin V, Warters D, *et al.* The endotracheal tube moves more often in obese patients undergoing laparoscopy compared with open abdominal surgery. *Anesth Analg* 2003; **96**: 278–82.

17. Wyner J, Merrell RC. Massive obesity and arterial oxygenation. *Anesth Analg* 1981; **60**: 691–3.

18. Watts RW. The influence of obesity on the relationship between body mass index and the distance to the epidural space from the skin. *Anaesth Intens Care* 1993; **21**: 309–10.

19. Todd N. Ultrasound guided femoral nerve block in an obese patient with a patellar tendon tear and severe obstructive sleep apnea. *Internet J Anesthesiol* 2007; **12** (1).

20. Collier B, Goreja MA, Duke BE. Postoperative rhabdomyolysis with bariatric surgery. *Obes Surg* 2003; **13**: 941–3.

21. Bostanjian D, Anthone GJ, Hamoui N, *et al.* Rhabdomyolysis of gluteal muscles leading to renal failure: A potentially fatal complication of surgery in the morbidly obese. *Obesity Surg* 2003; **13**: 302–05.

22. Elia M, Stroud M. Nutrition in acute care. *Clin Med* 2004; **4**: 405–7.

23. Sungurtekin H, Sungurtekin U, Balci C, *et al.* The influence of nutritional status on complications after major intraabdominal surgery. *J Am Coll Nutr* 2004; **23**: 227–32.

24. McCormack P. Undernutrition in the elderly population living at home in the community: A review of the literature. *J Adv Nurs* 1997; **26**: 856–63.

25. Hoffer LJ. Clinical nutrition: I. Protein-energy malnutrition in the inpatient. *Can Med Assoc J* 2001; **165**: 1345–9.

26. Royal College of Physicians. *Nutrition and Patients: A Doctor's Responsibility*. A report of a working party of the Royal College of Physicians. London, 2002.

27. Malnutrition Advisory Group of the British Association for Parenteral & Enteral Nutrition (BAPEN). *The "MUST" report. Nutritional Screening for Adults: A Multidisciplinary Responsibility*. BAPEN, 2003.

28. National Institute for Health and Clinical Excellence. Nutrition support in adults: Oral nutrition support, enteral tube feeding and parenteral nutrition. UK February 2006. www.nice.org.uk.

29. Tremblay A, Bandi V. Impact of body mass index on outcomes following critical care. *Chest* 2003; **123**: 1202–7.

30. Brown SC, Abraham JS, Walsh S, *et al.* Risk factors and operative mortality in surgery for colorectal cancer. *Ann R Coll Surg Engl* 1991; **73**: 269–72.

31. Andreyev HJ, Norman AR, Oates J, *et al.* Why do patients with weight loss have a worse outcome when undergoing chemotherapy for gastrointestinal

malignancies? *Eur J Cancer* 1998; **34**: 503–9.

32. Norman K, Lochs H, Pirlich M. Muscle dysfunction in malnutrition. *Curr Nutr Food Sci* 2005; **1**: 253–8.

33. Solomon SM, Kirby DF. The refeeding syndrome – A review. *J Parentr Enter Nutr* 1990: **14**: 90–7.

34. Crook MA, Hally V, Panteli JV. The importance of the refeeding syndrome. *Nutrition* 2001; **17**: 632–7.

35. World Health Organization. *Management of the Child with Severe Malnutrition: A Manual for Physicians and Senior Health Care Workers.* Geneva, WHO, 1999.

36. Sullivan DH, Walls RC. The risk of life-threatening complications in a select population of geriatric patients: The impact of nutritional status. *J Am Coll Nutr* 1995; **14**: 29–36.

37. Kurian J, Kaul V. Profound postoperative hypoglycaemia in a malnourished patient. *Can J Anesth* 2001; **48**: 881–3.

38. Detsky AS, McLaughlin JR, Baker JP, *et al.* What is subjective global assessment of nutritional status? *J Parenter Enteral Nutr* 1987; **11**: 8–13.

39. The Veterans Affairs Total Parenteral Nutrition Cooperative Study Group. Perioperative total parenteral nutrition in surgical patients. *N Engl J Med* 1991; **325**: 525–32.

40. Frisancho AR. New norms of upper limb fat and muscle areas for assessment of nutritional status. *Am J Clin Nutr* 1981; **34**: 2540–5.

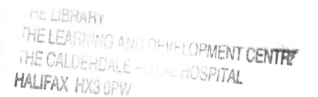

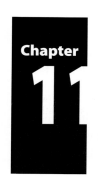

Chapter

1

Smoking, alcohol and recreational drug abuse

G. Evans and I. McConachie

This chapter outlines anesthetic implications of several, unfortunately common, recreational habits (both legal and illegal) which are known to increase anesthetic and perioperative risk.

This chapter can only provide a brief overview of these topics and the reader is encouraged to review the suggestions for Further reading.

Smoking

Oxygen delivery is impaired by carboxyhemoglobin and levels may exceed 10% in smokers. Carbon monoxide (CO) present in smoke reduces the amount of hemoglobin available to carry oxygen and also shifts the oxyhemoglobin dissociation curve to the left. These effects are important factors in exercise-induced angina and ventricular arrhythmias in smokers with coronary artery disease (CAD). Expired CO concentration has been correlated with the frequency of significant ST depression during general anesthesia [1].

Quitting smoking for patients with CAD decreases risk for all cause mortality by about one-third; however, it is estimated that several months are required to realize the full benefit [2].

Current evidence supports the safety of nicotine replacement therapy (NRT) in patients with CAD [3]. In addition, NRT does not affect the patency of bypass grafts. Therefore, the benefit of NRT in patients with CAD outweighs the risks of continuing to smoke.

Respiratory function

- COPD develops in almost 15% of smokers and up to another 50% have chronic bronchitis.
- Smokers produce greater amounts of mucous and clearance is impaired; also, immune function is decreased.
- Structural changes develop with chronic use leading to smooth muscle proliferation and fibrosis.
- Mucociliary clearance shows some improvement with abstinence after 1 week.
- Smokers are at higher risk of perioperative pulmonary complications (PPC), including: respiratory failure, pneumonia, need for post-op respiratory or aerosol therapy, airway events during induction (i.e. cough, laryngospasm), bronchospasm and increased airway secretions. Children exposed to smoke at home are also at increased risk of PPCs.
- Retrospective analysis has determined that the frequency of PPCs in smokers who had CABG and continued to smoke up until surgery was not different than those who quit within 8 weeks of surgery (48% vs. 56%). However, the rate of PPCs was significantly lower in those patients who quit more than 8 weeks prior the surgery (17%) and similar to the rate of PPCs in nonsmokers (11%) [4].

Anesthesia for the High Risk Patient, ed. I. McConachie. Published by Cambridge University Press.
© Cambridge University Press 2009.

- Some studies have suggested an increase in rates of PPC in the first month of abstinence, possibly in relation to increased mucous production; however, evidence is still lacking and most experts would continue to recommend to stop smoking preoperatively even if abstinence is for a period of less than 4 weeks.

- Long-term tobacco smoking increases the risk of postoperative admission to intensive care (in a dose-dependent fashion) with a trend towards increased mortality [5].

- Most perioperative problems due to smoking occur in the postoperative period but airway problems and, in particular, coughing during induction may vary with the anesthetic agent in use. For example, airway problems in smokers have been shown to be much commoner with isoflurane compared to sevoflurane [6].

- Postoperative nausea and vomiting are probably less in smokers compared with non-smokers [7], but this consideration does not outweigh the health benefits of encouraging smokers to quit before surgery.

Wound and bone healing

Bone healing may be impaired in smokers after orthopedic procedures [8]. Smoking cessation preoperatively dramatically decreases the rate of wound-related complications. The duration of cessation to realize this benefit is unknown but it appears to be at least 4 weeks [9].

Helping smokers quit

A primary recommendation from the US Public Health Service Guideline on Tobacco Use and Dependence is to strongly urge all smokers who come in contact with the health care system to quit smoking and aid them in doing so. This recommendation is based on the fact that physician advice to quit smoking increases abstinence rates even if the encounter is only brief, such as that in a preoperative clinic (i.e. < 3 min duration of counseling). However, more intensive and multiple counseling formats will further increase abstinence. The use of medications will approximately double abstinence rates [10]. Gum, inhalers, patches and lozenges are all effective methods to replace nicotine. Bupropion is also approved to promote cessation of smoking.

Many smokers are reluctant to quit smoking preoperatively as cigarettes are used as a stress reliever. However, some recent data demonstrate that smokers do not report greater stress in the perioperative period than nonsmokers, nor do they consistently develop withdrawal symptoms [11].

Alcohol

Ethanol is absorbed from the upper gastrointestinal track and reaches peak levels in blood within 30 min. Hepatic ADH (alcohol dehydrogenase) metabolizes ethanol to acetaldehyde which then is converted to acetate. Acetate is metabolized to acetylcoenzyme A, then eventually to carbon dioxide and water. Thiamine is an essential cofactor in the final step of metabolism and deficiency contributes to build up of metabolites.

Acetaldehyde directly impairs cardiac contractile function, disrupts cardiac excitation–contractile coupling, inhibits myocardial protein synthesis, interferes with phosphorylation and inactivates coenzyme A. ADH is saturated at relatively low blood levels, and this changes elimination from first-order to zero-order kinetics. Oxidative metabolism of ethanol indirectly results in lactate accumulation, ketone formation and impaired gluconeogenesis, secondary to an overall decrease in redox potential.

Table 11.1 Summary of medical problems associated with alcoholism.

Central nervous system	• Psychiatric disorders (depression) • Nutritional disorders (Wernicke–Korsakoff) • Withdrawal syndrome • Cerebellar degeneration • Cerebral atrophy • Peripheral neuropathy
Cardiovascular effects	• Dilated cardiomyopathy • Cardiac dysrhythmias • Systemic hypertension • Autonomic insufficiency
Gastrointestinal and hepatobiliary effects	• Esophagitis • Gastritis • Pancreatitis • Hepatic cirrhosis (portal hypertension leading to varices and hemorrhoids)
Skin and musculoskeletal effects	• Spider angiomas • Myopathy • Osteoporosis
Endocrine and metabolic effects	• Decreased serum testosterone • Decreased gluconeogenesis (hypoglycemia) • Ketoacidosis • Hypoalbuminemia • Hypomagnesemia
Hematologic effects	• Thrombocytopenia • Leukopenia • Anemia

Physical findings associated with long-term alcoholism are parotid enlargement, flushed faces, gynecomastia, cardiomyopathy, hepatomegaly, stigma of cirrhosis, testicular atrophy, palmar erythema, Dupyutren contractures, peripheral neuropathy, nutritional deficiencies and recurrent infections. Table 11.1 summarises medical problems associated with alcoholism.

Toxicity

- Gross motor control and orientation may be significantly affected at $50\,\mathrm{mg\,dl^{-1}}$ ($10.87\,\mathrm{mmol\,l^{-1}}$).
- Classic signs of intoxication include ataxia, dysarthia, mydriasis, and nystagmus.
- Initially, ethanol causes CNS stimulation via disinhibition, but then progresses to loss of protective reflexes, respiratory depression, and coma.

- Facial flushing associated with ethanol-induced vasodilation can lead to hypotension and tachycardia.
- In patients with cardiac disease, this may lead to decreased cardiac output, atrial fibrillation, nonsustained ventricular tachycardia and atrioventricular block.
- Hypoglycemia is generally seen in children, binge drinkers with poor carbohydrate intake, and those who are malnourished.

Withdrawal and its management [12]

Ongoing stimulation of inhibitory gamma-aminobutyric acid (GABA) receptor channel complex by ethanol leads to downregulation of this complex. Withdrawal is associated with a decrease in GABAergic activity and an increase in glutamatergic activity, which results in autonomic excitability and psychomotor agitation. Alcohol withdrawal may begin as early as 6 h after cessation of drinking and is characterized as autonomic hyperactivity including tachycardia, tremor, hypertension and psychomotor agitation.

Approximately 25% of patients with alcohol withdrawal syndrome (AWS) will develop hallucinations – as apposed to delirium tremens (DT), these hallucinations are associated with a clear sensorium. AWS seizures occur in about 10% of patients – 40% of these will be isolated seizures and 3% will develop status epilepticus. Benzodiazepines are the first-line treatment for AWS seizures (note there is no role for phenytoin in treatment or prevention of these seizures), i.e. Diazepam 5–10 mg iv every 5 min titrated to achieve sedation and seizure control.

DT is the most serious complication of AWS and is usually seen between 48 and 96 h after the last consumption of alcohol. They are associated with either a disturbance of consciousness or a change in cognition, or the development of a perceptual disturbance. DTs can last for up to 2 weeks. Initial management of DTs should include IV benzodiazepines for sedation aiming to maintain spontaneous respiration with normal vital signs. Diazepam is generally the first-line drug due to its long half-life – unless the patient has advanced liver disease, in which case, lorazepam may be a better choice due to its lack of active metabolites.

If patients fail to respond to high doses of diazepam, then a second GABAergic drug should be used, such as Phenobarbital or Propofol – these patients will generally require airway management and ICU admission.

All patients should be assessed for dehydration and appropriate volume resuscitation instituted. Nutritional deficiencies are common in chronic alcohol users and all should receive thiamine to prevent the development of Wernicke encephalopathy. Ideally this should be started before dextrose; however, it may be reasonable to co-administer dextrose with thiamine. Magnesium deficiency is common and should be corrected.

Although the mainstay of management of alcohol withdrawal remains the benzodiazepines, carbamazepine and valproic acid have been shown to increase the seizure threshold in alcohol withdrawal. These drugs may therefore be used as adjuncts to benzodiazepines [12]. In addition, the blunting of sympathetic activity by clonidine makes it an agent of potential value in alcohol withdrawal syndromes [13]. It is widely used for this purpose in Europe.

Anesthetic considerations for acute intoxication

- If possible, surgery and anesthesia should be delayed to allow the acute toxic effects to wear off and to allow rehydration and electrolyte corrections.

- If anesthesia is unavoidable, one should consider that there may be decreased MAC, decreased level of consciousness, hypoventilation, full stomach, hypotension, hypothermia, impaired autonomic responses and platelet dysfunction.
- Careful padding and positioning is essential as patients are at increased risk of peripheral nerve palsy.
- Consider Internal Medicine consultation for postoperative management of withdrawal.

Anesthesia for chronic alcohol abusers

- Chronic alcohol abusers may be on a downward spiral towards organ failure and death.
- Anesthesia requirements will vary. Initially there is increased tolerance due to a degree of cross-sensitization and enzyme induction. As the patient's general health fails, the patient may become very sensitive to usual induction doses of anesthesia.
- Nutritional disorders, cardiomyopathy, liver disease and frank cirrhosis may all develop.
- Cholinesterase levels may be reduced, but the clinical significance of this with regard to succinylcholine action is often small.
- The immune system will be impaired leading to increased wound infections.
- Coagulation disturbances will also lead to increased problems with perioperative bleeding.
- In patients with advanced liver disease, acute liver failure may occur postoperatively.
- The alcohol withdrawal syndrome and DT resulting from abstinence during perioperative admission is a significant factor in the increased morbidity seen in chronic alcohol abusers.
- However, as little as one month of preoperative abstinence can reduce postoperative morbidity in alcohol abusers [14]. This is likely due to improving organ function and a reduced surgical stress response.

Cocaine

Coca alkaloid cocaine was isolated and purified in 1860 by a Viennese chemist, Niemann. In South America, cocaine-filled saliva from chewed coca leaves was used as a local anesthetic for skull trephination over 1200 years ago.

In the 1870s, Carl Koller introduced cocaine as a local anesthetic for operative procedures on the eye. Abuse of cocaine entered the mainstream at the end of the nineteenth century and "crack" cocaine was introduced in the 1980s.

Pharmacology and physiology

Cocaine is an alkaloid benzoylmethylecgonine from the leaf of the *Erythroxylon coca* shrub. The hydrochloride salt forms a white crystalline compound, soluble in water, which may be absorbed through nasal mucosa. After being dissolved in ether and extracted via evaporation the "freebase" form is created, which can be inhaled.

"Crack" cocaine is formed after dissolving the hydrochloride salt in water and adding sodium bicarbonate and then heating the substance to a hard rock-like substance.

Cocaine powder is absorbed from the nasal mucosa with a time to onset of 1–3 min, with peak effect in 20 min. Inhalation or injection results in faster onset of only seconds and peak effect in 3–5 min. The half-life of cocaine is 0.5–1.5 h; however, the half-life of active metabolites ranges from 3.5 to 8 h. The fatal dose is 1 g of pure cocaine orally or as little as 10 mg IV.

Local anesthetic effects are via direct blockade of sodium channels and stabilization of axonal membrane. Type IA and IC anti-arrhythmic effects on myocardial cells decrease the rate of depolarization and amplitude of action potentials [15].

Cocaine causes an accumulation of catecholamines by interfering with the uptake of neurotransmitters by presynaptic sympathetic nerve terminals with a secondary effect of release of norepinephrine. This results in increased concentrations of norepinephrine and epinephrine causing vasoconstriction and tachycardia.

Psychostimulant effects are secondary to inhibition of dopamine reuptake into presynaptic neurons, resulting in euphoria and alertness. Other central affects include mydriasis, headache, vomiting and hallucinations.

Between 1 and 5% of cocaine is excreted in the urine unaltered. Thus, cocaine or its metabolites can be identified by immunochemical assay of the urine for up to 24–48 h after ingestion.

Cocaine and ethanol together produce cocaethylene, which has direct cardiac depressant effects.

Cardiac toxicity

- The most frequent complications are coronary ischemia, myocardial infarction, arrythmias and cardiomyopathy. Cocaine use leads to premature atherosclerosis.
- Aspirin should be given to all cocaine users complaining of chest pain. Of those with cocaine-related chest pain, 6% will have enzymatic evidence of myocardial infarction [16].
- Coronary vasoconstriction can produce vasospasm and decreases in vessel caliber by 10% [17].
- Acute toxicity can produce tachy- and bradydysrythmias, prolonged QRS, increased QTc, increased atrioventricular (AV) conduction time and refractory atrial periods.
- People abusing cocaine are at increased risk of ventricular fibrillation and sudden death because of increased sympathetic tone [18].
- Chronic cocaine use may result in myocarditis and left ventricular diastolic dysfunction.

Cerebrovascular toxicity

- Cocaine abuse is associated with generalized tonic–clonic or focal seizures.
- The increasing use of crack cocaine has led to increasing case reports of ischemic and hemorrhagic strokes [19].

Pulmonary toxicity

- As many as 25% of users experience pulmonary complications – most frequently associated with drug inhalation.
- Injury secondary to thermal injury generally involves the tracheobronchial tree.
- Damage to bronchial epithelium can stimulate vagal receptors and result in bronchospasm.
- Valsalva maneuver during inhalation or abrupt cough, resulting in increased intra-alveolar pressure, has been associated with pneumothorax, pneumomediastinum and pneumopericardium [20].

- Cocaine can also act as a hapten or antigen when inhaled, inducing a hypersensitivity pneumonitis (the so-called Crack Lung) – this pneumonitis is characterized by diffuse alveolar and interstitial infiltrates [21].
- Massive hemoptysis occurs secondary to diffuse alveolar hemorrhage. Etiology is likely vasoconstriction-induced anoxia of epithelium and endothelium [20].
- Direct injury to the pulmonary capillary endothelial wall resulting in increased permeability can lead to noncardiogenic pulmonary edema [20].
- Cardiogenic pulmonary edema is seen in the setting of left ventricular dysfunction associated with chronic use or acutely with increased sympathetic tone.

GI toxicity

- The most common serious gastrointestinal complication is mucosal ischemia and perforation.
- The anticholinergic properties of cocaine decrease gastric motility and increased acid exposure promotes ulcer formation [15].
- Infarction or hemorrhage of the spleen has been associated with cocaine abuse [22].

Renal toxicity

- Myocyte injury secondary to ischemia, seizures and direct myocyte injury may manifest as rhabdomyolysis and acute renal failure.
- Thrombosis and renal artery spasm have been described as a mechanism for renal infarction [22].
- Renal scleroderma, Henoch–Schönlien purpura and focal segmental glomerulosclerosis have all been associated with cocaine abuse [23].

Management

- Benzodiazepines appear to be the most effective in decreasing psychomotor agitation, seizures and hyperthermia; high doses may be required, i.e. diazepam titrated up to $1 \, mg \, kg^{-1}$ or more, starting with 5–10 mg and repeated every 3–5 min.
- Pure beta-blockers are contraindicated as they may precipitate unopposed alpha-adrenergic stimulation with catastrophic consequences (i.e. severe hypertension and vasospasm).
- Phentolamine, a pure alpha-adrenergic antagonist, is highly effective in reducing cocaine-induced vasoconstriction – dosage is 1–2.5 mg iv repeated until symptoms resolve or hypotension develops.
- Nitrates such as nitroglycerin or nitroprusside are effective in the treatment of chest pain associated with cocaine use.
- Sodium bicarbonate appears to be effective in treating wide-complex tachycardias [16].
- Lidocaine continues to be a first-line agent in the management of tachy-arrhythmias as per the American Heart Association, despite the concern over shared-type IA profiles of both cocaine and lidocaine.
- Amiodarone has been suggested as a safer choice by some; however, validation in prospective studies is lacking, and others suggest that its beta-blocking effects are of significant concern. Calcium channel blocking drugs have been shown in animal studies to enhance the occurrence of seizures [24].

Anesthesia considerations

- Potentiation of neuromuscular blockade has been demonstrated in patients receiving succinylcholine and cocaine [25]. This does not contraindicate its use in these patients, but caution should be used due to this possible interaction.

- Cocaine-intoxicated patients will require an increase in MAC and may experience severe hypertension with larnygoscopy.

- Increased risk of cardiac arrhythmias, such as ventricular tachycardia, frequent PVCs or torsades de pointes with use of potent volatile anesthetics (especially Halothane which should be avoided) [26].

- There may be concern over regional techniques if thrombocytopenia is present. One should consider requesting a platelet count in all prior to surgery.

- Treat intoxicated patients as full stomach.

- General anesthesia is considered by many to be safe [27] in nontoxic patients who present for elective surgery and have positive screen for metabolites in their urine (i.e. normal arterial pressure, normal heart rate, normothermic, a normal ECG including a QTc interval <500 ms), others would suggest that a one-week drug-free period is required before elective surgery [28].

- One should avoid using ketamine due to its sympathomimetic properties. Etomidate should be used with caution because of the risk of myoclonus, seizures and hyperreflexia. Thus induction of general anesthesia with propofol or thiopental is considered most appropriate by most authors.

- Patients may demonstrate hypotension unresponsive to ephedrine (in chronic users). Hypotension appears to respond well to low doses of phenylephrine.

Chronic abuse of opiates

History
Evidence of use in 1500 BC in the Ebers Papyrus' description of a poppy derivative used to soothe crying children. Morphine was later purified by a German pharmacologist in 1804. Heroin (diamorphine) was introduced in 1898 by Bayer and Company – initially used as an antitussive! The abusive properties of opiates led to the Harrison Narcotic Control Act of 1914 in the US. This restricted the sale of narcotics and led to a ban on heroin sale in 1924.

Pharmacology and pathophysiology

Opium is derived from the seedpod of the poppy plant *Somniferum*. Alkaloids derived directly from opium are referred to as opiates, i.e. morphine and codeine. Chemical alteration of these alkaloids is used to create semi-synthetic opioids such as heroin, naloxone and oxycodone. Methadone and fentanyl are examples of synthetic opioids.

Heroin

Due to its high lipid solubility, heroin is rapidly absorbed and crosses the blood brain barrier within 20 s. This rapid absorption contributes to its euphoric effect. In the central nervous system, heroin is locally hydrolyzed to the active metabolites monoacetylmorphine and morphine within 30 min. Heroin is more appropriately known as diamorphine and is still widely used as a narcotic analgesic in the UK.

Opiate toxicity

- Classic "toxidrome" consists of miosis, hypoventilation, lethargy and ileus.
- Chemoreceptor sensitivity to hypercarbia and hypoxia are decreased, resulting in decreased ventilatory drive.
- Alveolar ventilation is decreased secondary to decreased respiratory rate and tidal volume.
- Heroin has been reported to cause noncardiogenic pulmonary edema as far back as 1880 by Osler. Other similar reports have been described for virtually all opiates, although the etiology remains unclear.
- Heroin may stimulate status asthmaticus when inhaled. The likely mechanism is opiate-induced bronchial constriction compounded by histamine release; these attacks are often poorly or unresponsive to bronchodilators [29].
- Hypotension with opiates is secondary to arteriolar and venous dilation; this response is mediated by histamine release and increased vagal activity.
- Methadone can prolong QT interval and predispose the patient to torsades de pointes.
- Meperidine (pethidine in some countries), propoxyphene and tramadol may all be associated with decreased seizure threshold.
- Meperidine is metabolized to normeperidine and accumulation especially in patients with renal failure can cause delirium, tremors and seizures [30].

Naloxone

Acts as an antagonist at all opioid receptors. Naloxone's safety profile in opiate naïve patients has been well established. However, there is a small increase in the incidence of severe complications in opioid-dependent patients. These complications have been reported in approximately 2% of heroin users and include asystole, seizures, pulmonary edema and acute withdrawal [31]. Therefore, the initial dose in intoxication should be small and titrated to effect, e.g. starting with 0.04–0.05 mg IV.

Anesthesia considerations in the opioid-abusing patient

- Associated infections if IV user (i.e. HIV, hepatitis, syphilis, endocarditis).
- Potential difficult IV access.
- Co-ingestions of other agents of abuse.
- Full stomach, decreased LOC, respiratory depression.
- Potential for opiate "withdrawal".
- Exaggerated postoperative pain.
- Need for larger doses of intraoperative and postoperative opiates. It is suggested that regular base opiate requirements should be continued both preoperatively and post-operatively [32].

157

Cannabinoids

The earliest use of marijuana was in the fourth century in China, reaching Europe in 500 AD. Marijuana is the most commonly used illicit drug in North America. In fact, at least 40% of the population over the age of 12 has used the drug at least once.

Pharmacology and pathophysiology

Tetrahydrocannabinol (THC) binds to two specific cannabinoid-binding receptors, CB1 located throughout the brain and CB2 receptors located in immune system tissues (splenic macrophages), peripheral nerve terminals and the vas deferens. Binding at both receptors inhibits adenylyl cyclase and stimulates potassium channel conductance [33].

Between 10 and 35% of smoke containing THC is absorbed and peak plasma concentration occurs on average in 8 min with the onset of psychoactive effects within minutes. Ingestion of THC results in an unpredictable onset of psychoactive effects ranging from 1 to 3 h.

THC is nearly completely metabolized in the liver by hepatic microsomal hydroxylation and oxidation via the P450 (CPY) system. Metabolites can be detected in the urine several days after use (THC-COOH average excretion half-life 2–3 days, range 0.9–9.8 days). Thus, in chronic users, detection may remain possible for up to several weeks.

Clinical effects

- Psychological effects are variable, but most commonly involve relaxation, giddiness or laughter and increased appetite.
- Toxicity leads to decreased coordination, muscle strength, hand steadiness, lethargy, sedation, postural hypotension, inability to concentrate, slurred speech, and slow reaction times.
- Users may also experience distrust, dysphoria, fear or panic, and transient psychotic episodes.
- Common cardiovascular changes are increases in heart rate (mean baseline increase from 66 to 89 min^{-1}) and decreased vascular resistance (these changes last for 2–3 h). Repeated ingestion may, however, result in decreased heart rate and blood pressure [34].
- Inhalation or ingestion produces decreased airway resistance and increased airway conductance in both normal patients and asthmatics.
- Ocular effects include conjunctival injection and decreased intraocular pressure.

Management and anesthesia considerations

- Agitation, anxiety and transient psychotic episodes may be treated with benzodiazepines or antipsychotics.
- There are no specific antidotes.
- Co-ingestions or other illicit drug use should be identified so their effects can also be anticipated.
- It may be prudent to consider recent users as having a full stomach.
- If low or moderate doses of the drug have been consumed, an increase in sympathetic activity occurs, parasympathetic activity is reduced, and tachycardia with increased cardiac output is observed. Therefore, drugs that increase heart rate further should be avoided, e.g. ketamine, pancuronium, atropine and epinephrine [26].

- High doses result in inhibition of sympathetic activity but not parasympathetic activity, and this leads to hypotension and bradycardia; this may cause profound myocardial depression with induction and initiation of potent inhalational agents.

- Increased incidence of life-threatening arrhythmias has not been reported; however, an increase in ectopic activity (supraventricular or ventricular), ST-segment and T-wave changes can occur [35].

- Upper airway irritability may be increased and reports of oropharyngitis, acute upper airway edema and obstruction have been reported in these patients undergoing general anesthesia [26].

- Cannabinnoids are used in some countries as adjuncts for management of chronic pain.

Amphetamines

The first amphetamine was synthesized by Edeleano in 1887 and rediscovered in the 1920s when there was concern over the shortage of ephedrine for asthma treatment. Amphetamine abuse was recognized as early as 1936 with "designer" amphetamines surfacing in the 1980s with the most well-known examples being MDMA (methylenedioxymethamphetamine or "ecstasy") and MDEA (3,4-methylenedioxyethamphetamine). Amphetamines have been used to treat narcolepsy as far back as 1935.

Pharmacology

The primary mechanism of action of amphetamines is release of catecholamines from presynaptic terminals (particularly norepinephrine and dopamine). Binding affinity for select neurotransmitters largely determines pharmacological effects, i.e. MDMA has high affinity for serotonin transporters, resulting in primarily serotonergic effects [36]. Higher levels of norepinephrine at the locus ceruleus in the brain results in increased alertness, anorectic and locomotor stimulation. Increased levels of dopamine in the CNS mediates the stereotypical compulsive repetitive behaviors displayed by users. The effects of serotonin and dopamine on the mesolimbic system are responsible for altering perception and causing psychotic behavior.

As amphetamines are relatively lipophilic they cross the blood–brain barrier readily. Elimination is via multiple pathways, including hepatic transformation and renal excretion.

Toxicity

- Clinical effects are similar to cocaine; however, duration of effects tends to be longer (up to 24 h).

- Amphetamines are, however, less likely to result in seizures, dysrhythmias, and myocardial ischemia than cocaine [37].

- Psychosis is more common.

- Patients who present to hospital are often anxious, volatile, aggressive, have visual and tactile hallucinations and may progress to life-threatening agitation.

- Sympathetic findings include mydriasis, diaphoresis, hyperthermia, tachycardia, hypertension, vasospasm; severe complications include myocardial infarction, aortic dissection, ischemic colitis, acute lung injury and intracranial hemorrhage. Ecstasy use may present with hyperthermia as a predominant feature. Deaths from ecstasy may be idiosyncratic with fatal reactions claimed to occur on first use. Severe dehydration is also a feature in some reports.

- High levels of muscular activity and hyperthermia may result in metabolic acidosis, rhabdomyolysis, acute renal failure (ATN) and coagulopathy; multi-organ failure may then follow. Necrotizing vasculitis has also been associated with amphetamine use.
- Cardiomyopathy has been described as a complication of acute and chronic use.
- Death is most commonly secondary to hyperthermia, dysrhythmias and intracerebral hemorrhage.
- Chronic use of MDMA in animals has been reported to produce irreversible destruction of neurons effected by dopamine and serotonin transporters (possibly by generation of toxic oxygen free radicals).
- Co-ingestion of other agents of abuse should also be considered.

Management and anesthesia considerations

- Hyperthermia requires interventions to achieve cooling. Dantrolene anecdotally has been used in ecstasy poisoning [38].
- Restraints may be required for agitated patients in order to protect from self-harm or harm to staff.
- Sedation with benzodiazepines or other medication should be instituted early to decrease heat generation and rhabdomyolysis with rapid titration until the patient is calm (antipsychotics such as haloperidol are recommended to treat delirium).
- One may consider intubation and muscle relaxation in severe cases.
- Blood and urine investigations for co-ingestion agents, glucose, BUN, CK, coagulation screen and electrolytes should be sent.
- Patients may be significantly dehydrated and hyponatremia should be considered due to an increase in ADH secretion [39].
- Urine output should be maintained at $1-2\,\mathrm{ml\,kg^{-1}\,h^{-1}}$.
- Patients with acute renal failure may require urgent hemodialysis secondary to hyperkalemia and acidosis.
- Full stomach considerations if surgery are required.
- With general anesthesia, the risk of autonomic dysregulation is high – this may result in wide swings in blood pressure and tachycardia [26].
- Extreme caution should be used with administration of drugs such as ephedrine and ketamine, as these patients will exhibit exaggerated responses [26].
- In patients with a history of MDMA-induced hyperthermia, succinylcholine should not be used and avoidance of potent volatile agents should be considered [26].
- In MDMA users, drugs metabolized by the liver and eliminated by the kidneys will have prolonged effect (possibly secondary to fatty infiltration of the liver and acute renal failure).
- Chronic methamphetamine users have decreased anesthetic requirements if not intoxicated (due to decreased levels of catecholamines in the CNS).

Further reading

Cheng DC. The drug addicted patient. *Can J Anaesth* 1997; **44**: R101–11.

Hall AP, Henry JA. Illicit drugs and surgery. *Int J Surg* 2007; **5**: 365–70.

Kumar RN, Chambers WA, Pertwee RG. Pharmacological actions and therapeutic uses of cannabis and cannabinoids. *Anaesthesia* 2001; **56**: 1059–68.

Quasim S, Coleman JJ. Drugs of abuse – A review. *CPD Anaesth* 2007; **9**: 30–7.

Tonnesen H, Kehlet H. Preoperative alcoholism and postoperative morbidity. *Br J Surg* 1999; **86**: 869–74.

Warner DO. Perioperative abstinence from cigarettes: Physiologic and clinical consequences. *Anesthesiology* 2006; **104**: 356–67.

References

1. Woehlck HJ, Connolly LA, Cinquegrani MP, *et al*. Acute smoking increases ST depression in humans during general anaesthesia. *Anesth Analg* 1999; **89**: 856–60.

2. Lightwood JM, Glantz SA. Short-term economic and health benefits of smoking cessation: Myocardial infarction and stroke. *Circulation* 1997; **96**: 1086–97.

3. Benowitz NL, Gourlay SG. Cardiovascular toxicity of nicotine: Implications for nicotine replacement therapy. *J Am Coll Cardiol* 1997; **29**: 1422–31.

4. Warner MA, Divertie MB, Tinker JH. Preoperative cessation of smoking and pulmonary complications in coronary artery bypass patients. *Anesthesiology* 1984; **60**: 380–3.

5. Møller AM, Pedersen T, Villebro N, *et al*. A study of the impact of long-term tobacco smoking on postoperative intensive care admission. *Anaesthesia* 2003; **58**: 55–9.

6. Wild MR, Gornall CB, Griffiths DE. Maintenance of anaesthesia with sevoflurane or isoflurane effects on adverse airway events in smokers. *Anaesthesia* 2004; **59**: 891–3.

7. Chimbira W, Sweeney BP. The effect of smoking on postoperative nausea and vomiting. *Anaesthesia* 2000; **55**: 540–4.

8. Kwiatkowski TC, Hanley EN Jr, Ramp WK. Cigarette smoking and its orthopedic consequences. *Am J Orthop* 1996; **25**: 590–7.

9. Sorensen LT, Karlsmark T, Gottrup F. Abstinence from smoking reduces incisional wound infection. A randomized controlled trial. *Ann Surgery* 2003; **238**: 1–5.

10. Warner DO. Helping surgical patients quit smoking: Why, when and how. *Anesth Analg* 2005; **101**: 481–7.

11. Warner DO, Patten CA, Ames SC, *et al*. Smoking behavior and perceived stress in cigarette smokers undergoing elective surgery. *Anesthesiology* 2004; **100**: 1125–7.

12. Mayo-Smith MF. Pharmacological management of alcohol withdrawal. A meta-analysis and evidence-based practice guideline. American Society of Addiction Medicine Working Group on Pharmacological Management of Alcohol Withdrawal. *JAMA* 1997; **278**: 144–51.

13. Dobrydnjov I, Axelsson K, Berggren L, *et al*. Intrathecal and oral clonidine as prophylaxis for postoperative alcohol withdrawal syndrome: A randomized double-blinded study. *Anesth Analg* 2004; **98**: 738–44.

14. Tonnesen H, Rosenberg J, Nielsen HJ, *et al*. Effect of preoperative abstinence on poor postoperative outcome in alcohol misusers: Randomised controlled trial. *BMJ* 1999; **318**: 1311–16.

15. Boghdadi MS, Henning RJ. Cocaine: Pathophysiology and clinical toxicology. *Heart Lung* 1997; **26**: 466–83.

16. Lange RA, Hillis LD. Cardiovascular complications of cocaine use. *N Engl J Med* 2001; **345**: 351–8.

17. Karch SB. Cocaine cardiovascular toxicity. *South Med J* 2005; **98**: 794–9.

18. Frishman WH, Del Vecchio A, Sanal S, *et al*. Cardiovascular manifestations of substance

abuse part 1: Cocaine. *Heart Dis* 2003; **5**: 187–201.

19. Daras M. Neurologic complications of cocaine. *NIDA Res Monogr* 1996; **163**: 43–65.

20. Haim DY, Lippmann ML, Goldberg SK, *et al.* The pulmonary complications of crack cocaine. A comprehensive review. *Chest* 1995; **107**: 233–40.

21. Laposata EA, Mayo GL. A review of pulmonary pathology and mechanisms associated with inhalation of freebase cocaine ("crack"). *Am J Forensic Med Pathol* 1993; **14**: 1–9.

22. Shanti CM, Lucas CE. Cocaine and the critical care challenge. *Crit Care Med* 2003; **31**: 1851–9.

23. Crowe AV, Howse M, Bell GM, *et al.* Substance abuse and the kidney. *Quant J Med* 2000; **93**: 147–52.

24. Derlet RW, Albertson TE. Potentiation of cocaine toxicity with calcium channel blockers. *Am J Emerg Med* 1989; **7**: 464–8.

25. Jatlow P, Barash PG, Van Dyke C, *et al.* Cocaine and succinylcholine sensitivity: A new caution. *Anesth Analg* 1979; **58**: 235–8.

26. Hernandez M, Birnbach DJ, Van Zundert AA. Anaesthetic management of the illicit-substance-using patient. *Curr Opin Anaesthesiol* 2005; **18**: 315–24.

27. Hill GE, Ogunnaike BO, Johnson ER. General anaesthesia for the cocaine abusing patient. Is it safe? *Br J Anaesthesia* 2006; **97**: 654–7.

28. Vagts DA, Boklage C, Galli C. Intraoperative ventricular fibrillation in a patient with chronic cocaine abuse – A case report. *Anaesthesiol Reanim* 2004; **29**: 19–24.

29. Cygan J, Trunsky M, Corbridge T. Inhaled heroin-induced status asthmaticus: Five cases and review of the literature. *Chest* 2000; **117**: 272–5.

30. Stone PA, Macintyre PE, Jarvis DA. Norpethidine toxicity and patient controlled analgesia. *Br J Anaesth* 1993; **71**: 738–40.

31. Osterwalder JJ. Naloxone – for intoxications with intravenous heroin and heroin mixtures – harmless or hazardous? A prospective clinical study. *J Toxicol Clin Toxicol* 1996; **34**: 409–16.

32. Balasubramanian S, Hadi I. Perioperative pain management in patients with chronic pain. *CPD Anaesthesia* 2006; **8**: 109–13.

33. Onaivi ES, Leonard CM, Ishiguro H, *et al.* Endocannabinoids and cannabinoid receptor genetics. *Prog Neurobiol* 2002; **66**: 307–44.

34. Benowitz NL, Jones RT. Cardiovascular effects of prolonged delta-9-tetrahydrocannabinol ingestion. *Clin Pharmacol Ther* 1975; **18**: 278–97.

35. Kuckowski KM. Marijuana in pregnancy. *Ann Acad Med Singapore* 2004; **33**: 336–9.

36. Green AR, Mechan AO, Elliott JM, *et al.* The pharmacology and clinical pharmacology of 3,4-methylenedioxymethamphetamine (MDMA, "ecstasy"). *Pharmacol Rev* 2003; **55**: 463–508.

37. Zagnoni PG, Albano CZ. Psychostimulants and epilepsy. *Epilepsia* 2002; **43** (Suppl 2): 28–31.

38. Watson JD, Ferguson C, Hinds CJ, *et al.* Exertional heat stroke induced by amphetamine analogues. Does dantrolene have a place? *Anaesthesia* 1993; **48**: 1057–60.

39. Wolff K, Tsapakis EM, Winstock AR, *et al.* Vasopressin and oxytocin secretion in response to the consumption of ecstasy in a clubbing population. *J Psychopharmacol* 2006; **20**: 400–10.

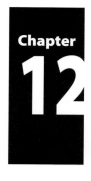

Chapter 12

Identification of the deteriorating patient in the perioperative period

P. Dean, J. Cupitt and I. McConachie

The problem

Today's surgical wards operate with a high throughput of cases of increasing complexity and in patients with multiple co-morbidities. In addition many institutions face problems with:

- inadequate funding;
- staff recruitment problems;
- less senior, experienced staff (both medical and nursing) on the floor;
- less continuity of medical care due to the introduction of shift systems; and
- inability of junior staff to recognize a deteriorating patient and/or seek senior help.

There is a consistent body of evidence which shows that patients who become, or who are at risk of becoming, acutely unwell on general hospital wards receive inadequate care [1–3].

- In the UK, the National Confidential Enquiry into Patient Outcome and Death (NCEPOD) identified the prime causes of this as being both delayed recognition and the institution of inappropriate therapy that subsequently culminated in a late referral to critical care [3].
- Admission to an intensive care unit (ICU) was thought to have been avoidable in 21% of cases, and suboptimal care contributed to about a third of the deaths that occurred.

The potential for deterioration is perhaps much higher than in the past. Perhaps the most valuable indicator is a high index of clinical suspicion. A careful consideration of the progress of each patient and a review of their vital signs charts should reveal those patients who are failing to progress. However, those of us involved in caring for patients after admission to ICU realize that, only too often, deteriorating vital signs have been diligently charted without either recognition of their significance or appropriate intervention. While there remains a place for clinical acumen, there is an essential need for more comprehensive observations and objective assessments.

Possible solutions

- Increased funding and more staff.
- More high care beds in the hospital.
- Education of staff.
- Shared care, staff rotations and skill sharing.

Anesthesia for the High Risk Patient, ed. I. McConachie. Published by Cambridge University Press.
© Cambridge University Press 2009.

- Early recognition and intervention of deteriorating patients.
- Medical emergency and/or critical care outreach teams.

This chapter will address the last two possible solutions.

The role of the anesthetist

Prior to surgery, the opportunity exists to recognize the at-risk patient. Preoperative assessment and early recognition of those patients who are likely to deteriorate through their own co-morbidities or through the complexity of the surgical procedure is vital. This enables appropriate investigations and risk stratification to be carried out, and improves awareness of those caring for the sick patient.

Anesthetists are acutely aware of patients who deteriorate on the operating table during surgical procedures. It is vital that this information is assimilated during the procedure and attempts made to remedy the problem. Such information should be conveyed to receiving ward staff, either in critical care units or general wards, as intraoperative events can have a significant impact on a patient's postoperative course. Unanticipated events, e.g. more complex surgery of longer duration, prolonged aortic cross-clamp times, uncontrolled bleeding, emergency splenectomy, fat emboli, damage to surrounding structures, can influence outcome. They need to be recognized, communicated and their implications monitored in the postoperative period.

Patient factors during surgery can also suggest those who are likely to develop postoperative complications, e.g.:

- increasing oxygen requirements,
- increasing ventilator pressures,
- failure to respond to fluids,
- vasopressor support,
- difficult temperature control with subsequent hypothermia,
- acidemia and/or increasing lactate levels,
- poor intraoperative urine output,
- poor glycemic control,
- ST segment or T wave changes on the ECG,
- the use of blood products in the intraoperative period.

Identification of deterioration

Clinical deterioration can occur at any stage of a patient's illness. However, there are certain periods when patients are at their most vulnerable:

- the onset of their illness,
- during surgical intervention,
- discharge from critical care.

The postoperative period is when close observation and monitoring are crucial in order to detect deterioration. Physiological systems are subjected to significant challenges:

- oxygen supply and demand imbalances,
- fluid and electrolyte shifts,
- pain and anxiety,
- gastrointestinal ileus,
- catabolism,
- energy supply and demand imbalance,
- infection and sepsis.

Patients who fail to meet expected goals must be identified and treatment instigated in order to prevent further decline. There are many subtle warning signs which suggest impending problems and these parallel many of those found intraoperatively (see patient factors above).

Beyond these subtle, often nonspecific signs, changes in physiological observations made by healthcare staff may enable those inexperienced in the identification of the critically ill to recognize the at-risk patient. It is well established that abnormal physiology is associated with adverse clinical outcomes.

- A multi-center, prospective, observational study found that the majority (60%) of primary events (deaths, cardiac arrests and unplanned ICU admissions) were preceded by documented abnormal physiology, the most common being hypotension and a fall in Glasgow coma score [4].
- In the UK NCEPOD report of 2007, the majority (66%) of inpatients who had been in hospital for more than 24 h before ICU admission exhibited physiological instability for more than 12 h [5].
- Mortality has been shown to increase with the number of abnormal physiological parameters ($p < 0.001$), being 0.7% with no abnormalities, 4.4% with one, 9.2% with two and 21.3% with three or more [6].
- Delays in ICU referral and admission and length of stay in hospital prior to ICU admission have been shown to be factors in poor outcome [6]. This implies that early diagnosis, referral and intervention may improve outcome.

Once recognition of critical illness has occurred, contact with appropriately skilled personnel can follow. This is the basis on which early warning scoring systems have been developed. It is important to note that these systems should be used in conjunction with clinical expertise and not as a replacement for it.

Physiological track and trigger systems

There are essentially three different types of systems, commonly referred to as physiological track and trigger systems (Table 12.1).

Physiological track and trigger systems rely on periodic observation of selected basic physiological signs ("tracking") with predetermined calling or response criteria ("trigger") for requesting the attendance of staff who have specific expertise in the management of acute illness and/or critical care. These systems allow a large number of patients to be monitored, and effectively screened, for deterioration without a large increase in workload. A number of systems have been developed internationally.

Table 12.1 Comparison of physiological track and trigger systems.

Track and Trigger System	Advantages	Disadvantages
Single parameter (Medical Emergency Team or MET calling criteria)	• Simple system with better reproducibility • Does not allow a patient's progress to be tracked	• Does not allow a graded response strategy • Current evidence suggests that the system has low sensitivity, low positive predictive value but high specificity. This could potentially cause increased triggers that are not related to an adverse event • Not widely adopted in UK hospitals
Multiple parameter (Patient at Risk Team or PART)	• Allows for a graded response strategy • Widely used in UK hospitals	• May lack reproducibility and reliability because systems are prone to human calculation errors • These systems have high sensitivity but low specificity when one abnormal observation is present, but sensitivity reduces and specificity increases as the number of abnormal variables increase
Aggregate scoring system (Early Warning Score or EWS)	• Simple to use • Allows monitoring of clinical progress • Allows for a graded response strategy • Widely used in UK hospitals	• May lack reproducibility and reliability because systems are prone to human calculation errors • A range of sensitivities and specificities depending on the cut-off score used, but it is possible to achieve high sensitivity and specificity at defined cut-off point

- The appropriate response pathway in the UK is initially via the ward medical staff and then the critical care outreach service.
- In Australia it may be via a Medical Emergency Team (MET). Much of the available studies on outreach come from Australia.
- In the USA, Rapid Response Teams are a key component of the Institute for Healthcare Improvement 100 000 Lives Campaign [7]. The International Partnership for Acute Care Safety initiative, endorsed by the World Health Organization, is shortly to commence a global study to investigate antecedents to cardiac arrest, death and emergency intensive care admission.
- Whilst much of the available evidence comes from the UK and Australia, there are also teams emerging in other parts of Europe.
- Critical Care Outreach is also developing in Canada [8].

Early warning scores

In the UK, predominately aggregate scoring systems have been developed. The original, basic Early Warning Score (EWS) was developed at the James Paget Hospital in Norfolk [9]

Table 12.2 Basic Early Warning Score [11].

Early Warning Score							
Score	3	2	1	0	1	2	3
HR		<40	41–50	51–100	101–110	111–130	130
BP	<70	71–80	81–100	101–199			
RR		<8		9–14	15–20	21–29	>30
Temp		<35	35.1–36.5		36.6–37.4	>37.5	
CNS				A	V	P	U

A = alert; V = response to voice; P = response to pain; U = unresponsive

Table 12.3 Modified Early Warning Score [12].

MEWS scoring table								
Score	3	2	1	0	1	2	3
RR		<8		9–14	15–20	21–29	>30
HR		<40	41–50	51–100	101–110	111–130	>130
BP (%)	<45	<30	<15	Normal for patient	>15	>30	>45
CNS				A	V	P	U
TEMP		<35		35–38.4		>38.4	
URINE		<0.5 ml kg^{-1} h^{-1}			>3 ml kg^{-1} h^{-1}		

(see Table 12.2) and other hospitals have taken the template idea and modified it for local use. The Modified Early Warning System (MEWS) is probably the most widely adopted variant in the UK [10] (see Table 12.3).

In 2007, the Worthing Physiological Scoring System (PSS) (see Table 12.4) was introduced following a derivation and validation study in a medical assessment unit.

- It utilizes physiological variables which are considered to be important predictors of hospital mortality.
- Multi-variate logistic regression analysis was used to identify the value of these physiological variables at which mortality is increased.
- Using this modeling technique, they have shown that this system performs better than the existing aggregate scoring systems [11].

Aggregated weighted scoring systems score every parameter of a set of bedside observations and add the scores to give a final figure. The more abnormal a single parameter, the higher the weighting and therefore the higher the aggregate score. If the score reaches a predetermined value, nursing staff trigger the appropriate response. The assistance requested is proportional to the severity of the score; low scores require a junior doctor response, higher scores require a more senior review or referral to critical care outreach services.

Table 12.4 Worthing Physiological Scoring System [13].

The Worthing PSS				
Score	0	1	2	3
RR	<19	20–21	>22	
HR	<101	>102		
Systolic BP	>100		<99	
TEMP	>35.5			<35.3
SpO2 on air	96–100	94–<96	92–<94	<92
AVPU	ALERT			OTHER

Table 12.5 The Medical Emergency Team [13].

MET primary calling criteria
Airway Respiratory distress Threatened airway
Breathing RR > 30 min^{-1} RR< 6 min^{-1} SaO$_2$< 90% on oxygen Difficulty speaking
Circulation Blood pressure < 90 mmHg despite treatment HR > 130 min^{-1}
Neurology Any unexpected decrease in consciousness Agitation or delirium Repeated or prolonged seizures
Other Concern about patient Uncontrolled pain Failure to respond to treatment Unable to obtain prompt assistance

The calling criteria for both Medical Emergency Teams (MET) and Patient At Risk Teams (PART) use single-parameter systems – the presence of one or more criteria triggering a response in the form of a specific team rather than the graded response associated with the EWS.

Medical Emergency Team

The concept of the MET was introduced by Lee *et al.* in 1995 [12]. The aim of the team was to provide assistance in the peri-arrest situation. The team could be triggered by a patient meeting set criteria (see Table 12.5) or simply a patient causing concern. The team would consist of nursing and medical staff with appropriate resuscitation skills.

Table 12.6 Patient At Risk Team [14].

PART primary calling criteria
Any 3 or more of:
RR > 25 or < 10 breaths per minute
Arterial systolic pressure < 90 mmHg HR > 130 min^{-1}
NOT fully orientated and alert
Oxygen saturation < 90%
Urine output < 100 ml over 4 h
Or a patient who is not fully orientated and RR > 35 breaths per min OR HR > 140 min^{-1}
PART can also be called if the above criteria pertain and a prompt response cannot be secured from the parent team or if the patient fails to respond to primary management by the parent team. The PART can also be called by any doctor of registrar grade or above in relation to any patient who is seriously ill and causing concern

Patient at Risk Team

PART consists of a critical care consultant, senior nurse and duty surgical or medical registrar. Their aim is to recognize deteriorating patients at an earlier stage and prevent or expedite admission to level 2 or 3 critical care beds. Whilst the PART criteria (Table 12.6) would trigger an initial assessment by the patient's surgical doctors, if this failed to improve the patient's condition the team would be alerted. The PART concept also allows for direct referral from registrar (senior resident level or above) [13].

In July 2007, the UK National Institute for Health and Clinical Excellence published a document entitled "Acutely ill patients in hospital – recognition of and response to acute illness in adults in hospital" [5]. They concluded that patients who are, or become, acutely unwell in hospital may receive suboptimal care. This may be because their deterioration is not recognized, is not appreciated, or not acted upon sufficiently rapidly. In an extensive literature review, they make a number of conclusions regarding physiological track and trigger systems.

- Physiological track and trigger systems, as currently used in the NHS in England and Wales, have low sensitivity and positive predictive values but high specificity and negative predictive values. The low sensitivity can be improved by reducing the trigger threshold.

- Single-parameter systems, as used by MET systems, have low sensitivity, low positive predictive values but high specificity.

- Multiple-parameter systems require the presence of one or more abnormal physiological variables. These systems have comparatively high sensitivity but relatively low specificity when one abnormal observation is present (that is, at low scores). Sensitivity reduces and specificity increases as the number of abnormal variables increase.

- Aggregate weighted scoring systems demonstrate a range of sensitivities and specificities depending on the cut-off score used. It is possible to achieve high sensitivity and specificity at defined cut-off scores.

Table 12.7   Parameters for aggregate scoring systems [8].

Multiparameter or aggregated weighted scoring systems used for physiological track and trigger
 should measure:
Heart rate
Respiratory rate
Systolic BP
Conscious level
Oxygen saturation
Temperature

In specific circumstances, measure additional parameters such as:
Hourly urine output
Biochemical analyses, lactate, blood glucose, base deficit, arterial pH
Pain assessment

The guidance recommends that multiple-parameter or aggregate scoring systems should use a minimum data set of observations with additional parameters being considered under specific circumstances (Table 12.7).

These recommendations raise a number of issues.

- Do track and trigger systems work?
- Why do they have such low statistical values?
- Should they continue to be introduced into clinical practice worldwide?
- Are they fit for purpose?
- Intuitively, physiological tract and trigger systems should work, but they are only able to predict with variable sensitivity and specificity those patients who are likely to deteriorate.

Evaluation of outreach systems

- The available track and trigger scores were not designed to predict outcome but to alert staff to potential problems in individual patients.
- In those studies which purport to show improved outcome with some variant of an outreach system, it is difficult to try and distinguish (and may be inappropriate to do so) between the role of the scoring trigger system used and any triggered interventions and resultant changes in outcomes.
- Few studies are randomized and adequately powered. Rigorous evaluation of the published studies in this field, e.g. Cochrane reviews, criticize the majority of studies published as being of poor methodological value [14]. They did not believe that meta-analysis was possible.

Accuracy of predictions

Prediction of cardiac arrest, ICU admission and of mortality have been examined.

- In one case control study the ability of a track and trigger system to predict in-hospital cardiac arrest based on 10 "MET" parameters was assessed. A receiver operating characteristic (ROC) analysis determined that a score of 4 has 89% sensitivity and 77% specificity for cardiac arrest; a score of 8 has 52% sensitivity and 99% specificity. Only 1% of patients who do not have a cardiac arrest score of 8 or more, and all patients scoring greater than 10 suffered a cardiac arrest [15].

- The ability of a PART to predict admission to ICU in hospital ward patients (patients triggered the system if they had three out of six abnormal physiological variables or reduced consciousness with increased heart or respiratory rate) had a sensitivity and specificity for patients with three abnormal observations of 27% and 57%, respectively. For patients with one abnormal observation, the sensitivity was 97% and specificity 18%. The presence of two abnormal observations had a sensitivity of 80% and specificity of 41% [16].

- In a third study, also based on the PART calling criteria, stepwise multiple regression identified five significant predictors of 30-day mortality (consciousness, heart rate, age, blood pressure and respiratory rate) – sensitivity and specificity were 7.7% and 99.8%, respectively [4].

- With regard to aggregate scoring systems, and MEWS in particular, a trigger score was associated with an increased risk of death (odds ratio [OR] 5.4, 95% confidence interval [CI] 2.8–10.7) and ICU admission (OR = 10.9, 95% CI 2.2–55.6) [17].

- The use of the early warning score (EWS) to predict mortality in a sample of 110 patients admitted with acute pancreatitis had sensitivities on days 1, 2 and 3 following admission of 85.7%, 71.4% and 100%, respectively. Specificities were 28.3%, 67.4% and 77.4%, respectively [18].

- The Worthing PSS has shown that the use of rigorous statistical methods in identifying both physiological parameters and abnormal physiological values has enabled the sensitivities and specificities of the system to be increased over older, existing EWS. At an intervention score of 2, its sensitivity and specificities are 78% and 57%, respectively [11].

It would seem that these systems have problems with diagnostic accuracy. This may be due to the nature by which the choices of parameter and trigger points are determined, i.e. through clinical intuition rather than rigorous methodologies.

Whilst having reasonable sensitivity and specificity in tightly controlled conditions, in clinical practice concern over their utility exists. In some part, this is due to calculation errors by healthcare workers and also by inter- and intraobserver reliability [19].

Improvements in outcome with outreach systems

Improvements in outcome could arise from reductions in cardiac arrest and better survival from cardiac arrests, avoidance of ICU admission and/or improved overall mortality. Full assessment of the effect of outreach systems on outcome is difficult due to different systems studied (EWS, METs, outreach teams, etc.), different hospitals, countries and patient population types and often lack of randomization or controlling for other changes in practice. Many of the published studies are underpowered or study too short a time period. Many of the studies of cardiac arrests recorded cardiac arrest calls rather than specific cardiac arrests. The Hawthorne effect in "control" groups is another possible confounding factor.

- Reductions in the incidence of cardiac arrest may be due to better education of ward staff in caring for patients and new "Do Not Attempt Resuscitation" or DNAR orders being made on sick patients as well as due to improvements in care of pre-arrest patients. All are arguably of benefit.

- Parr et al. in Australia identified the opportunity to reduce the incidence of cardiac arrest by the issuing of DNAR orders [20].

- However, Bellomo et al. [21], also in Australia, showed that the introduction of a MET system reduced the number of cardiac arrests and also the deaths from cardiac arrest when comparing the time period before the introduction of the system and the time period after its introduction. This was not found to be due to increased DNAR orders. They also demonstrated reduced overall inpatient mortality even after adjusting for other factors contributing to long-term surgical mortality.

- Buist et al. in a 6-year audit, found that the introduction of a MET system, after adjustment for case mix, was associated with a 50% reduction in the incidence of cardiac arrest [22].

- Using a nonphysician-based model, chiefly composed of physician assistants given extra training, Dacey et al. were able to demonstrate a reduction in the incidence of cardiac arrests, unexpected ICU admissions, and also reduced the in-hospital mortality from 2.82% to 2.35% (not statistically significant) [23]. New limitations of care were made following the input of the team such that all ICU admissions were reduced.

- Jones et al. assessed the effect of a MET service on patient mortality in the 4 years since its introduction into a teaching hospital [24]. They found fluctuating and variable effects on overall mortality, with apparent increases in mortality in medical patients perhaps reflecting differences in degree of disease complexity and reversibility between medical and surgical patients.

- One of only two "proper" RCTs in this field was the MERIT (Medical Early Response Intervention and Therapy) study from Australia [25]. This multi-center trial randomized 23 hospitals without a MET system to introduce such a system or maintain current practices. Results were disappointing for MET enthusiasts. The number of emergency calls for sick patients greatly increased over the course of the study period in the MET hospitals. However, both groups of hospitals showed a reduction in overall mortality over the study period with no statistically significant difference in outcome seen in the MET hospitals. Using their call-out criteria, many patients were not identified until less than 15 min before either cardiac arrest or intensive care admission. It appears that the study was underpowered.

- The other published RCT from the UK randomized the wards in a single, large hospital. Priestley et al. [26] found that the interventions associated with an outreach team reduced hospital mortality (OR 0.52) and length of stay. They also found a possible increased length of stay associated with outreach which, after further analysis, may not have been statistically significant.

- Ball et al. [27] found that the introduction of a critical care outreach team improved survival to discharge from hospital after discharge from critical care by 6.8%. Readmission to critical care decreased by 6.4% (0.48).

- Finally, Pittard [28] showed that, in his hospital, following the introduction of an outreach service the emergency admission rate to intensive care fell from 58% to 43% with a shorter length of stay (4.8 days vs. 7.4 days) and a lower mortality (28.6% vs. 23.5%, $p = 0.05$). The readmission rate also fell from 5.1% to 3.3% ($p = 0.05$).

The introduction of an ICU outreach program in a hospital is an opportunity for increased education and support of ward staff, both nursing and medical. It would seem that where outreach services are specifically designed to actively manage deteriorating patients at a ward level and prevent or expedite their critical care admission, improvements in outcome measures can be seen. Where outreach services are purely educational, supportive or in place to review discharged patients, service level improvements may be difficult to prove.

Specific postsurgical studies

- In a surgical ward population in the UK, 17% of patients triggered a MEWS response with a threshold of 4 for a call. MEWS in surgical patients was found to be 75% sensitive and 83% specific for admission to a high care area with a threshold of 4 or more [29].

- The introduction of a nurse-based outreach system in a large Australian hospital led to a reduction in the incidence of serious adverse events and myocardial infarction in the first 3 days after surgery [30].

- Also in Australia, the introduction of an ICU-based MET into a University hospital also seemed of benefit to patients having major surgery [31]. Although not a randomized trial the results are of interest. The introduction of the MET team was associated with reductions in several adverse events:

Adverse event	Relative risk reduction (%)
Overall adverse events	57.8
Respiratory failure	79.1
Renal failure	88.5
Emergency ICU admissions	44.4
Postoperative deaths	36.6

The average length of stay after major surgery was also reduced.

- A combined critical care outreach and anesthesia-based acute pain team [32] reviewed high-risk patients on the wards during the first 3 days after surgery. They were also able to demonstrate a reduction in the incidence of adverse events and 30 day mortality (from 9% to 3%).

- Introduction of a MET service in a teaching hospital in Australia was associated with increased long-term survival in surgical patients (65.8% in the control period and 71.6% during the MET period ($P = 0.001$)) even after adjusting for other factors that contribute to long-term surgical mortality [33].

The future

- Further work needs to be done both on the introduction of more rigorously determined systems and in improving, possibly through computer-based systems, data collection and analysis. Hospital-wide automated data collection systems may ensure that patient data or deterioration is not missed and possibly include an automated alerting system to the outreach team [34].

- The Cochrane reviewers [14] and others have called for large RCTs to fully evaluate aspects of outreach. Some may believe that it is unfortunate that outreach has been introduced worldwide despite little objective proof of benefit. Cuthbertson [35] has highlighted potential broad areas of concern requiring investigation:

  > Existing scoring systems may not allow early recognition.
  > Outreach teams do not always enable early intervention.
  > Maybe the wrong people are doing outreach.
  > Maybe outreach interventions may be ineffective.
  > Outreach teams may not be cost-effective.

- In the UK, the Government has invested heavily in outreach (although uptake amongst hospitals has been patchy [36]). Cynics may question whether this is an alternative to funding ICU beds in numbers comparable to other European Union countries.

- The early management of patients who may be developing critical illness is being targeted by other UK government bodies through similar simple assessment tools and basic clinical management skills.

- The National Institute for Health and Clinical Excellence in the UK has advocated the following graded response based on a track and trigger system [15].

  > Low-score group:
  > Increased frequency of observations and the nurse in charge alerted.
  >
  > Medium-score group:
  > Urgent call to team with primary medical responsibility for the patient.
  >
  > Simultaneous call to personnel with core competencies for acute illness. These competencies can be delivered by a variety of models at a local level, such as a critical care outreach team, a hospital-at-night team, or a specialist trainee in an acute medical or surgical specialty.
  >
  > High-score group:
  > Emergency call to team with critical care competencies and diagnostic skills. The team should include a medical practitioner skilled in the assessment of the critically ill patient, who possesses advanced airway management and resuscitation skills. There should be an immediate response.

- Prevention of clinical deterioration, avoidance of admission to intensive care, and improvement in patient outcome do not solely rely on the identification of patients at risk. An appropriate response, which is fit for purpose, is also required. It is recognized that junior medical and nursing staff are often unable to recognize and initiate treatment of the critically ill. Standard textbooks on clinical examination are poorly equipped to help students understand the principles of assessing the critically ill patient [37]. In order to fill this gap, in the UK the ALERT (Acute Life-threatening Events, Recognition and Treatment) and AIM (Acute Illness Management) courses have been developed. These multi-disciplinary courses are aimed at addressing suboptimal ward care often seen prior to admission to critical care units. Attendance at ALERT courses has been shown to improve junior doctors' knowledge of critical illness [38] and to improve their skills and confidence in managing the deteriorating high-risk patient [39].

Conclusion

Patients will continue to deteriorate whilst in hospital. The challenge remains to identify those patients early using detailed preoperative assessments, intraoperative observation, robust physiological track and trigger systems and, undoubtedly, sound clinical judgment. Identification is only useful if appropriate and skilled assistance is available through either a graded response or MET/PART depending on the individual needs of the institution.

Further reading

Esmonde L, McDonnell A, Ball C, *et al.* Investigating the effectiveness of critical care outreach services: A systematic review. *Intens Care Med* 2006; **32**: 1713–21.

Gao H, McDonnell A, Harrison DA, *et al.* Systematic review and evaluation of physiological track and trigger warning systems for identifying at-risk patients on the ward. *Intens Care Med* 2007; **33**: 667–79.

Smith GB, Prytherch DR, Schmidt PE, *et al.* Review and performance evaluation of aggregate weighted "track and trigger" systems. *Resuscitation* 2008; **77**: 170–9.

Winters BD, Pham JC, Hunt EA, *et al.* Rapid response systems: A systematic review. *Crit Care Med* 2007; **35**: 1238–43.

References

1. McQuillian P, Pilkington S, Allan A, *et al.* Confidential enquiry into quality of care before admission to intensive care. *BMJ* 1998; **316**: 1853–8.

2. McGloin H, Adam SK, Singer M. Unexpected deaths and referrals to intensive care of patients on general wards. Are some cases potentially avoidable? *J R Coll Phys Lond* 1999; **33**: 255–9.

3. NCEPOD. *An acute problem? A report of the National Confidential Enquiry into Patient Outcome and Death (NCEPOD).* London, NCEPOD, 2005.

4. Kause J, Smith G, Prytherch D, *et al.* A comparison of antecedents to cardiac arrests, deaths and emergency intensive care admissions in Australia and New Zealand, and the United Kingdom – the ACADEMIA study. *Resuscitation* 2004; **62**: 275–82.

5. National Institute for Health and Clinical Excellence. Acutely ill patients in hospital. *Recognition of and response to acute illness in adults in hospital.* CG250 London, UK July 2007.

6. Goldhill DR, McNarry AF. Physiological abnormalities in early warning scores are related to mortality in adult inpatients. *Br J Anaesthesia* 2004; **92**: 882–4.

7. Berwick DM, Calkins DR, Mc-Cannon CJ, Hackbarth AD. The 100,000 Lives Campaign. *JAMA* 2006; **295**: 324–7.

8. Baxter AD, Cardinal P, Hooper J, *et al.* Medical emergency teams at The Ottawa Hospital: The first two years. *Can J Anaesth* 2008; **55**: 223–31.

9. Morgan RJM, Williams F, Wright MM. An early warning scoring system for detecting developing critical illness. *Clin Inten Care* 1997; **8**: 100.

10. Stenhouse C, Coates S, Tivery M, *et al.* Prospective evaluation of a modified early warning score to aid earlier detection of patients developing critical illness on general surgical wards. *Br J Anaesthesia* 2000; **84**: 663.

11. Duckitt RW, Buxton-Thomas R, Walker J, *et al.* Worthing physiological scoring system: Derivation and validation of a physiological early-warning system for medical admissions. An observational, population-based single centre study. *Br J Anaesthesia* 2007; **98**: 769–74.

12. Lee A, Bishop G, Hilman KM. The Medical Emergency Team. *Anaesth Intens Care* 1995; **23**: 183–6.

13. Goldhill DR, Worthington L, Mulcahy A, *et al.* The patient-at-risk team: Identifying and managing seriously ill ward patients. *Anaesthesia* 1999; **54**: 853–60.

14. McGaughey J, Alderdice F, Fowler R, *et al.* Outreach and Early Warning Systems (EWS) for the prevention of intensive care admission and death of critically ill adult patients on general hospital wards. *Cochrane Database Syst Rev* 2007; **3**: CD005529.

15. Hodgetts TJ, Kenward G, Vlachonikolis IG, *et al.* The identification of risk factors for cardiac arrest and formulation of activation criteria to alert a medical emergency team. *Resuscitation* 2002; **54**: 125–31.

16. Goldhill DR, McNarry AF, Mandersloot G, *et al.* A physiologically based early warning score for ward patients: The association between score and outcome. *Anaesthesia* 2005; **60**: 547–53.

17. Subbe CP, Davies RG, Williams E, *et al.* Effect of introducing the Modified Early Warning score on clinical outcomes, cardio-pulmonary arrests and intensive care utilisation in acute medical admissions. *Anaesthesia* 2003; **58**: 797–802.

18. Garcea G, Jackson B, Pattenden CJ, *et al.* Early warning scores predict outcome in acute pancreatitis. *J Gastroint Surg* 2006; **10**: 1008–15.

19. Cuthbertson BH, Smith GB. A warning on early warning score. *Br J Anaesthesia* 2007; **98**: 704–6.

20. Parr MJ, Hadfield JH, Flabouris A, *et al.* The Medical Emergency Team: 12 month analysis of reasons for activation, immediate outcome and not-for-resuscitation orders. *Resuscitation* 2001; **50**: 39–44.

21. Bellomo R, Goldsmith D, Uchino S, *et al.* A prospective before-and-after trial of a medical emergency team. *Med J Australia* 2003; **179**: 283–7.

22. Buist M, Harrison J, Abaloz E, *et al.* Six year audit of cardiac arrests and medical emergency team calls in an Australian outer metropolitan teaching hospital. *BMJ* 2007; **335**: 1210–2.

23. Dacey MJ, Mirza ER, Wilcox V, *et al.* The effect of a rapid response team on major clinical outcome measures in a community hospital. *Crit Care Med* 2007; **35**: 2076–82.

24. Jones D, Opdam H, Egi M, *et al.* Long-term effect of a Medical Emergency Team on mortality in a teaching hospital. *Resuscitation* 2007; **74**: 235–41.

25. Hillman K, Chen J, Cretikos M, *et al.* Introduction of the medical emergency team (MET) system: A cluster-randomised controlled trial. *Lancet* 2005; **365**: 2091–7.

26. Priestley G, Watson W, Rashidian A, *et al.* Introducing Critical Care Outreach: A ward-randomised trial of phased introduction in a general hospital. *Intens Care Med* 2004; **30**: 1398–404.

27. Ball C, Kirkby M, Williams S. Effect of the critical care outreach team on patient survival to discharge from hospital and readmission to critical care: non-randomised population based study. *BMJ* 2003; **327**: 1014.

28. Pittard AJ. Out of our reach? Assessing the impact of introducing a critical care outreach service. *Anaesthesia* 2003; **58**: 882–5.

29. Gardner-Thorpe J, Love N, Wrightson J, *et al.* The value of Modified Early Warning Score (MEWS) in surgical in-patients: A prospective observational study. *Ann R Coll Surg Engl* 2006; **88**: 571–5.

30. Story DA, Shelton AC, Poustie SJ, *et al.* The effect of critical care outreach on postoperative serious adverse events. *Anaesthesia* 2004; **59**: 762–6.

31. Bellomo R, Goldsmith D, Uchino S, *et al.* Prospective controlled trial of effect of medical emergency team on postoperative morbidity and mortality rates. *Crit Care Med* 2004; **32**: 916–21.

32. Story DA, Shelton AC, Poustie SJ, *et al.* Effect of an anaesthesia department led critical care outreach and acute pain service on postoperative serious adverse events. *Anaesthesia* 2006; **61**: 24–8.

33. Jones D, Egi M, Bellomo R, *et al.* Effect of the medical emergency team on long-term mortality following major surgery. *Crit Care* 2007; **11**: R12.

34. Smith GB, Prytherch DR, Schmidt P, *et al.* Hospital-wide physiological surveillance – a

new approach to the early identification and management of the sick patient. *Resuscitation* 2006; **71**: 19–28.

35. Cuthbertson BH. Lecture, Manchester, UK, 27 April 2006.

36. McDonnell A, Esmonde L, Morgan R, *et al.* The provision of critical care outreach services in England: Findings from a national survey. *J Crit Care* 2007; **22**: 212–8.

37. Cook CJ, Smith GB. Do textbooks of clinical examination contain information regarding the assessment of critically ill patients? *Resuscitation* 2004; **60**: 129–36.

38. Smith GB, Poplett N. Impact of attending a 1-day multi-professional course (ALERT) on the knowledge of acute care in trainee doctors. *Resuscitation* 2004; **61**: 117–22.

39. Featherstone P, Smith GB, Linnell M, *et al.* Impact of a one-day inter-professional course (ALERT) on attitudes and confidence in managing critically ill adult patients. *Resuscitation* 2005; **65**: 329–36.

Chapter 3

Perioperative renal insufficiency and failure

R. Kishen

Kidneys are robust organs and will function normally under a variety of physiological and pathological conditions. In the perioperative period, renal dysfunction sometimes occurs, which is usually multi-factorial in origin. Development of renal dysfunction prolongs patients' hospital stay and increases mortality and morbidity.

Introduction

The main functions of the kidneys are maintenance of fluid and electrolyte balance, excretion of waste products of metabolism, control of vascular tone, maintenance of blood pressure, and regulating hematopoiesis and bone metabolism. Kidneys are robust organs and will function under many adverse conditions. However, surgery and, to some extent, anesthesia do affect renal function, and perioperative renal dysfunction does occur. Perioperative renal dysfunction increases morbidity, length of intensive care unit (ICU) and hospital stay as well as mortality, not to mention increased cost of health care both immediately and in the long term. Thus it is imperative for the anesthetists, surgeons, intensivists and all those looking after postoperative patients to understand the pathophysiology and risk factors for development of perioperative renal dysfunction as well as its prevention and treatment. Clinicians should also appreciate that ultimately all patients with perioperative renal dysfunction will become critically ill, and the boundaries between patients with perioperative renal dysfunction and acute kidney injury in the critically ill become vague, and both categories of patients are managed on same clinical principles.

The importance of recognition of patients at risk and prevention of perioperative renal dysfunction has been designated an important public health priority by the Department of Health (DH) in the UK. The Renal Advisory Group of DH conducted a workshop in March 2006, gathering expert opinion and best practice together. The deliberations of the Group have been published, and pathways for prevention of postoperative acute renal failure in the perioperative period have been outlined [1].

Basic applied anatomy and physiology [2]

In order to appreciate the various mechanisms and processes involved in renal dysfunction in the peri- and postoperative period, it is important to go over some basic physiological principles.

- Kidneys receive about 20–25% of cardiac output – the highest blood supply per unit weight of any tissue in the body.
- Distribution of this blood flow in the kidney is not uniform, with the cortex receiving about 90% of the total blood flow. Renal medulla, metabolically very active, receives only

Anesthesia for the High Risk Patient, ed. I. McConachie. Published by Cambridge University Press.
© Cambridge University Press 2009.

about 10% of this blood flow. The low blood flow in the medulla is to maintain the high osmolality in the medullary interstitium.

- Oxygen delivery to the kidney is about 80 ml min^{-1} 100 g^{-1} of tissue. Thus kidneys, on the whole, are the best perfused organs in the body.

- There are complex blood supply patterns in the kidney. The renal artery divides into segmental arteries which are "end arteries" in that there is no collateral circulation between them. These segmental arteries, in turn, divide into interlobular arteries.

- Afferent arterioles (each arteriole has a sphincter) arise from the interlobular arteries and supply blood to the glomerular tuft of capillaries. These drain into efferent arterioles (which also have a sphincter) and then proceed on to become peritubular capillaries (for cortical nephrons) or vasa recta (for juxtamedullary nephrons). Afferent arteriolar sphincter regulates blood flow to the glomerular capillaries in response to various stimuli, especially tubulo-glomerular feedback (TGF).

- Under normal physiological conditions, total renal blood flow (TRBF) is maintained despite variations in mean arterial pressure (MAP). However, this may not be so under pathological conditions.

- The nephron is the metabolically active unit of the kidney. Most of the sodium reabsorption takes place in the proximal convoluted tubule (PCT) and the medullary thick ascending part of the loop of Henlé (mTAL). Sodium reabsorption (against medullary interstitial osmotic gradient) is an energy-consuming process (involving Na/K-ATPase carrier) and accounts for about 80–90% of the kidney's oxygen consumption.

- Although the kidney has high oxygen delivery, its overall oxygen extraction is low, there being regional differences in oxygen extraction within the kidney. Renal cortex extracts about 18% of oxygen delivered to it (as it has a very high blood supply) whereas the medulla extracts about 79% (which has a low blood supply). Thus medullary structures like the descending and ascending parts of the loop of Henlé work virtually at the verge of hypoxia. It is therefore obvious that these metabolically active medullary structures (e.g. loop of Henlé) are highly vulnerable to hypoperfusion and tissue hypoxia.

- Various regulatory mechanisms exist in the kidneys for preserving local blood flow and oxygen delivery to the kidney structures. These include:
  - elaboration of local nitric oxide (NO), various dilating prostaglandins (e.g. prostaglandin E$_1$, prostacyclin – PGI$_2$), dopamine, urodilatin (urinary analogue of atrial natriuretic factor).

  - formation of vasoconstrictors like endothelins, angiotensin II.

  - TGF: a mechanism that can feed back to the afferent (and efferent) arterioles to regulate glomerular filtrate (decrease or increase it) depending on hydration, perfusion and other factors. At times of low perfusion, TGF causes afferent arteriolar sphincter constriction, reduced filtration pressure in the glomerulus and thus less filtrate to come down the tubule; this reduces tubular function (as less sodium needs to be reabsorbed), reducing tubular oxygen consumption and preserving tubular cell integrity at times of hypoperfusion.

  - Medullary tubular growth factors like insulin-like growth factor I, epidermal growth factor are elaborated as well – however, their role in pathogenesis or renal recovery in humans has not been fully studied.

It must be appreciated that the large proportion of the cardiac output received by the kidneys is designed to produce large amounts of glomerular filtrate (necessary to filter out adequate quantities of toxins and metabolic waste) that is subsequently modified in the tubules and collecting ducts to form urine – most (99%) of the glomerular filtrate being reabsorbed.

Under conditions of hypovolemia (whether hypotension is present or not), dehydration and reduced cardiac output, TGF and other mechanisms come into play to preserve body fluid which clinically manifests as oliguria.

Thus oliguria is not always a sign of renal dysfunction [3].

What is acute renal failure (ARF)? Quantifying perioperative renal insufficiency and failure and defining ARF

The definition of the syndrome of perioperative renal insufficiency and failure (PORIF) and indeed that of ARF in the critically ill patient has suffered from inconsistency and wide variation. This has confounded the clinicians, as it is difficult to make sense of published literature, make informed decisions and advance research in prevention and treatment of this condition [4].

- It is generally accepted that an abrupt cessation of urine formation and rise in uremic toxins (urea and creatinine) in blood is indicative of "renal failure" [5].

- Clinicians should be aware that sudden, absolute and total anuria is a blocked urinary catheter unless proven otherwise.

- Acute renal failure in the perioperative period (and in the critically ill) is now called Acute Kidney Injury (AKI). AKI describes a continuum of the process rather than a single stage of the disease. The term AKI is an important step forward because it encompasses even those patients in whom total (oligo/anuric) failure of kidneys has not yet set in. Furthermore, not all patients with PORIF progress to failure or end-stage disease.

- More than 30 definitions of AKI appear in the literature; this makes it very difficult to analyze the literature and to compare the treatment strategies meaningfully [6, 7].

- Definitions based on glomerular filtration rate (GFR) and creatinine clearance are difficult to use clinically in the perioperative period. These tests are better suited to patients in a "steady state" and take time to organize and report (e.g. 24 h urine collection for creatinine clearance). Critically ill patients are not in a steady state, and the time required for the tests makes them unsuitable for use in operating theaters or sometimes even in the ICU or high-dependency unit (HDU).

- Work is ongoing to assess the feasibility and diagnostic utility of biomarkers of renal injury. Thus cystatin C, neutrophil gelatinase-associated lipocalin (NGAL, lipocalin 2) [8], interleukin 18 (IL 18) and kidney injury molecule 1 (KIM1) are being studied extensively. Any or all of these markers may become available as easy bedside tests in the future; at present, they are not/cannot be recommended for routine use in clinical settings [9].

- Measurement of serum creatinine and urine output (UO) have their own problems. Serum creatinine is influenced by age, sex, muscle mass, etc., and UO is affected by the state of patient's hydration, MAP, cardiac output and use of diuretics. However, serum creatinine and UO are the two easily measurable parameters by the bedside or in the operating theater. Hence any definition incorporating these two parameters is easy to

Table 13.1 RIFLE criteria for AKI

	GFR criteria	UO criteria	
Risk	↑ in serum creatinine × 1.5 or ↓ in GFR > 25%	UO < 0.5 ml kg^{-1} h^{-1} over 6 h	
Injury	↑ in serum creatinine × 2 or ↓ in GFR > 50%	UO < 0.5 ml kg^{-1} h^{-1} over 12 h	High sensitivity
Failure	↑ in serum creatinine × 3 or ↓ in GFR > 75% or serum creatinine > μmol l^{-1} or an acute rise of 48 μmol l^{-1}	UO < 0.3 ml kg^{-1} h^{-1} over 24 h or anuria for 12 h (oliguria)	
Loss	Persistent AKI – complete loss of renal function > 4 weeks.		
ESKD	End-stage kidney disease (>3 months)		High specificity

Table 13.2 Staging criteria for AKI

Stage	Creatinine	UO
1	≥ 26 μmol l^{-1} or 1.5–2-fold increase	< 0.5 ml kg^{-1} h^{-1} > 6 h
2	Increase by ×2-fold to ×3-fold	< 0.5 ml kg^{-1} h^{-1} > 12 h
3	Increase by >3-fold	< 0.3 ml kg^{-1} h^{-1} or anuria > 12 h

employ by the bedside or in the operating theater in the absence of easily available biomarkers of kidney injury.

- In patients with pre-existing renal dysfunction, serum creatinine rises disproportionate to kidney injury and therefore does not accurately reflect the extent of new or emerging AKI.

- Emerging data have shown that even small or modest rises in serum creatinine are highly associated with an adverse outcome in hospitalized patients [10, 11]. Studies in patients with cardiac surgery and other cardiac conditions have also shown a similar pattern [12]. Hence new definitions based on relatively small changes in serum creatinine and UO have been proposed.

- Acute Dialysis Quality Initiative (ADQI) [13] proposed RIFLE criteria for AKI. The RIFLE (Risk, Injury, Failure and outcome of Loss and End-stage kidney disease) criteria define AKI severity grades based on GFR and/or serum creatinine, UO and clinical outcome (Table 13.1) [14]. This definition will inevitably increase the "prevalence" of PORIF/AKI in that more patients will be identified that have AKI who hitherto would not have been classified as having "acute renal failure". The majority of the studies suggest that the use of RIFLE criteria convey significant prognostic information, at least in ICU setting. These criteria need to be further evaluated to be applicable universally.

- More recently, the Acute Kidney Injury Network [15] has suggested a simplified definition which depends on a smaller rise of creatinine (>25 μmol l^{-1} or a >50% rise from base line) or development of oliguria as defined by a UO of <0.5 ml kg^{-1} h^{-1} for > 6 h (Table 13.2). These have simply been called "Staging Criteria for AKI".

- However, as with the RIFLE criteria, the Staging Criteria need to be validated extensively in terms of universal applicability. Staging Criteria may also "increase the prevalence" of AKI as do ADQI RIFLE criteria.

- Neither the RIFLE nor Staging Criteria define the points at which renal replacement therapy (RRT) should be commenced (if required) or stopped.
- The author has used a simple working definition (very close to RIFLE or Staging Criteria but antedating them) based on serum creatinine and UO for clinical decision-making [16]. Thus, a patient with a precipitating etiological factor ± risk factors (see below), who is adequately fluid-loaded and has a normal or near-normal MAP and cardiac output (whether measured or clinically judged) with:
  - a urine UO <0.25 ml kg^{-1} h^{-1} for 6 h (<500 ml day^{-1} in a 80 kg adult),
  - a rise of 50% in serum creatinine in 12–24 h,
  - development of metabolic acidosis – not explained by clinical condition (e.g. severe sepsis, hyperchloremia, etc.),

fulfills a clinical definition indicating that renal function has "failed" (Criterion F of RIFLE criteria and Stage III in Staging AKI). This is also helpful in making the clinical decision for starting RRT. It has to be emphasized that the definition is only applied when all causes of "prerenal azotemia or failure" have been eliminated (see under management) and irreversibility of AKI established.

Types, pathophysiology, diagnostic test and incidence of AKI: types of "renal failure"

Traditionally, textbooks have taught generations of doctors that renal failure (now called AKI) is of three types: prerenal, renal and postrenal. It is still in popular teaching.

- Prerenal renal failure, i.e. "before blood arrives into the kidneys for purification", e.g. hypovolemia, hypotension, low cardiac output, hemorrhage, etc.
- Intrinsic-renal or simply renal failure is due to "intrinsic pathology" of the renal parenchyma caused by a variety of conditions, e.g. various nephropathies (vasculitides, pigment-induced renal damage, contrast-induced nephropathy, interstitial nephritides, etc.), classical acute tubular necrosis (ATN – rarely seen clinically), antibiotic-induced AKI.
- Postrenal: obstruction to collecting system within the kidney (e.g. renal pelvis) or outside (ureteric obstruction).
- Prerenal implies etiological factors "outside the kidney" affecting kidney function (but does not include obstruction to urinary excretory pathways – postrenal failure). It is not too difficult to imagine why this classical and attractive but simplistic view gained popularity, withstood the passage of time, and has been a popular paradigm for the last half a century [17].
- The term is "neat" and helps organize some of the causes of oliguria as separate and distinct entities.
- It is also easy to suggest that this prerenal state if not "treated" progresses to the next phase – the renal (or intrinsic renal) phase – the so-called acute tubular necrosis (ATN), as it is assumed that untreated prerenal situation progresses to renal damage by ischemia (a natural consequence of prolonged hypovolemia, hypotension, or low cardiac output).
- However, as discussed below, the term ATN does not convey the true pathophysiology of PORIF or AKI in the critically ill.

- Consider the example of a patient with severe diarrhea and oliguria (due to dehydration, and who may even exhibit raised serum creatinine) who will be classified as having prerenal renal failure. In this case, prerenal failure is not actually a failure of the kidney function: the kidneys are actually working very well in preserving the body's fluid; it is simply *physiological oliguria* (author's personal observation) and it is implied that fluid therapy will restore kidney function (e.g. normal UO) – so the kidneys have not actually failed. However, as the term prerenal failure is still popular and in vogue, we need to rethink the utility of this term in the clinical context of PORIF/AKI.

- It can also be argued that we cannot classify a syndrome (emerging AKI) whose pathology we do not really know as yet [17] (see below under pathophysiology).

- It is also difficult to define the point at which prerenal failure progresses to intrinsic renal failure when, pathologically, the distinction would be almost impossible to make.

- Thus, as far as PORIF and AKI in the critically ill are concerned, the classical subdivisions of AKI no longer explain or represent the true clinical situation (except in postrenal or obstructive AKI).

- It can also be argued that, in simple clinical terms, prerenal AKI is unrecognized resuscitation failure (author's personal observation).

- Future studies on pathology of AKI may shed more light on this subject. It is however, useful to remember that prerenal AKI should prompt evaluation of fluid and hemodynamic status of the patient, and postrenal should prompt evaluation of the renal outflow tract, as the management of obstructive AKI is dramatically different from other "forms" of AKI. As the following section on pathophysiology will show, the three forms of AKI can be present at the same time in patients with PORIF/AKI.

Whereas the term postrenal failure is a useful and distinct clinical entity, the above discussion argues that the term prerenal may be flawed in the context of PORIF/AKI in the critically ill.

Pathophysiology

Traditionally, PORIF is thought to be mostly prerenal in origin and it is suggested that if left untreated, this prerenal stage progresses to the intrinsic or renal stage and ATN. This view has been perpetuated by animal studies and the belief that most of the PORIF is due to ischemia–reperfusion. Animal models have enhanced our understanding of renal physiology, but have done little to advance our knowledge of PORIF or AKI in the critically ill.

- The usual animal model of AKI is a small animal where, after sedation/anesthesia one or both renal arteries are clamped, the renal blood flow being restored after a suitable interval. In this situation, there is no blood flow, nor are the kidneys carrying out any of their functions – a situation far removed from the clinical situation [18].

- Clinically, renal blood flow (RBF) may be low but is never zero; thus kidneys are functioning, albeit under a state of low perfusion.

- Furthermore, a few blood flow studies undertaken in humans and animals have shown that in the critically ill (especially with sepsis), RBF is either normal or increased, but not always low as is generally assumed [19, 20].

- That the ultimate pathophysiological picture is that of necrosis (so-called ATN) has also been challenged with newer insights into this condition. It is also unusual to have biopsy specimens from these critically ill patients. The few biopsy specimens that are available to us do not show necrosis; on the contrary, in patients with previously normal kidneys, the renal architecture looks remarkably normal [21].

- Thus the true pathophysiology of PORIF and AKI in the critically ill is mostly ill understood.

- It is also a common observation that, with appropriate care, renal function in survivors returns to normal within a few days unless there has been background (and often unrecognized) renal dysfunction before surgery.

- Abnormalities in renal parenchyma do occur; however, glomerular and tubular cell destruction and necrosis are rare or non-existent and the histology of such kidneys shows absence of glomerulopathy (cf. vasculitic renal disorders) [21, 22].

- There is reversal of polarity in the tubular cells (Na–K ATPase carrier pump relocates to the luminal side of the cell from its baso-lateral site), cell swelling and disruption of tight junctions causing back-leak of tubular luminal fluid into medullary and cortical paren- chyma [22]. Tubular cells may come off the basement membrane, and this phenomenon together with cell swelling causes tubular obstruction. Tubular obstruction along with disruption of tight junctions and back-leak of tubular fluid back into renal parenchyma manifests as oliguria.

- Disrupted tubular cells may undergo apoptosis (programmed cell death) which may be accelerated by hypoxia, cytokines and other by-products of inflammation. However, it must be appreciated that apoptosis is an oxygen-consuming process (as opposed to necrosis, which results from total anoxia) and goes through various programmed stages; cell swelling, etc., is a part of this process [22].

- Thus the true pathophysiological picture of PORIF and AKI in the critically ill (especially sepsis-induced AKI) seems to be that of nonfunctioning but structurally relatively normal kidney.

- Therefore, it is also suggested that the term ATN is a misnomer, and its use in describing PORIF and AKI in the critically ill should be abandoned [23].

The above discussion, although not detailed, argues that the pathophysiology of PORIF and AKI in the critically ill is not fully understood. It also argues that AKI in the critically ill (which includes PORIF) is a different disease entity from that seen on the nephrology wards (i.e. medical AKI) [16]. It then follows that management of this condition is different from that employed in other forms of AKI. It must also be remembered that this type of AKI may be superimposed on pre-existing renal dysfunction in many patients. In patients with pre-existing renal dysfunction even slight insults (that would not affect normal kidneys) can cause PORIF/AKI.

With the above discussion on pathophysiology of PORIF and AKI, it should also be clear that with hypovolemia, shock, hypotension, possible cardiac dysfunction (one or more may be present perioperatively) and histological changes in the kidney (cell swelling, back-leak, etc.) the so-called prerenal, intrinsic or renal, and postrenal situations co-exist in the dysfunctioning kidney at the same time.

Renal function tests

The classical tests of renal function such as measurement of glomerular filtration rate (GFR) and creatinine clearance are established and time-honoured tests in patients with renal failure.

- However, these tests are usually performed in patients who are stable and in whom creatinine or renal function do not change quickly over short periods of time.

- Critically ill patients are different in that they do not have stable metabolic function; biochemical markers for kidney injury (urea and creatinine) are not stable, and there is an ever-changing fluid balance, at least in the initial period of critical illness.

- Creatinine clearance also requires urine collection over 24 h, making the test tedious in postoperative and critical care setting. Although collections over shorter periods (2 h) have been shown to be equally valid in some studies [24], others have challenged their accuracy and validity in the critically ill [25].

- Various tests like urine microscopy, fractional excretion of sodium and urine/plasma ratios are equally not applicable in these patients.

- That kidney dysfunction is present and can be defined (according to RIFLE or AKI Staging Criteria) is enough to make clinical decisions in these patients, little being gained from performing the classical renal function tests.

- Classical renal function tests performed in the preoperative period to evaluate renal function in patients are useful in assessing the patients and their existing renal function preoperatively; however, they will not be discussed here.

Incidence

- Until recently, it has been difficult to estimate accurately the true incidence of PORIF in the perioperative period and AKI in the critically ill simply because of varying definitions of acute renal failure.

- PORIF (AKI in the perioperative period) has variously been estimated at 0.7–35% depending on the definition used.

- In a uniform population of patients undergoing cardiac surgery, it is estimated that 1–15% of patients suffer from PORIF [4]. In other studies in patients undergoing cardiopulmonary bypass, PORIF was found to occur in around 7–8% with about 1–2% requiring renal replacement therapy [26, 27].

- However, with recently acceptable definitions (RIFLE and AKI Staging Criteria), it should be now possible to estimate the true incidence of this syndrome.

- In the UK, data from the Intensive Care National Audit and Research Centre (ICNARC) show that in patients admitted to critical care areas after major surgery, the incidence of acute renal failure is around 0.5% (with an ICU mortality of 25% and hospital mortality of about 38%) [28]. This certainly is an underestimate, as many patients who develop AKI postoperatively (but remain on the general wards) are not counted in these numbers, and milder forms of renal injury may not be reported as ARF. Defining kidney injury based on RIFLE criteria (creatinine rise by 50%) with a minimum serum creatinine $\geq 180\,\mu mol\,l^{-1}$ on admission from theater, the AKI rate goes up to 10.5% (with ICU mortality of 32.7% and hospital mortality of 46.3%) [28].

What causes renal dysfunction perioperatively, and what are the risk factors?

Perioperative renal dysfunction is multi-factorial in origin. Generally, the incidence is higher in patients undergoing complex surgery and prolonged operations. Certain situations are more prone to result in AKI as well. The factors that are responsible for renal dysfunction in surgical populations are given as follows.

Effect of anesthesia on renal function

- Anesthesia, per se, has little effect on renal function [2].
- Most anesthetic agents (both intravenous as well as inhalational) cause vasodilatation and depress cardiac output. Thus anesthesia indirectly affects renal perfusion. Whereas this may not matter in otherwise healthy patients with normal renal function, such hypoperfusion may be detrimental to the kidneys of patients at risk especially and in those with pre-existing renal dysfunction [2].
- Positive pressure ventilation can reduce cardiac output and renal perfusion especially in dehydrated and shocked patients [2].
- Certain fluorinated anesthetic agents have been known to cause renal dysfunction due to liberation of fluoride ion. Of these agents, methoxyflurane is no longer in clinical use. Methoxyflurane caused high output renal failure with elevation of serum creatinine and urea. This toxicity was related to production of fluoride by metabolism of methoxyflurane and started with fluoride levels of 50–80 mM; however, other fluorinated volatile anesthetic agents such as enflurane, isoflurane and sevoflurane are not clinically nephrotoxic despite fluoride levels higher than 50 mM obtained during their use [29]. Unlike methoxyflurane which is metabolized to a significant degree in the kidneys, these latter agents are relatively insoluble in body tissue and also undergo biotransformation in the liver. It is suggested that the site of biotransformation/metabolism is crucial for occurrence of nephrotoxicity [29].
- Renal toxicity is also caused by haloalkenes produced by the inhalation of anesthetic agents by reacting with CO_2 absorbents. Halothane, enflurane, isoflurane and sevoflurane are all known to react with CO_2 absorbents. Halothane nephrotoxicity with haloalkenes occurred in rats, but was never demonstrated clinically.
- Sevoflurane reacts with CO_2 absorbents to form a haloalkene, the compound A, especially when high concentrations of the agents are being used, with low fresh gas flows, with baralyme (instead of soda lime), higher CO_2 absorbent temperatures and higher CO_2 production. Despite this, sevoflurane anesthesia with low flows has been found as safe as other agents with low flows, and renal toxicity has never been demonstrated convincingly in humans.
- Suxamethonium has been known to cause rhabdomyolysis and may contribute to PORIF in exceptional circumstances, e.g. suxamethonium-induced hyperpyrexia [30].

- Epidural anesthesia has been found as safe as general anesthesia for renal transplant surgery [31].
- Most other anesthetic agents and other drugs used in anesthesia do not demonstrate any significant nephrotoxicity, although drug and drug metabolite excretion may be affected when renal dysfunction presents/occurs perioperatively.

Effect of surgery on development of AKI

- Type of surgery can affect renal function in the perioperative period. Thus major surgery can cause renal dysfunction. Specific types of surgery, e.g. cardiac and vascular surgery, are especially associated with a higher risk of renal dysfunction in the perioperative period.
- AKI is more common after cardiac than any other surgery. Up to 15% of patients may experience elevation of serum creatinine at some point in the postoperative period. AKI following cardiac surgery increases morbidity, length of hospital stay and mortality ($\approx$ 60%) [26, 27]. AKI is particularly associated with reduced cardiac output, increased cardiopulmonary bypass (CPB) time, diabetes requiring therapy, pre-existing renal dysfunction and age > 70 years. Cytokine release by CPB, oxidant stress due to stimulation of neutrophils by CPB and possible pigment nephropathy (due to release of hemoglobin during CPB) are additional factors responsible for AKI in cardiac surgery [32]. The incidence of AKI may be less after off-pump compared to on-pump heart operations [33].
- Major vascular surgery and operations on the liver are other important surgical causes of AKI. Aortic surgery is a bigger risk factor than operations on peripheral vessels [34]; the risk of AKI is enhanced by advanced age, increased preoperative serum creatinine, large volume blood transfusion, duration of aortic cross-clamping and requirement of inotropes in the postoperative period. Suprarenal cross-clamping is more of a risk than infrarenal cross-clamping; however, AKI is still related to the total duration of cross-clamping, whatever the site. There is an increased incidence of AKI in emergency aortic surgery than in planned operations [35].
- Any major surgery is a risk factor for development of AKI, especially if the risk factors are present (see below).
- Prolonged surgery is another important factor in development of AKI, particularly where there is a large loss of blood and this has not been appropriately replaced by fluids or blood.
- Emergency surgery, especially in patients not adequately resuscitated in the preoperative period.

Other factors influencing/causing AKI in the perioperative period

There are other factors that cause or increase the incidence of PORIF.

- Anesthetists should not forget that nonanesthetic drugs used before, during or after an operation may adversely affect renal function. In this regard nephrotoxic antibiotics, nonsteroidal analgesic drugs in patients at risk, combination of nephrotoxic antibiotics and diuretics (e.g. a combination of furosemide and gentamicin) will all increase the risk of PORIF [36].
- Special mention must be made of contrast media used in imaging techniques. These drugs can cause severe renal impairment, especially if followed by major surgery shortly

afterwards. Mechanisms of contrast-induced nephropathy (CIN) are not fully understood; however, local renal vasoconstriction, direct tubular toxic effect of drugs used and contrast osmolality have all been implicated [37].

- Multiple trauma, especially where large volumes of blood are transfused, is associated with high incidence of PORIF and AKI.
- Rhabdomyolysis due to crush injuries, long bone fractures and limb swelling after trauma are additional factors responsible for the development of AKI in trauma victims. Mechanisms of tubular injury by myoglobin are still being debated. The commonest accepted mechanism of cause of AKI in this situation, i.e. that of tubular obstruction by precipitated myoglobin casts in acidic urine [38], is being challenged constantly and alternative explanations offered. One such explanation is that in acidic urine (pH < 5.6) myoglobin dissociates into ferrihemate and globulin. Ferrihemate causes impairment of renal tubular transport mechanisms, cell death and deterioration of renal function [39].
- Abdominal compartment syndrome is an additional factor in postoperative patients or in victims of multiple trauma. Increased intra-abdominal pressure may be caused by ileus, large intra-abdominal hematomata, abdominal organ edema and intra-abdominal packs. Increased intra-abdominal pressure directly compresses renal parenchyma, reduces renal perfusion, increases release of ADH and aldosterone (by stimulation of abdominal wall stretch receptors), thus reducing GFR and causing oligo/anuria.

Risk factors predisposing patients to AKI during the perioperative period [40, 41]

There are a variety of risk factors that predispose patients to development of AKI in the perioperative period.

- Age – there is increased risk of PORIF/AKI in the elderly. This probably reflects reduced GFR, reduced NO production and associated co-morbidities like hypertension, diabetes and other degenerative vascular disorders in the elderly, although in a multi-variate analysis age did not appear to be significant [40].
- Chronic kidney disease is a major risk factor. In patients with chronic renal dysfunction, a more pronounced rise in serum creatinine for the same degree of kidney dysfunction is observed than in those with previously normal renal function.
- Low cardiac output states, cardiogenic shock, use of balloon pump and need for inotropes after cardiac surgery.
- Diabetes, especially requiring treatment.
- Cirrhosis, acute or chronic liver dysfunction.
- Pregnancy, pre-eclampsia or frank eclampsia.
- Chronic NSAIDs use preoperatively. Inadvertent NSAIDs, COX-1 and COX-2 inhibitor use postoperatively, especially in patients with risk factors (high risk in diabetes).
- Intravascular volume reduction (dehydration, reduced cardiac output, cirrhosis, sepsis, etc.).
- Sepsis is a major risk, because of hypovolemia, hemodynamic instability and the effects of endotoxin and various cytokines on renal tubules.

- Risk is increased in sodium-depleted patients, those receiving concomitant diuretics and other nephrotoxic drugs.
- Multiple myeloma, acid base disturbance and hypoalbuminemia may increase risk as well.

How can renal function be preserved during the peri- and postoperative periods?

Most instances of the renal dysfunction in the perioperative period are due to lack of adequate fluid loading, less than adequate perfusion pressure or low cardiac output – the so-called prerenal failure. Less than adequate hydration can creep in on the patients insidiously and must be addressed as a first priority. The same is true of inadequate perfusion (blood) pressure and cardiac output. The following section addresses these issues, although the discussion is general, without elaborating each process for sake of brevity.

- There are no definitely proven strategies that prevent development of PORIF in the perioperative period or in the critically ill [42].
- A urine flow of at least $0.5 \, \mathrm{ml \, kg^{-1} \, h^{-1}}$ should be the clinical aim during and after surgery. Although there are no randomized controlled trials to suggest that this strategy prevents PORIF, it seems logical and also ensures that the patients are reasonably well hydrated.
- Adequate hydration: although specific evidence of the preventative benefits of hydration in PORIF is lacking, it seems logical that adequate hydration is the first step in ameliorating oliguria and the so-called prerenal failure. As has been pointed out above, fully functioning kidneys under normal (and even under abnormal) physiological conditions will preserve fluid in conditions of dehydration and low fluid states – this always manifests as oliguria (which does not necessarily mean PORIF or AKI).
- Evidence of the benefits of fluid resuscitation is seen daily in our clinical practice. However, the most definitive evidence is seen in studies involving radiocontrast media and CIN. One of the most important conclusions drawn from these studies is that precontrast hydration reduces the incidence of CIN.
- Fluid resuscitation expands intravascular volume, increases cardiac output, raises blood (hence perfusion) pressure, and improves oxygen delivery, all designed to improve renal perfusion, RBF and glomerular filtration, thus overcoming oliguria and prerenal failure.
- Central venous pressure (CVP) monitoring may well be adequate in routine surgery in monitoring fluid therapy, but it has its limitations. In complex patients and/or surgery, more invasive monitoring (e.g. a pulmonary artery catheter despite the controversy about its use, or other flow monitoring devices such as esophageal Doppler, transthoracic echocardiography, etc.) may be required.
- What fluid should be used to resuscitate the dehydrated or underperfused kidney? There is little evidence in the literature as to what fluid is ideal. The debate on colloids vs. crystalloids has not died yet neither has the debate given us any clear direction.
- Use of solutions containing large amounts of chloride (e.g. 0.9% saline) should be avoided in excessive amounts. Hyperchloremia causes metabolic acidosis and increases metabolic load and oxygen requirement of the underperfused renal tubular cells. There are also some data indicating that saline-based fluids in both man and experimental animals may

adversely affect renal function [43, 44]. Studies in dogs have shown that a raised serum chloride can reduce renal blood flow, GFR, and urine formation [45].

- Bennett-Guerrero and colleagues examined the results of different infusion solutions in 200 patients undergoing coronary artery bypass grafting (namely 5% albumin in saline; 6% hetastarch in saline; Hextend, a colloid and compound sodium lactate) on the serum creatinine at 1 week postsurgery. The highest postoperative plasma creatinine concentrations were seen in the albumin and hetastarch groups (both made up in saline); furthermore, six patients needed postoperative hemodialysis – again all six had received saline-based solution [46].

- Volume expansion, avoiding operations shortly after angiography, and using low-osmolality contrast media are suggested interventions that reduce CIN [47].

- Avoiding nephrotoxins in perioperative periods in patients at risk cannot be overemphasized. Clinicians should be aware that nephrotoxin use in the perioperative period can creep upon their patients by zealous but well-intentioned desire to provide pain relief (e.g. use of NSAIDs for pain relief in a patient who has just had an angiographic procedure).

Preserving renal function with pharmacological agents: what works and what does not?

Every day in their clinical practice, anesthetists and intensivists face kidney dysfunction, PORIF or AKI in their patients. It is every clinician's endeavor to keep urine flowing! To this end, various renal protective strategies are used. Unfortunately, these protective strategies are mostly based on anecdotes, opinion, tradition and animal experiments that have no relationship to clinical situations. Smaller, double-blind randomized controlled trials favor various strategies; however, convincing evidence that one strategy is superior to another or indeed any strategy works at all is lacking. There has always been a crusade to find a simple, single pharmacological magic bullet for prevention of AKI; unfortunately, this penicillin of AKI has eluded us thus far.

- Many pharmacological agents have been used to either prevent or ameliorate established PORIF/AKI.

- In this regard agents like furosemide, low-dose dopamine, dopexamine, mannitol and other newer agents have all been tried.

Dopamine

- Low-dose dopamine stimulates DA-1 and DA-2 receptors causing renal arteriolar vasodilatation and increase in RBF. This has been clearly demonstrated in well-hydrated animals (rats) and healthy human volunteers. It also inhibits proximal tubular sodium re-absorption thus causing natriuresis [48, 49]. Higher doses stimulate α- and β-adrenergic receptors and increase cardiac output and systemic vascular resistance.

- On the basis of these hemodynamic and diuretic effects on animals and normal humans it has always been thought that low (renal) dose dopamine affords considerable protective effects in patients at risk of AKI [50]. This view still prevails widely.

- Two large, multi-center randomized controlled trials in patients with early signs of renal dysfunction failed to show any beneficial effect on prevention or outcome [51, 52].

- More than 200 articles, 60 studies, 17 randomized controlled trials, many meta-analyses, reviews and one Cochrane Systematic Review have been performed since 1966. None of them show any benefit of low or 'renal' dose dopamine in either prevention of AKI/ PORIF or amelioration after AKI/PORIF has set in [42, 53].

- By causing diuresis, low-dose dopamine may worsen hypovolemia as well as increase metabolic load on the mTAL segment of the nephron due to its natriuretic effect. Thus low-dose dopamine may worsen kidney injury in certain situations.

- Besides the lack of proven beneficial effects on failing renal function or in prevention of AKI, dopamine in low doses has some adverse effects of its own. Dopamine is prone to cause arrhythmias, has some undesirable neuroendocrine effects, and preferentially increases renal cortical blood flow without enhancing renal medullary blood flow [54].

- Low-dose dopamine has also been found to have a direct adverse effect on renal vascular resistance (RVR). Whereas low-dose dopamine reduces RVR in the normal kidney, it has the opposite effect in a dysfunctioning kidney, thus causing worsening hemodynamics in the very situation it is thought to be useful in [55].

There is strong evidence in the literature that low or renal dose dopamine has no beneficial effect in either preventing or treating PORIF/AKI. Instead there seems to be potential for harm in that the kidney function may worsen with this strategy.

Furosemide

- Furosemide is the commonest drug used to prevent PORIF/AKI, increase urine output, convert oliguria into polyuria and to treat these conditions.

- Furosemide reduces sodium absorption by the renal tubule at mTAL level, thus reducing tubular oxygen consumption and increasing urine output.

- Increases in urine output may dislodge tubular obstruction and augment RBF. It also induces cyclo-oxygenases and thereby increases release of vasodilatory prostaglandins [56].

- Furosemide may also cause COX-2 inhibition, which in turn inhibits TNF-induced apoptosis in tubular cells, especially in renal mesangial cell [57].

- Along with this it is thought that its use helps manage fluid balance in patients with failing or failed kidneys.

- Many studies with furosemide in at-risk patients and in those with established acute renal failure have failed to show any real benefit in terms of prevention of PORIF/AKI, need for reduced RRT, or reduced mortality. Besides this, studies in patients with AKI after cardiac surgery, CIN and other forms of AKI have been equally disappointing [58].

- Recent meta-analyses as well as other reviews have failed to show any tangible benefits from furosemide use in PORIF/AKI other than increased urine production [59, 60]. The latter study also showed that there was a tendency to increased mortality with the use of higher doses of furosemide, probably due to immunosuppression [60].

Mannitol

- Mannitol is an osmotic diuretic and has been used in various clinical situations to improve urine output and prevent kidney injury.

- It increases urine output, is a free-radical scavenger, induces dilatory prostaglandin synthesis and may thus improve RBF (as has been shown in animal studies).
- Along with sodium bicarbonate, it has been specifically recommended for prevention of AKI that accompanies rhabdomyolysis by promoting diuresis and "flushing myoglobin and preventing its precipitation in renal tubules" [61].
- Mannitol has also been recommended for prophylaxis in surgery in obstructive jaundice and major vascular surgery.
- Unfortunately, subsequent studies have shown that mannitol is of no benefit in AKI induced by rhabdomyolysis [62], obstructive jaundice [63], or major vascular surgery [64, 65].
- Mannitol can cause endothelial and epithelial cell apoptosis, hypernatremia, as well as hyperosmolar renal failure. Tubular cells also take up the osmotic agent molecules by pinocytosis and cause cellular damage, thus perpetuating renal injury and failure. Mannitol may also cause renal vasoconstriction [66] and if the diuretic response is small, volume expansion and hyponatremia may result [66].

Other pharmacological agents

Many other pharmacological agents have been tried in the hope of preventing AKI or treating emerging PORIF/AKI. However, there is little evidence that any of these agents work.

- Fenaldopam, another DA-1 agonist, causes natriuresis and increase in RBF and UO. The RBF increase is dose-dependent and linear and almost equally distributed to cortex and medulla. It is safe if infused peripherally, but causes hypotension and reflex tachycardia. In various studies with small numbers of patients, fenaldopam has been shown to be reno-protective in CIN [67, 68] and after CPB [69] and major vascular surgery [70].
- A recent meta-analysis of RCTs on the reno-protective effects of fenaldopam suggested that it affords renal protection in a variety of clinical situations, including PORIF/AKI [71]. However, the authors also state that the study qualities were substandard, and randomization was not obvious in many studies, most of which were underpowered.
- Other agents that have been tried are: atrial natriuretic peptide, calcium channel blockers, growth factors, N-acetylcysteine – all have shown varying degrees of success, but none have proven to be useful [42].
- Adenosine antagonists, endothelin inhibitors, modulators of complement system and NO, antioxidants and various other agents like dobutamine and dopexamine have been tried. None can be recommended as reno-protective in PORIF/AKI [66].

Managing PORIF/AKI in at-risk surgical patients

It is clear from the above discussion that there are few pharmacological means available to us to treat or prevent emerging PORIF. However, other steps can be taken to prevent or minimize its emergence. The following are acceptable strategies as preventative measures.

- The first step is to identify patients at risk. In this context, it has been found that pre-existing renal dysfunction is the single best predictor of PORIF/AKI. Thus identification of such patients cannot be overemphasized. Particularly at risk are diabetic patients scheduled for cardiac or major vascular surgery.

- In the UK, almost all chemical pathology laboratories report estimated GFR (eGFR) based on a simplified Modification of Diet in Renal Disease (MDRD) equation [72]. Although it does not accurately predict GFR in all patients, it is an indicator of existing renal dysfunction in the general population.

- As PORIF/AKI results from multiple factors, it is imperative to take note of factors causing PORIF and avoid them, especially in patients at risk.

- Thus, as an example, close proximity of angiographic studies and surgery should be avoided. If surgery cannot be avoided, then patients should be well-hydrated before the operation is begun.

- Other nephrotoxins should be avoided. Examples of this are nephrotoxic antibiotics, diuretics, combination of nephrotoxic antibiotics and diuretics, NSAIDs (even if used by patients before operation), hyperosmolar contrast media, etc.

- In all patients, but especially in patients at risk, renal (indeed whole body) perfusion should be optimized. For the kidney, this is mainly determined by cardiac output (CO), renal perfusion pressure (RPP), proportional to and dependent on mean arterial pressure (MAP), glomerular hemodynamics (primarily afferent and efferent arteriolar tone), cortico-medullary blood flow distribution, and renal tubular oxygen consumption.

- Fluid loading is of the utmost importance. As has been suggested above, there is no consensus agreement on the type of fluid that is better at preventing PORIF/AKI. However, excess use of 0.9% saline should be avoided as it causes metabolic acidosis due to narrowing of the strong ion difference (usually called hyperchloremic acidosis).

- Optimizing CO is essential. Poor CO means poor perfusion. There are various ways of assessing and improving CO in surgical patients; a detailed description of these techniques is outside the scope of this chapter. Suffice it to say that fluid resuscitation, inotropes and vasoactive drugs all have their place in appropriate situations. Clinicians should be cautious in using inotropes like dopamine, dobutamine and vasoactive drugs like metaraminol and norepinephrine unless they are sure that the patients are adequately fluid-loaded.

- MAP should be adequate for the patient; hypertensive patients may well require higher MAP to maintain adequate RPP. Remember, autoregulation of RBF may well be disrupted.

- Patients with established PORIF/AKI need monitoring and management in a critical care setting.

- Steps should be taken to establish the reversibility of AKI. This may include, but is not limited to, careful fluid challenges, optimization of cardiovascular status and MAP, stopping of all nephrotoxic drugs if at all possible (including low-dose dopamine, furosemide, etc.) and re-evaluation of the patient's clinical condition.

- Sepsis must be treated (if necessary by surgical drainage), and appropriate antibiotics started and fractures fixed and stabilized.

- In established AKI, renal replacement therapy (RRT) should be started without unnecessary delay; if necessary and depending on the institutional protocols, advice from nephrologists used to dealing with the critically ill should be sought.

- Detailed description of RRT specific to the critically ill is outside the scope of this chapter. Continuous forms of RRT (CRRT) are preferred in the UK. CRRT should be delivered by

193

health care workers familiar with the techniques and equipment management. Detailed standards for delivering CRRT in the critically ill have recently been described which contain up-to-date information [73].

Conclusions

Although anesthetic agents have little direct effect on renal function per se, surgery and anesthesia do affect renal function, especially in patients at risk. There are no definitely proven strategies or pharmacological agents that prevent PORIF/AKI in the perioperative period. Awareness of patients at risk going for surgery, avoiding the use of nephrotoxins if at all possible and good hemodynamic management along with adequate fluid loading are the key to prevention of PORIF/AKI. Such patients should be monitored in critical care areas. In established AKI, RRT may be required, which should be provided without undue delay in critical care settings.

References

1. http://www.dh.gov.uk/en/ Publicationsandstatistics/Publications/ PublicationsPolicyAndGuidance/ DH_077251 (accessed 3 November 2007).

2. Wagener G, Berntjens TE. Renal disease: The anesthesiologist's perspective. *Anesthesiol Clin* 2006; **24**: 523–47.

3. Thurau K, Boylan JW. Acute renal success. The unexpected logic of oliguria in acute renal failure. *Am J Med* 1976; **61**: 308–15.

4. Sadovnikoff N. Perioperative acute renal failure. *Int Anesthesiol Clin* 2001; **39**: 95–109.

5. Nolan C, Anderson R. Hospital-acquired acute renal failure. *J Am Soc Nephrol* 1998; **9**: 710–18.

6. Mehta RL, Chertow GM. Acute renal failure definitions and classification: Time for change? *J Am Soc Nephrol* 2003; **14**: 2178–87.

7. Farley SJ. Acute kidney injury/acute renal failure: Standardizing nomenclature, definitions and staging. *Nature Clin Pract Nephrol* 2007; **3**: 405.

8. Mori K, Nako K. Neutrophil gelatinase-associated lipocalin as the real-time indicator of active kidney damage. *Kidney Int* 2007; **71**: 967–70.

9. Devarajan P. Emerging biomarkers of acute kidney injury. *Contrib Nephrol* 2007; **156**: 203–12.

10. Chertow GM, Burdick E, Honour M, *et al.* Acute kidney injury, mortality, length of stay

and costs in hospitalized patients. *J Am Soc Nephrol* 2005; **16**: 3365–70.

11. Himmelfarb J, Ikizler TA. Acute kidney injury: Changing lexicography, definitions and epidemiology. *Kidney Int* 2007; **71**: 971–6.

12. Lassnigg A, Schmidlin D, Mouhieddine M, *et al.* Minimal changes of serum creatinine predict prognosis in patients after cardiac surgery: A prospective cohort study. *J Am Soc Nephrol* 2004; **15**: 1597–1605.

13. www.adqi.net (accessed 15 November 2007).

14. Bellomo R, Ronco C, Kellum JA, *et al.* Acute renal failure – definitions, outcome measures, animal models, fluid therapy and information technology needs: The Second International Consensus Conference of the Acute Dialysis Quality Initiative (ADQI) Group. *Crit Care* 2004; **8**: R204–10.

15. Ronco C, Levin A, Warnock DG, *et al.* Improving outcomes from acute kidney injury (AKI): Report on an initiative. *Int J Artif Org* 2007; **30**: 373–6.

16. Kishen R. Acute renal failure. In: McConachie I, ed. *Handbook of ICU Therapy*. London, Greenwich Media. 1999; 161–72.

17. Bellomo R, Bagshaw S, Langenberg C, *et al.* Pre-renal azotemia: A flawed paradigm in critically ill septic patients? *Contrib Nephrol* 2007; **156**: 1–9.

18. Rosen S, Heyman SN. Difficulties in understanding human acute tubular

necrosis: Limited data and flawed animal models. *Kidney Int* 200; **60**: 1220–4.

19. Di Giantomasso D, Morimatsu H, May CN, *et al.* Intra-renal blood flow distribution in hyperdynamic septic shock: Effect of norepinephrine. *Crit Care Med* 31: 2509–13.

20. Langenberg C, Bellomo R, May C. Renal blood flow in sepsis. *Crit Care* 2005; **9**: R363–74.

21. Solez K, Racusen C. Role of the renal biopsy in acute renal failure. *Contrib Nephrol* 2001; **132**: 68–75.

22. Sheridan AM, Bonventre JV. Pathophysiology of ischaemic acute renal failure. *Contrib Nephrol* 2001; **132**: 7–21.

23. Bock HA. Pathogenesis of acute renal failure: new aspects. *Nephron* 1997; **76**: 130–42.

24. Sladen RN, Endo E, Harrison T. Two-hour versus 22-hour creatinine clearance in critically ill patients. *Anesthesiology* 1987; **67**: 1013–16.

25. Cherry RA, Eachempati SR, Hydo L, *et al.* Accuracy of short-duration creatinine clearance determinations in predicting 24-hour creatinine clearance in critically ill and injured patients. *J Trauma* 2002; **53**: 267–71.

26. Mangano CM, Diamonstone LS, Ramsay JG, *et al.* Renal dysfunction after myocardial revascularisation: Risk factors, adverse outcomes and hospital utilisation. *Ann Intern Med* 1998; **128**: 194–203.

27. Conlon PJ, Stafford-Smith M, White WD, *et al.* Acute renal failure following cardiac surgery. *Nephrol Dial Transplant* 1999; **14**: 1158–62.

28. ICNARC – Case Mix Patients Database; November 2007 (1996–2006).

29. Mazze RI. Fluorinated anaesthetic nephrotoxicity: An update. *Can J Anaesthesia* 1984; **31**: S16–22.

30. Coco TJ, Klasner AE. Drug-induced rhabdomyolysis. *Curr Opin Paediatr* 2004; **16**: 206–10.

31. Akpek EA, Kayhan Z, Dönmez A, *et al.* Early postoperative renal function following renal transplant surgery: Effect of anaesthetic technique. *J Anesth* 2002; **16**: 114–18.

32. Haase M, Haase-Fielitz A, Bagshaw SM, *et al.* Cardio-pulmonary bypass-associated acute kidney injury: A pigment nephropathy? *Contrib Nephrol* 2007; **156**: 340–53.

33. Loef BG, Epema AH, Navis G, *et al.* Off-pump coronary revascularisation attenuates transient renal damage compared with on-pump coronary revascularisation. *Chest* 2002; **121**: 1190–4.

34. Tallgren M, Niemi T, Pöyhiä R, *et al.* Acute renal injury and dysfunction following elective abdominal aortic surgery. *Eur J Vasc Endovasc Surg* 2007; **33**: 550–5.

35. Braams R, Vossen V, Lisman BA, *et al.* Outcome in patients requiring renal replacement therapy after surgery for ruptured and non-ruptured aneurysm of the abdominal aorta. *Eur J Endovasc Surg* 1999; **18**: 323–7.

36. Kishen R. Drug-induced nephropathy and acute renal injury in the critically ill. In Nayyar V, Peter JV, Kishen R, Srinivas S, eds. *Critical Care Update 2006*. New Delhi, Jaypee Brothers. 2006; 68–75.

37. Thomsen HS, Morcos SK. Contrast media and the kidney: European Society of Urogenital Radiology (ESUR) guidelines. *Br J Radiol* 2003; **76**: 513–18.

38. Prendergast BD, George CF. Drug-induced rhabdomyolysis: Mechanisms and management. *Postgrad Med J* 1993; **69**: 333–6.

39. Thompson PD, Clarkson P, Karas R. Statin-associated myopathy. *JAMA* 2003; **289**: 1681–90.

40. Novis BK, Roizen MF, Aronson S, *et al.* Association of preoperative risk factors with postoperative renal failure. *Anesth Analg* 1994: **78**: 143–9.

41. Chertow GM, Lazarus JM, Christiansen CL, *et al.* Perioperative renal risk stratification. *Circulation* 1997; **95**: 878–84.

42. Zacharias M, Gilmore ICS, Herbison GP, *et al.* Interventions for protecting renal function in the perioperative period. *Cochrane Database of Systematic Reviews* 2005, Issue 3. Art. No.: CD003590. DOI: 10.1002/14651858.CD003590.pub2.

43. Wilkes NJ, Woolf R, Mutch M, *et al.* The effects of balanced versus

saline-based hetastarch and crystalloid solutions on acid–base and electrolyte status and gastric mucosal perfusion in elderly surgical patients. *Anesth Analg* 2001; **93**: 811–16.

44. Wilcox CS. Regulation of renal blood flow by plasma chloride. *J Clin Invest* 1983; **71**: 726–35.

45. Heidemann HT, Jackson EK, Gerkens JF, *et al.* Intrarenal hypertonic saline infusions in dogs with thoracic caval constriction. *Kidney Int* 1987; **32**: 488–92.

46. Bennett-Guerrero E, Frumento RJ, Mets B, *et al.* Impact of normal saline based versus balanced-salt intravenous fluid replacement on clinical outcomes: A randomized blinded clinical trial. *Anesthesiology* 2001; **95**: A147.

47. Solomon R, Deray G. How to prevent contrast-induced nephropathy and manage risk patients: Practical recommendations. *Kidney Int* 2006; **69**(Suppl 100): S51–3.

48. McDonald R, Goldberg I, McNay J, *et al.* Effects of dopamine in man: Augmentation of sodium excretion, glomerular filtration rate and renal plasma flow. *J Clin Invest* 1964; **43**: 1116–24.

49. Hollenberg MK, Adams DF, Mendall P, *et al.* Renal vascular responses to dopamine: Haemodynamic and angiographic observations in normal man. *Clin Sci* 1973; **45**: 733–42.

50. Cuthbertson BH, Noble DW. Dopamine in oliguria. *Br Med J* 1997; **314**: 690–1.

51. Chertow GM, Sayegh MH, Allgern RL, *et al.* Is the administration of dopamine associated with adverse or favourable outcome in acute renal failure? Auriculin Anaritide Acute Renal Failure Study Group. *Am J Med* 1996; **101**: 49–53.

52. Bellomo R, Chapman M, Finer S, *et al.* Low dose dopamine in patients with early renal dysfunction: A placebo-controlled randomised trial. Australian and New Zealand Intensive Care Society (ANZICS) Clinical Trials Group. *Lancet* 2000; **356**: 2139–43.

53. Kellum JA. Use of dopamine in acute renal failure: A meta-analysis. *Crit Care Med* 2001; **29**: 1526–31.

54. Tang IY. Prevention of perioperative acute renal failure: What works? *Best Pract Res Clin Anaesthesiol* 2004; **18**: 91–111.

55. Lauschke A, Teichgräber MA, Frei U, *et al.* "Low-dose" dopamine worsens renal perfusion in patients with acute renal failure. *Kidney Int* 2006; **69**: 1669–74.

56. Liguori A, Casini A, Di Loreto M, *et al.* Loop diuretics enhance the secretion of prostacyclin in vitro, in healthy persons, and in patients with chronic heart failure. *Eur J Clin Pharmacol* 1999; **55**: 117–24.

57. Ishaque A, Dunn MJ, Sorokin A. Cyclooxygenase-2 inhibits tumour necrosis alpha-mediated apoptosis in renal glomerular mesangial cells. *J Biol Chem* 2003; **278**: 10 629–40.

58. Schetz M. Should we use diuretics in acute renal failure? *Best Pract Res Clin Anaesthesiol* 2004; **18**: 75–89.

59. Ho KM, Sheridan DJ. Meta-analysis of frusemide to prevent or treat acute renal failure. *Br Med J* 2006; **333**: 420–3.

60. Sampath S, Moran JL, Graham PL, *et al.* The efficacy of loop diuretics in acute renal failure: Assessment using Bayesian evidence synthesis techniques. *Crit Care Med* 2007; **35**: 2516–24.

61. Better OS, Rubinstein I. Management of shock and acute renal failure in casualties suffering from the crush syndrome. *Renal Failure* 1997; **19**: 647–53.

62. Homsi E, Barreiro MF, Orlando JM, *et al.* Prophylaxis of acute renal failure in patients with rhabdomyolysis. *Renal Fail* 1997; **19**: 283–8.

63. Gubern JM, Sancho JJ, Simo J, *et al.* A randomized trial on the effect of mannitol on postoperative renal function in patients with obstructive jaundice. *Surgery* 1988; **103**: 39–44.

64. Pass LJ, Eberhart RC, Brown JC, *et al.* The effect of mannitol and dopamine on the renal response to thoracic aortic cross-clamping. *J Thor Cardiovasc Surg* 1988; **95**: 608–12.

65. Baker AB, Lloyd G, Fraser TA, *et al.* Retrospective review of 100 cases of endoluminal aortic stent-graft surgery from

an anaesthetic perspective. *Anaesth Intens Care* 1997; **25**: 378–84.

66. Jarnberg P-O. Renal protection strategies in the perioperative period. *Best Pract Res Clin Anaesthesiol* 2004; **18**: 645–60.

67. Tumlin JA, Wang A, Murray PT, *et al.* Fenaldopam mesylate blocks reduction in renal plasma flow after radiocontrast dye infusion: A pilot trial in the prevention of contrast nephropathy. *Am Heart J* 2002; **143**: 894–903.

68. Kini AS, Mitre CE, Kamran M, *et al.* Changing trends in incidence and predictors of radiographic contrast nephropathy after percutaneous coronary intervention with use of fenaldopam. *Am J Cardiol* 2002; **89**: 999–1002.

69. Halpenny M, Lakshmi S, O'Donnell A, *et al.* Fenaldopam: Renal and splanchnic effects in patients undergoing coronary artery bypass grafting. *Anaesthesia* 2001; **56**: 953–60.

70. Halpenny M, Rushe C, Breen P, *et al.* The effect of fenaldopam on renal function in patients undergoing elective aortic surgery. *Eur J Anaesthesiol* 2002; **19**: 32–9.

71. Landoni G, Biondi-Zoccai GG, Tumlin JA, *et al.* Beneficial effects of fenaldopam in critically ill patients with or at risk for acute renal failure: A meta-analysis of randomised clinical trials. *Am J Kidney Dis* 2007; **49**: 56–68.

72. Levey A, Greene T, Kusek J, Beck G, MDRD Study Group. A simplified equation to predict glomerular filtration rate from serum creatinine. *J Am Soc Nephrol* 2000; **11**: A0828.

73. Kishen R, Blakeley S, Bray K. Intensive Care Society – Standards for renal replacement therapy. Available at: http://www.ics.ac.uk/icmprof/standards.asp?menuid=7 (accessed 16 November 2007).

The critically ill patient undergoing surgery

I. McConachie

Anesthetic management of the critically ill patient who requires operative intervention remains a significant challenge and source of anesthetic mortality. The goal of the anesthetist has always been to facilitate surgery (which is often potentially life-saving) in these patients but, in addition, choices and techniques chosen by the anesthetist may have a significant effect on long-term outcome. This chapter will also review selected aspects of anesthesia for the high-risk patient with relevance to the critically ill patient.

Source

Critically ill patients present to the anesthetist from three main areas within the hospital.

1. The Emergency Department
   Victims of major trauma requiring immediate operative intervention fall into two categories.

   - Major hemorrhage of any source that cannot be controlled by simple resuscitative measures such as pressure dressing and splinting may transfer to the operating room (OR) while active fluid resuscitation is ongoing.

   - Patients with traumatic intracranial hemorrhage resulting in increased intracranial pressure will need urgent decompression if they are to avoid medullary "coning". Again such patients may require operative intervention prior to instituting full resuscitative measures.

   Patients presenting with acute general surgical pathology of a nontraumatic nature may occasionally proceed from the emergency department straight to the OR; however, it is more likely that there will be time for some degree of resuscitation and investigation on the general ward or ICU prior to surgery.

2. The general hospital
   Patients who have already been admitted to the general hospital may deteriorate during the course of their management. This may necessitate a more precipitous trip to the operating theater than had originally been anticipated. It is, however, likely that a degree of resuscitative intervention will already have occurred.

3. The Intensive Care Unit
   This group of patients have the advantage to the anesthetist that, provided they have spent a number of hours on the unit, they are most likely to have all resuscitative measures in place. Mechanical ventilation has usually been instituted, together with invasive lines for both monitoring and the administration of drugs and fluid.

   Clearly the corollary of this situation is that this group of patients may be profoundly "sick" and receiving multi-system support on the intensive care unit, support that should ideally continue during any trip to the operating room.

Anesthesia for the High Risk Patient, ed. I. McConachie. Published by Cambridge University Press.
© Cambridge University Press 2009.

Regardless of the source of both patient and surgical pathology, the issues and principles of anesthesia surrounding any operative procedure remain the same. The individual patient and his or her pathology merely alter the emphasis.

The remainder of this chapter will consider these principles in some detail.

The patient with multiple injuries

- Traumatic injury is the leading cause of death under the age of 40 and the third leading cause overall.
- Many patients are intoxicated.
- Injuries are often multi-system in nature.

Deaths from trauma follow a trimodal distribution.

- Immediate deaths in the first minutes at the scene are either due to massive hemorrhage or crush injuries, massive CNS trauma or (potentially avoidable) airway obstruction.
- Early deaths are often due to the effects of hemorrhage or hypoxia and may be preventable.
- Late deaths are chiefly due to sepsis and organ failures. Many of these may be preventable by prompt recognition of injuries and their physiological significance and definitive intervention.

Assessment of the trauma patient

- A system for evaluation of trauma victims results in faster, more effective resuscitation, fewer life-threatening injuries missed, and a greater appreciation of priorities.
- The Advanced Trauma Life Support system, as promoted by the American College of Surgeons since 1979, is one such system which has gained widespread acceptance.
- Assessment, diagnosis and initial treatment should be carried out simultaneously.
- This is facilitated by a team approach with a "team leader".
- The patient needs to be completely undressed and examined thoroughly as blunt, high-velocity injury can result in injury to virtually any part of the body.
- The first priorities are to detect and treat immediately life-threatening conditions while second priorities are to detect other injuries (none should be missed).
- Radiological investigations should not take priority over resuscitation.
- Relevant senior specialists should be involved at an early stage.
- The abdomen should be evaluated. Peritoneal lavage may be performed where doubt exists regarding the presence of an intra-abdominal injury. Abdominal ultrasound or CT scanning have their advocates.
- One must not forget to administer appropriate antibiotics and tetanus toxoid.
- All dislocations and fractures should be splinted and reduced if possible. This eases nursing, reduces pain and bleeding, and may reduce the incidence of Acute Respiratory Distress Syndrome (ARDS).

Airway and cervical spine protection

- The airway must be clear or permanent neurological damage or death may occur within minutes.

- The cervical spine should be assumed to be at risk and protected from further damage until proven by radiological screening to be intact. A hard cervical collar is mandatory.
- Unless immediate intubation is required, the cervical spine should be assessed by adequate radiological views of all seven cervical vertebrae. One should look for:
  - normal soft tissue shadows,
  - normal vertebral alignment, and
  - normal cervical lordosis.
- Cervical spine injuries are not uncommon in multiply-injured patients and may be missed, or the radiography misinterpreted.
- If intubation is required, the technique of choice is preoxygenation followed by oral intubation with manual in-line stabilization of the cervical spine by an assistant. Cricoid force to reduce the risk of aspiration of stomach contents should be applied (cricoid force controversies are discussed in Chapter 18).
- It is difficult to find good evidence that this technique, properly performed, has resulted in additional neurological impairment in any trauma patient with cervical spine injury. Neurological signs should be documented before intubation, if possible.
- If the patient cannot be intubated then a surgical airway should be created.

Breathing/ventilation

- High-flow O_2 should be administered to all patients.
- Clinically obvious pneumothoraces should be drained.
- There should be a low threshold for immediate tracheal intubation on clinical grounds – even before the result of arterial blood gases.
- Indications for immediate intubation and ventilation include gross respiratory distress, obvious hypoventilation and severe shock.
- Delayed ventilation by promoting tissue hypoxia results in an increased incidence of organ failures.

Circulation

- External hemorrhage must be controlled.
- Large bore catheters ×2 are inserted and volume infused.
- All multiply injured patients should have large volumes of warmed IV fluids, administered quickly (see below for more detail on fluid therapy).
- One is far more likely to run into problems of inadequate infusion than problems of excess infusion. The concept of permissive hypovolemia for trauma patients is discussed later in this chapter.
- As soon as possible, blood should be sent for blood gases and cross-matching.

Operative intervention in the trauma patient

- Many trauma patients will need surgery.

- In general, all the required surgical procedures should be performed acutely, i.e. during one anesthetic, providing the patient has been appropriately resuscitated and is hemodynamically stable.

- The rationale is that, once the patient is resuscitated, the patient may be in the best condition that he will be in for some time, i.e. before the development of sepsis, tissue edema, malnutrition and metabolic complications.

- Delayed fixation of long bone fractures may increase the incidence of ARDS [1]. The mechanisms are uncertain, but probably include ongoing bleeding, increased pain and physiological stress response and possible fat embolus.

- Conversely, if the patient undergoing surgery *is* unstable, with developing hypothermia, coagulopathy and acidosis, prolonged surgery has a high mortality. Many surgeons now accept that the best way to manage these patients is to "bail out", e.g. pack the abdomen to stop bleeding, bring out bowel ends on to the abdominal wall, etc., and take the patient to ICU for stabilization and further resuscitation. Further surgical intervention is deferred to a later date. This has been described as "damage control surgery" [2].

- Blood clots, packing the abdomen, ileus and tissue edema all, however, contribute to the development of an abdominal compartment syndrome where the increase in pressure literally squeezes the kidney. This causes a reduction in renal blood flow, GFR, direct compression of the renal parenchyma and increased release of ADH and aldosterone from stimulation of abdominal wall stretch receptors. In general, intra-abdominal pressures of 15–20 mmHg are associated with oliguria, while pressures greater than 30 mmHg may be associated with anuria. Interestingly, the use of large volumes of fluids in an attempt to achieve supranormal resuscitation goals has been shown to be associated with an increased incidence of abdominal compartment syndrome [3]. This variant of abdominal compartment syndrome has been called secondary compartment syndrome.

Management of the critically ill or injured patient in the OR

Patient transfer to and from the OR

The safe transfer of any patient within a hospital requires organization and planning. Even the most urgent of transfers to the OR must not be undertaken until all steps to ensure that the patient will not be harmed by the transfer have been addressed. One needs to guard against complacency because one is "only going down the corridor".

The principles of safe patient transfer are the same regardless of the distance involved. There are a number of texts devoted to this topic. The Association of Anaesthetists of Great Britain and Ireland and the Intensive Care Society have published guidelines for safe patient transfer (see further reading). These include the following.

- The patient's airway must be adequately secured.

- Ventilation must be adequate, either spontaneous or mechanical. It has been shown that manual ventilation with a bag is unpredictable and unreliable compared with a portable mechanical ventilator. Ventilate with the same modes as in ICU. Modern portable ventilators can supply PEEP and vary the I:E ratio.

- Lifting of patients on and off stretchers is a cause of inadvertant extubation. It is probably safest to temporarily disconnect the ventilator for a few seconds during movement.

- Blood pressure must be maintained with a combination of fluids and inotropic agents. Stabilize patient before transfer, if possible.
- Patient monitoring must be appropriate to ensure safe transfer.
- Consideration should be given to pharmacological sedation and muscle relaxation as indicated by the clinical condition.
- Communication between transferring and receiving staff should ensure safe receipt of the patient.
- One must avoid last-minute panic and rush. Planning should be such as to minimize delays and waiting in OR reception areas. Check the availability of equipment in the X-ray department before the transfer commences. Check that adequate porter services are available.
- Appropriate equipment required during the transfer includes a portable ventilator, full oxygen cylinder, equipment for reintubation, drugs – e.g. sedation, paralysis, cardiac resuscitation, self-inflating bag or equivalent in the event of ventilator/oxygen supply failure and battery-powered syringe pumps if required. There is no excuse for battery-powered equipment becoming exhausted, oxygen cylinders emptying or drug syringes running out.

Pitfalls and problems
- Inadequate resuscitation. Beware of occult injuries in multiple-trauma patients.
- Staff and equipment problems. Inexperienced medical or nursing staff should not be used for transferring critically ill patients.
- Appropriate technical support should be available and take responsibility for the necessary equipment.
- Transfer of ventilated patients out of the ICU has been shown to increase those patient's risk of developing nosocomial pneumonia [4], and increased infection surveillance and preventative strategies (out of the scope of this chapter) may be warranted postoperatively.

As important as ensuring the safety of the patient to be transferred is the importance of not delaying the transfer to the OR by undertaking procedures that can be performed later during the operation. For example, if a patient is exsanguinating and needs a laparotomy for abdominal trauma, there is little to be gained by spending time in the Emergency department inserting an arterial line. This procedure can be performed during the laparotomy when the surgeon has begun to effect hemostasis. There is no merit in delivering a corpse with an arterial line to the operating table.

Patient positioning

When positioning the critically ill patient there are a number of points that merit emphasis.

- The number of lines, tubes and bags increases with the severity of the patient's condition. Every piece of equipment inserted into the patient is there for a reason (or time should not have been wasted inserting it) and it therefore must be accessible during an operative procedure.
- Patients who have come to OR as a result of trauma may well not have had a full primary and secondary survey (as the operative procedure may constitute "C" of the primary survey). In such cases it is vital that the presence of as yet undiagnosed fractures to any

part of the spine is taken into account when moving and positioning the patient. In particular, the cervical spine should stay fixed with head blocks and strapping and the patient should not be moved without a formal log-rolling technique being used.

- Patients who have been critically ill on the ICU and have a significant sequestration of fluid into the extra-vascular compartments will have edematous skin that is weakened and is prone to tearing, bruising and vulnerable to pressure injury. Every effort should be made to minimize any damage done to the skin in such cases by providing adequate support and padding to the patient's exposed extremities.

Perioperative hypothermia

Maintenance of body temperature is important. Although there is some limited evidence that heat generation may occur following certain types of acute injury, it is far more common for the traumatized patient to present to the OR cold and peripherally "shut down". The reasons for this are as follows.

- Following acute blood loss the cardiovascular response is profound peripheral vaso-constriction resulting in maintained perfusion of vital organs, brain, heart, lungs and kidneys at the expense of other vascular beds.
- During acute traumatic injury, central mechanisms of thermoregulation are disrupted. Thus shivering is diminished or absent. Whether this is secondary to reduced oxygen delivery or a response to altered hormonal activity in the thermoregulatory center in the brain stem is unclear.
- In order to fully assess the extent of injury in the traumatized patient, it is necessary to remove clothing and leave the patient exposed during repeated examination. This is compounded by the infusion of unwarmed intravenous fluid and blood worsening the relative hypothermia.

In addition to the above problems in trauma patients, all patients undergoing major surgery are at risk of becoming hypothermic (core temperature $< 36°C$). Reasons include:

- reduced metabolic rate associated with anesthesia,
- vasodilation under anesthesia,
- abolished subclinical shivering,
- exposure,
- cold fluids used for skin preparation – which are usually allowed to evaporate,
- inadequately warmed IV fluids.

Adverse effects of perioperative hypothermia
Postoperative hypothermia has become recognized in recent years as a significant, and common, problem.

- Delayed awakening due to decreased clearance of anesthetic agents.
- Most organ function is depressed by hypothermia.
- Hemodynamic instability during rewarming – increased fluids often needed as the patient vasodilates during rewarming. The hypotension thus produced can be confused with continued bleeding.

- Oxygen consumption is increased by about 140% by shivering during rewarming. If oxygen delivery to the tissues is not able to match this increase, the oxygen debt is prolonged.
- Wound infection rates may be increased by reductions in skin blood flow.
- Cell-mediated immune function may be reduced.
- Hypothermia causes coagulopathy and a decrease in platelet count. Intra- and post-operative blood loss is increased with hypothermia; for example, the typical decrease in core temperature during hip replacement significantly increases blood loss [5]. Normalization of clotting problems may require normalization of temperature as well as giving clotting factors.
- Adrenergic responses are increased postoperatively in hypothermic patients – responsible for increased cardiac morbidity. There is a 55% less relative risk of adverse cardiac events when normothermia is maintained [6]. Unintentional hypothermia is associated with increased incidence of myocardial ischemia in the postoperative period.

Note:

1. The degree of hypothermia in many of the studies cited was not that severe – 35°C. Thus, development of hypothermia after prolonged surgery is highly significant and warrants serious attention to its prevention and mangagement.
2. Laboratories perform coagulation studies at 37°C – regardless of the temperature of the patient at the time the sample was taken. Thus, these studies may underestimate the degree of impairment of coagulopathy in the hypothermic patient – what is, after all, a dynamic problem in vivo rather than in vitro.

Prevention of hypothermia

All practical measures should be undertaken to minimize heat loss and maintain the patient's body temperature.

- Circle system ventilation with carbon dioxide absorber and heat and moisture exchanger in the patient circuit.
- Fluid warmer for all intravenous fluids.
- Warmed patient mattress.
- Insulation of all areas of the patient that do not need to be exposed for either surgical or anesthetic access.
- Use of a forced air warming system.
- Use of heat-retaining insulating materials is less effective at maintaining patient temperatures than forced air warming systems [7] which add energy to the system.

Ventilation and airway management

Most critically ill patients presenting to the OR will already have some form of definitive airway control in place. Under most circumstances it would be prudent to leave this airway alone for fear of losing control in a patient who may have acquired abnormalities with their airway due to tissue swelling or trauma. If the airway is not secure, one should assume a full stomach and take appropriate precautions – and assume a cervical spine injury in all trauma patients.

Under certain circumstances it is appropriate to use the trip to the OR as an opportunity to alter airway management. For example, patients who require ventilation on the ICU for an extended period may benefit from the insertion of a tracheostomy. Although it is often possible to do this via the percutaneous route in the ICU, on occasions where technical difficulties preclude this it may be possible to combine an operative event in the OR with insertion of a tracheostomy, thus limiting patient transfers.

Ventilation of the critically ill patient should always be controlled using appropriate drugs for anesthesia and muscle relaxation. There is no place for spontaneous ventilation because the patient's work of breathing is usually increased, causing "rapid, shallow breathing" which will result in the development of atelectasis.

Where possible, the ventilatory strategy undertaken should attempt to avoid volutrauma and barotrauma, both of which may serve to worsen any degree of ARDS from which the patient may be suffering. Ideally the mode of ventilation in the OR and, indeed, in transit to and from the ICU or emergency department should be of the same standard as can be delivered in the ICU. Pressure control ventilation with the ability to alter (reverse) the inspiratory:expiratory ratio and to apply positive end expiratory pressure (PEEP) is ideal. Lack of ongoing ventilation with PEEP and the other lung recruitment maneuvers taken in the ICU will result in loss of recruitment of alveoli and hypoxia.

Occasionally, to ensure minimal deterioration in respiratory physiology, it may be necessary to move a static ICU ventilator to the OR and ventilate the patient with it throughout the procedure. Under this circumstance it would be necessary to adopt a total intravenous anesthetic technique.

For some time now there has been a need for transport ventilators capable of delivering appropriate modes of gas delivery for critically ill patients. Recently a number of genuinely portable machines with these facilities have become available.

Practical points
Critically ill patients under anesthesia are different from "normal" patients.

- Most critically ill patients presenting for anesthesia have significant acute lung injury.

- Preoperative presence of increased pulmonary vascular resistance (PVR) is common in critically ill patients.

- Shallow breathing can increase PVR, partly by collapsing alveoli causing a reduction in the diameter of extra-alveolar pulmonary blood vessels, and partly by development of hypoxic pulmonary vasoconstriction. The worsening PVR exacerbates the development of hypoxia and acidosis, which further worsens PVR! Work of breathing is also increased.

- Any condition increasing work of breathing requires oxygen and energy. This requires increased blood flow and, in essence, the heart has to work harder. The potential for myocardial ischemia is present especially when there is associated tachycardia and hypoxemia.

- In critically ill patients, the usual presence of injured lungs with reduced compliance results in greater increases in peak and mean airway pressures compared to "normal" patients under anesthesia.

- In severe shock, the reduced blood flow to the diaphragm coupled with the increased minute volume and respiratory energy expenditure causes respiratory failure – even in normal lungs. This is convincingly demonstrated in animal studies, e.g. much of the lactic acid accumulating in shock comes from the respiratory muscles [8]. Controlled ventilation, by reducing the work of breathing, lessens the blood lactate levels compared with spontaneous breathing. Thus, controlling ventilation during anesthesia will be essential in the shocked patient.

- Many practitioners apply PEEP to anesthetized patients in the OR undergoing long surgery to attempt to minimize atelectasis. PEEP of 10 cm has been shown in one study to prevent intraoperative atelectasis even when high inspired oxygen concentrations are given [9].

- High ventilatory tidal volumes in the ICU have been shown to contribute to ventilator-induced lung injury (VILI) – chiefly due to release of inflammatory mediators from the injured lung. These mediators are not released during ventilation and anesthesia for high-risk surgery, implying that the healthy lung is less susceptible to the damaging effects of high tidal volumes [10].

- Nevertheless, many now recommend applying lung protective strategies (e.g. PEEP, low tidal volumes, low peak and plateau airway pressures, permissive hypercapnia) during anesthesia and ventilation of high-risk patients in the OR. A full discussion of this subject is beyond the scope of this chapter, but can be found in the review article by Schultz listed in Further reading.

- Decreased venous return and therefore decreased cardiac output with IPPV is the major hemodynamic effect of ventilation in most patients. As it is related to intrathoracic pressure (ITP) it is worse if the ventilator is set to provide either a high TV (high peak ITP) or a prolonged inspiratory time (high mean ITP). PEEP also exacerbates the fall in venous return.

- Venous return and cardiac output can be restored by either fluid infusion or sympathetic drugs, both of which restore the gradient for venous return despite further increases in RA pressure.

- With IPPV, the increased ITP decreases the gradient across the left ventricle that the left ventricle has to work against – one aspect of afterload. In other words, decreased transmural pressure decreases left ventricular afterload. Any beneficial effect on afterload in the normal heart is limited by the fall in venous return. In the failing heart, the cardiac output is relatively insensitive to changes in preload, but exquisitely sensitive to small reductions in afterload. Thus in patients with heart failure undergoing surgery there may be beneficial effects on cardiac output from increases in ITP with ventilation.

- Conversely, at the end of surgery, patients with failing hearts may deteriorate during attempts to rapidly wean off IPPV for extubation. This is as a result of increased LV afterload and increased venous return due to the fall in ITP with spontaneous ventilation and also the tachycardia, myocardial ischemia and release of catecholamines during spontaneous breathing and awakening.

- Therefore, patients with heart failure undergoing surgery may require a period of post-operative respiratory support and a more gentle return to spontaneous ventilation.

Inspired oxygen concentration

- High inspired oxygen concentrations may be required during anesthesia and surgery due to pulmonary pathology.

- Oxygen (100%) causes absorption atelectasis and other problems – even when given for brief periods at the end of surgery prior to awakening [11].

- Increased oxygen levels may worsen reperfusion injury following temporary ischemia.

- In animal models increased oxygen inspired concentrations prolong survival in hemorrhagic shock [12].

- High inspired oxygen levels may lead to a reduction in tachycardia postoperatively [13] and, more worryingly, a reduction in cardiac index [14]. The exact significance of this is unclear, especially where overall oxygen delivery to the tissues is maintained or even improved.

- Oxygen (100%) intraoperatively has been shown to improve alveolar macrophage function postoperatively [15]. Whether lesser increases in inspired oxygen will have similar effects is uncertain.

- High inspired oxygen concentrations perioperatively may have other benefits, e.g. possible reduction of wound infections after colonic surgery [16]. See Chapter 18.

Anesthetic agents

Every available technique and drug combination has been used to anesthetize the critically ill patient. To some extent the reader must distil his or her own technique. The way a drug is used, e.g. dose, speed of injection, etc., may be more important in many patients than the absolute choice of drug.

Notes on individual agents

Induction agents

1. Thiopental (thiopentone). A rapidly effective drug for the induction of general anesthesia. Many believe that thiopental is still the best choice of induction agent for rapid sequence induction for the purposes of securing the airway due to a slightly faster onset than, for example, propofol. Thiopental is the induction agent that most reduces the brain's metabolic requirement for oxygen and is hence neuroprotective. It produces depression of myocardial contractility together with vasodilatation resulting in a fall of blood pressure. It is noteworthy that in the hypovolemic or shocked patient the sleep dose of thiopental is greatly reduced as compared to the healthy patient.

2. Etomidate (carboxylated imidazole). Etomidate shares many common properties with other anesthetic induction agents – namely, a predictable, rapid onset of anesthesia, relatively short emergence time and falls in cerebral blood flow, cerebral metabolic rate and intracranial pressure. Cerebral perfusion pressure is usually maintained. Etomidate is discussed in detail later in this chapter.

3. Propofol (di-isopropyl phenol). Rapid onset (although a little slower than thiopentone) and obtunds pharyngeal and glottal reflexes to a greater extent than thiopentone. Widely used for total intravenous anesthesia and ICU sedation. The hypotension produced is chiefly secondary to vasodilation rather than myocardial depression.

4. Ketamine (phencyclidine derivative). Sympathomimetic effects maintain blood pressure, but the increases in HR and stroke volume increase myocardial work. Profoundly analgesic and an effective analgesic agent at subanesthetic doses. Despite its sympathomimetic effects, ketamine may cause cardiac depression, myocardial ischemia and collapse in shocked patients in whom catecholamine stores may be exhausted. Ketamine increases intracranial pressure and is usually considered contraindicated in head injuries. Animal studies have raised concerns that ketamine may have some neurotoxic effects due to its antagonism at the NMDA receptor [17].

   A novel combination of ketamine and propofol (nicknamed ketofol) has been used by physicians in some emergency departments and may be worth exploring further in the OR [18].

Opioids

1. Remifentanil. The cautious use of short-acting agents is important in critically ill patients unless, of course, postoperative ventilation is planned or anticipated. The shortest available is Remifentanil, which is metabolized by esterases. Remifentanil produces no postoperative analgesia and may increase postoperative pain by a process of acute tolerance at the opioid receptors or by sensitization at other pain receptors [19]. The lack of a postoperative effect of Remifentanil and its titratability cause many anesthetists to prefer its use for all high-risk patients. Of course, additional measures must be taken for postoperative analgesia, e.g. epidural anesthesia.

2. Fentanyl. Minimal effect on the cardiovascular system in the stable, calm, patient undergoing cardiac surgery. In shocked patients exhibiting high sympathetic tone, abolition of this with fentanyl results in a fall in BP.

3. Morphine should be used with great care in the critically ill patient as it has pharmacologically active metabolites and is reliant on the liver and kidneys for its elimination. Morphine is still a very useful drug for postoperative analgesia in the critically ill patient and is widely used for sedation of the postoperative ventilated patient.

Muscle relaxants

There are four main factors governing the choice of muscle relaxant for anesthesia.

1. Onset. All critically ill patients are assumed to have a full stomach. Despite recent introduction of faster onset nondepolarizing drugs such as Rocuronium, Succinylcholine (suxamethonium) remains the "gold standard" for rapidly securing the airway. If cardiac instability is a major concern, Rocuronium may be a better choice.

2. Cardiovascular effects. Rocuronium has the least cardiac effects of the relaxants followed by Vecuronium. However, the vagolytic and sympathomimetic effects of Pancuronium may make it an appropriate choice in shocked patients.

3. Termination of effect and excretion. Agents not dependent on the kidney or liver for termination of effect sound attractive in the critically ill patient, but from a practical point of view few critically ill patients are "reversed" at the end of the operation due to planned ongoing ventilatory support. Thus, an effect of reduced elimination of muscle relaxants is not a big problem.

4. Duration. In a similar manner, short or long duration is not usually an issue.

Inhalational agents

1. Enflurane – greatest degree of myocardial depression for equivalent MAC amongst all volatile agents. Limited use in many countries.

2. Sevoflurane – less increase in cerebral blood volume. Rapid onset and rapid recovery.

3. Halothane – rarely used nowadays. Long-acting with more active metabolites retained in the body than other volatile agents, with potential for liver toxicity. Sensitizes the heart to endogenous and exogenous catecholamines with the potential for arrhythmias.

4. Isoflurane – impressive safety profile in large numbers of patients. Hypotension chiefly by vasodilation rather than myocardial depression. Early concerns regarding coronary steal are unfounded in conventional usage.

5. Desflurane – specialized delivery systems required. Very short-acting. Some residual concerns regarding coronary steal.

6. Nitrous oxide (N_2O) – due to low blood gas solubility has very fast uptake and onset. Limited anesthetic efficacy due to low potency, but speeds uptake of other volatile agents due to second gas effect. In some countries its useful analgesic properties maintain its role in analgesia in the field when administered by paramedics for, for example, extrication of trauma patients. The longest history of any inhalational anesthetic still in routine usage in the western world, but under increasing scrutiny and controversy in recent years (see below).

Adverse effects of anesthesia

In addition to the usual adverse effects of anesthesia, the critically ill and high-risk surgical patient may be at additional risk from exposure to anesthesia.

- Anesthesia modifies the normal compensatory response to hypoxia in animals [20]. The normal compensatory increase in cerebral and coronary blood flow does not occur under volatile anesthesia. Thus, in the critically ill patient who becomes hypoxic, anesthesia potentially further compromises oxygenation of the vital organs.

- Again in animals, Enflurane attenuates the sympathetic responses to hemorrhage, resulting in worse hemodynamics than the nonanesthetized state [21].

Choice of anesthetic agent in the shocked patient

Controlled studies on shocked patients undergoing anesthesia are problematic due to:

- differences in severity of injury or shock,
- differences in fluids administered,
- adequacy of resuscitation prior to surgery,
- hemodynamic state and degree of cardiovascular support, and
- previous health, most notably cardiac reserve.

Thus one must take guidance from basic anesthetic and pharmacological principles including guidance from the notes summarized above. In addition, studies on animal models are available, case studies and series may be of interest, and there are reports on the use of anesthesia in military situations.

A major dilemma is how to provide any anesthesia for the profoundly shocked patient. Thiopental is said, almost certainly incorrectly [22], to have killed more Americans at Pearl Harbor than the Japanese! Many patients suffering from an exsanguinating injury may be so "shocked" as to be thought to not require or be able to tolerate any anesthetic administration. While the intent to save life in this situation is laudable, the absence of recordable blood pressure *does not guarantee lack of awareness*. It is strongly recommended that, at the very least, small amounts of midazolam are given to the patient, as this will reduce the incidence of recall [23]. As the patient's condition improves, e.g. as hemorrhage is controlled, judicious amounts of opioids and other anesthetic agents may be introduced.

Ketamine may be a useful option in the above circumstances, but the profoundly shocked patient whose endogenous catecholamine stores have been exhausted may still suffer profound falls in blood pressure on induction. Indeed, ketamine has negative inotropic effects on human heart muscle in vitro and reduces the heart's ability to respond to β stimulation.

There are some animal studies to guide choice of anesthesia in the shocked patient.

- Ketamine was associated with significantly increased survival compared with other agents in a model of hemorrhagic shock [24]. In that study the animals anesthetized with ketamine had better preservation of cell structure in the splanchnic organs.

- Ketamine was associated with increased cardiac output compared to thiopental in another animal hemorrhagic shock model [25]. Vital organ blood flow was also improved in the ketamine group. The percentage of blood volume loss required to cause significant hypotension was significantly less in the thiopental group. In critically ill patients the use of ketamine is more unpredictable.

- Hemorrhagic shock alters the pharmacokinetics and pharmacodynamics of propofol [26], suggesting that less propofol is required to achieve its desired effect in hemorrhagic shock.

- Conversely, animal studies suggest minimal adjustment in the dose of etomidate [27] to achieve the same drug effect in hemorrhagic shock.

- Hemorrhagic shock altered the pharmacokinetics of remifentanil [28], suggesting that less remifentanil would be required to maintain a target plasma concentration. However, due to its rapid metabolism, hemorrhagic shock does not result in accumulation of remifentanil during infusion.

Choice of anesthetic agent in the septic patient

There are no controlled studies of septic patients from the ICU undergoing surgery in the OR. What guidance is available comes from case reports and animal studies.

- The sympathetic stimulation associated with the use of ketamine may result in improved hemodynamics, diuresis and reduction in the degree of cardiovascular support required in patients with septic shock [29].

- In animals with septic shock, volatile agents are associated with increases in serum lactate, while ketamine was associated with reductions in lactate. Ketamine preserved SVR and blood pressure best [30]. To summarize a complex paper, ketamine best preserved cardiac function and tissue oxygenation.

- Isoflurane resulted in less cytokine release in septic mice compared with pentobarbital-anesthetized mice [31].

- Ketamine directly suppresses proinflammatory cytokine production [32].

- An in vitro study demonstrated that ketamine suppressed cytokine production in human whole blood [33].

- The beneficial effect of even low-dose ketamine on cytokine function has been shown in patients to persist into the postoperative period [34]. Thus ketamine may be of value in preventing immune function alterations in the early postoperative period.

- Many anesthetists have experience of continuing propofol sedation from ICU into the OR. Propofol, after endotoxin injection, reduced the mortality rate of rats and attenuated their cytokine responses [35]. These findings suggest that propofol administration may be beneficial during sepsis.

- The beneficial effects of propofol treatment may, in part, be due to reductions in the overproduction of nitric oxide in sepsis [36].

- Sevoflurane pretreatment decreased mortality rate, severity of hypotension, and acidosis, and inhibited cytokine responses in rats injected with endotoxin, suggesting that sevoflurane may also be an appropriate anesthetic choice in sepsis [37].

It seems that most anesthetic agents have potentially beneficial effects on the inflammatory response to sepsis and could be recommended for the septic patient – assuming that clinical studies corroborate these findings. Hemodynamic effects may favor ketamine over volatile agents.

Thus, animal studies and case reports support the use of ketamine in shocked and septic patients undergoing anesthesia, but caution is still advised. Falls in blood pressure and cardiac output may still occur. Unfortunately there is a shortage of convincing comparative patient studies, and the above animal studies are not necessarily directly transferable into clinical practice. Most anesthetists use the techniques they are most familiar with, either total intravenous anesthesia or inhalational anesthesia, for the critically ill patient in the OR. Few have much experience of ketamine. Therefore, despite its strong theoretical advantages it is not commonly used. Further clinical studies in this patient group are urgently needed.

The etomidate controversy

Although not widely used for routine anesthesia, many believe etomidate's properties enable it to occupy a specific niche in anesthetic practice for the high-risk and critically ill patient. Its use by nonanesthetists, e.g. in the emergency department in many countries, seems to be expanding and this, and its unique properties, have resulted in renewed interest (and controversy) in recent years.

The chief advantageous property of etomidate is its remarkable cardiovascular stability, even in patients with cardiac disease. However, other properties of etomidate are not so desirable: namely, adrenal suppression, pain and thrombophlebitis and myoclonus.

Etomidate hemodynamics

- Careful recent studies suggest that (at least in vitro) the effects of different induction agents on the heart are less different than previously believed. In isolated human atrial muscle, no significant inhibition of cardiac contractility is produced by propofol, midazolam or etomidate, in contrast to thiopental which showed strong and ketamine weak negative inotropic properties [38].

- The cardiac effects in vivo will depend on more than the inotropic properties of agents, and it is of interest that animal studies suggest that etomidate may act as an agonist at alpha2-adrenoceptors [39], perhaps contributing to its cardiovascular stability.

- Recent reviews still recommend etomidate for induction of anesthesia in the high-risk cardiac patient owing to its cardiovascular stability [40] and, in the UK, Mackay et al. [41] have suggested that etomidate is the agent of choice for trauma patients requiring a rapid sequence induction due to its lesser cardiovascular depression compared to other agents.

- It is not, however, universally accepted that etomidate is the safest agent in either high-risk or shocked patients. Many practitioners believe they can achieve equal hemodynamic stability in such patients by careful titration of the dose of other induction agents.

Current controversy in ICU

- It has long been accepted that etomidate infusions have a negative effect on the outcome of ICU patients despite preservation of hemodynamics. Whether avoidance of hypotension at induction by the use of etomidate is worth a "trade off" with adrenal suppression is now openly being questioned.

- There have been numerous studies over the years convincingly demonstrating that even a single induction dose of etomidate has a reversible inhibitory effect on cortisol production lasting up to 24 h. It has always been assumed that the transient adrenal suppressant effect of a single etomidate bolus for intubation would not have a significant effect on overall ICU outcome and, indeed, it is even conceivable that modification by etomidate of the normal "stress response" to surgery (in part due to elevations in serum cortisol levels) may be desirable in some patients.

- However, evidence is appearing suggesting that the single induction dose of etomidate given to patients entering ICU, e.g. either following etomidate given during anesthesia for, say, peritonitis or following intubation in the emergency department, may indeed influence eventual survival. In one recent study [42], adrenal depression in septic shock was, perhaps not surprisingly, associated with a worse outcome. The authors suggest, but by no means prove, that etomidate exposure could be a major risk factor for mortality in septic shock. A recent review article [43] and editorials in the anesthetic [44] and ICU literature [45] have called for a moratorium on the use of etomidate in ICU patients and patients who will be going to ICU. Others [46] have long suggested that each time etomidate is administered, hydrocortisone should be administered to prevent adrenal dysfunction.

Thus, the use of etomidate for induction of anesthesia of critically ill patients is increasingly controversial [47].

The nitrous oxide controversy

In normal patients mild indirect sympathetic stimulation reduces any myocardial depressant actions of N_2O. Following hemorrhage this protective effect is lost and N_2O may have the same depressant effects on the heart as halothane.

With the additional concerns regarding lesser inspired oxygen concentrations and the potential for expansion of air spaces, e.g. pneumothoraces, it is difficult to see a major role for N_2O in critically ill patients. In recent years additional concerns have been raised.

- Is N_2O a neurotoxin in usual clinical circumstances? An increasing body of animal work supports the concept that N_2O is neurotoxic [17].

- Does N_2O cause myocardial ischemia? N_2O inhibits methionine synthase, which aids in the conversion of homocysteine to methionine. Hyperhomocysteinemia is a risk factor for coronary artery and cerebrovascular disease. Use of N_2O during carotid artery surgery has been shown to cause increases in postoperative plasma homocysteine concentration and increased postoperative myocardial ischemia [48].

- Does N_2O worsen outcome in high-risk patients? A large, multi-center randomized trial (ENIGMA) examined the effect of N_2O on outcome in major surgery. Unfortunately the inspired oxygen levels in the two groups were widely different (80% in the N_2O-free group and 30% in the N_2O group). The N_2O group had an increased incidence of complications after major surgery, but no significant difference in length of hospital stay [49].

The definitive answer to this last question may perhaps be provided by the ENIGMA 2 study but, already, many anesthetists no longer use N_2O in critically ill patients.

Intraoperative management of head injuries and other causes of raised intracranial pressure (ICP)

Trauma patients frequently have concomitant head injury. The principles of anesthesia for trauma patients with head injury are well established and covered fully in the standard anesthesia and neuroanesthesia texts. Important principles worth emphasizing include the following.

- Factors causing increases in ICP should be avoided.
- Encourage venous drainage and therefore minimize ICP by
  - neck maintained in neutral position,
  - minimize the use of PEEP where possible,
  - nurse with head up by 10°.
- Avoid hypotension. There is a loss of normal BP/cerebral blood flow (CBF) autoregulation. Hyperventilation reduces ICP and brain volume and permits surgical access to the brain. Ideally, hyperventilation would be monitored by jugular venous oxygen content in view of the potential for ischemia if CBF is reduced excessively.
- All volatile agents may increase CBF and ICP. Hyperventilation is essential if volatile agents are used.
- Propofol infusions are increasingly popular.
- Ketamine may increase BP and ICP and should be avoided.
- Full muscle relaxation is essential to avoid straining and coughing-induced increases in ICP.

Practical conduct of anesthesia in the critically ill patient

- Conventional assessments of fitness for anesthesia and surgery may not be helpful. The bleeding patient may not be able to be stabilized until the bleeding is controlled.
- Many of these patients require ongoing resuscitation. The ABC system is widely followed:

  A = airway including cervical spine protection,
  B = breathing,
  C = circulation.

  The less well known system of VIP (Ventilation, Infusion and Perfusion) is perhaps equally appropriate for surgical and trauma patients, as it emphasizes the interrelationship between ventilation and perfusion in overall oxygen transport and because it reminds us that the cornerstone of resuscitation in these patients is fluid infusion.

- It is an important principle that inotropes and vasopressors should not be given as a substitute for fluids in the hypovolemic patient, but perfusion of the coronary and cerebral circulations must be maintained. It is therefore appropriate to use such drugs to maintain perfusion of the heart and brain in the short term while one "catches up" with blood loss. Many anesthetists routinely follow injection of, for example, propofol for induction with a phenylephrine "chaser" in order to prevent falls in blood pressure being precipitated by the induction agent. Although a useful approach to this problem, this should not result in overconfidence!

- Many patients coming to the OR from the ICU will already be receiving hemodynamic support with infusions of inotropes and/or vasopressors. These should obviously be continued and, indeed, usually require to be increased to compensate for the effects of the anesthetic agents.

- Intraoperative control of blood sugar and other aspects of optimization are discussed in that specific chapter.

- Critically ill patients do not always tolerate movement. Many will already be intubated. Therefore, in those countries where there are induction rooms, it seems logical to transfer these patients direct into the OR rather than via the induction room. In addition, in many hospitals monitoring standards remain higher in the OR than in an induction room.

- Portable monitors with full invasive monitoring facilities are commonplace and will be used for transfer of patients from ICU or the emergency department to the OR. It may be sensible to continue to use this monitor rather than risk confusion swapping over all the lines and cables. (Do not forget to plug in the portable monitor to maintain battery life for the journey back!)

- If invasive monitoring is not in situ it may be prudent (time permitting) to establish this using local anesthesia prior to induction for beat-to-beat monitoring of this period of the anesthetic (see below).

- Ruptured aneurysms and other cases of massive hemorrhage should be "prepped" on the table prior to induction as discussed in the chapter on vascular anesthesia.

- Communication and timing with theater staff, surgeons, porters, etc., should eliminate delays in potentially difficult circumstances and environments.

Intraoperative monitoring

Full monitoring according to local and national protocols should be employed in all patients. In addition, critically ill patients will require invasive monitoring with an indwelling arterial line for:

- beat-to-beat monitoring of blood pressure,
- sampling of blood for blood gas measurement,
- control of inotrope and vasopressor infusions,

and a central venous catheter for:

- measurement of filling pressure, i.e. preload of the right ventricle,
- guide to fluid requirements, and
- infusion of irritant drugs, e.g. inotropes, vasopressors and IV nutrition.

CVP reflects Right Atrial Pressure which is usually taken to reflect RV end diastolic pressure. It does *not* necessarily reflect LV preload, and also poorly correlates with blood volume. CVP is often used as a guide to LV function. Directional changes in CVP may reflect alterations in LV performance. However, if either ventricle becomes selectively depressed, or if there is severe pulmonary disease, changes in CVP will *not* reflect changes in LV function.

Such patients may require a pulmonary artery flotation catheter (PAFC) to enable measurements of the filling pressures at the left side of the heart (estimated by the pulmonary capillary wedge pressure (PCWP) as the inflated balloon at the catheter tip is "wedged" in the pulmonary artery) and cardiac output and derived hemodynamic variables.

A urinary catheter is required for hourly urine volume measurement. Temperature should be monitored for all long procedures because of the dangers of perioperative hypothermia as discussed above.

Monitoring strategies in the high-risk surgical patient

- Invasive monitoring of elderly surgical patients has revealed a high incidence of "hidden" abnormalities reflecting their reduced physiological reserve even in patients "cleared" for surgery. Invasive monitoring during anesthesia and in the postoperative period may result in early recognition of problems, "fine tuning" of cardiovascular parameters, and in some studies, an improved outcome [50].

- Perioperative optimization (discussed elsewhere) of cardiac function and oxygen transport will obviously require invasive monitoring of cardiac function – most commonly with the aid of a PAFC.

- Broad indications currently for the use of a PAFC are patients with severe disease of either ventricle, but most commonly patients with severe LV dysfunction, in order to optimize preload prior to the use of inotropes.

- In addition, the PAFC may enable early diagnosis of cardiac ischemia if there are sudden increases in PCWP, guide hemodynamic management of septic patients and monitor pulmonary artery pressures where these are elevated.

- Paradoxically, the PAFC is not always helpful in shocked or bleeding patients in the operating theater in whom the main aim of the anesthetist is often to administer sufficient fluids to enable the patient to survive the necessary "damage control" surgery – followed by fine tuning of the hemodynamic state in the ICU.

- Perioperative use of the PAFC is controversial, with studies casting doubt on the role of the PAFC in elective high-risk surgery. For example, routine use of PAFCs during aortic surgery is not beneficial and may lead to increased complications [51]. Similarly there is no benefit from the PAFC for routine CABG surgery [52]. Even in ICU patients there is no convincing evidence of benefit (but no convincing evidence of harm either) arising from the use of the PAFC [53]. The American Society of Anesthesiologists has published guidelines for its perioperative use [54].

Fluid therapy

The crystalloid versus colloid debate

- There has been controversy over the best type of fluid for resuscitation, i.e. crystalloids or colloids. Part of the problem is the lack of studies showing a sufficiently clear superiority of one fluid type over another, sufficient to convert its opponents, and without reasonable criticisms of study methodology. There are several problems with most of the available studies, e.g. different species, fluids, injuries, illnesses, complications studied.

- It is not widely appreciated that many of the original studies of crystalloids versus colloids were flawed. This was because most patients in both groups were given blood transfusions. At that time, many patients were commonly given *whole* blood (as opposed to packed red cells) so that both groups received colloid from the whole blood, i.e. there was no such thing as a pure crystalloid group. Perhaps it is not surprising that few differences in outcome were detected.

- However, in most studies there is probably a skewed distribution of severity of sickness with a large group of patients who will do all right whichever fluid is given and a smaller group of patients who will die regardless of which fluid is given. These patients may mask (statistically speaking) a group of patients in whom choice of fluid may be critical. This possibility has been seized upon by the colloid enthusiasts!

- However, recent systematic reviews have failed to uncover any survival benefit from the use of colloids [55].

- There are certain statements regarding the colloid/crystalloid controversy which can be made which are reasonably accepted by both groups:

- Crystalloids replace interstitial losses. Colloids are superior at replacing plasma volume deficits – more quickly and lasting longer – giving greater increases in cardiac output and oxygen delivery. Crystalloid administration may also produce such increases, but approximately three times as much will be needed with consequent delays in achieving goals of resuscitation.

- Crystalloids are cheap. Colloids are more expensive. Many centers use crystalloids almost exclusively.

- In most situations, e.g. routine surgery, both potentially give excellent results if appropriate amounts are used. Many studies show similar effects on respiratory function. Overdose of either may produce respiratory failure. Fluid overload may be a polite term for drowning!

- Most reasonable people do not take extreme positions in the debate. In most situations close monitoring, especially with regard to fluid overload, is more important than absolute choice of fluid.

- However, many believe in the "Golden Hour" for resuscitation and that, therefore, speed of resuscitation is crucial. Therefore, when restoration of blood volume, cardiac output and tissue perfusion is urgent colloids may be preferable to crystalloids.

Saline-induced metabolic acidosis and choice of crystalloid

- In elderly surgical patients, the use of crystalloids and colloids containing balanced electrolyte solutions prevented the development of hyperchloremic metabolic acidosis and improved indices of gastric mucosal perfusion compared with saline-based crystalloid and colloid fluids [56].

- A study of saline versus Ringer's lactate in aortic aneurysm surgery showed higher perioperative blood loss in the saline group [57].

- However, the infusion of large volumes of Ringer's lactate solution during major surgery leads to postoperative mild hyponatremia and respiratory acidosis [58].

Intraoperative fluid loading or fluid restriction?

- Some studies show benefits from fluid loading in the high-risk or critically ill patient, e.g. in one study fluid loading after induction of anesthesia to a maximum stroke volume led to a reduction in the incidence of low pHi (an index of gastric mucosal perfusion) from 50% to 10% [59]. In a more recent study of patients undergoing major elective surgery, goal-directed volume loading resulted in earlier return of bowel function and a decreased length of stay [60].

- This approach must be tempered with caution in the elderly or patients with known heart failure due to the potential risk of fluid overload precipitating pulmonary edema. Perioperative invasive monitoring may be indicated.

- However, inadequate fluid therapy is dangerous if resulting organ hypoperfusion leads to organ failure, e.g. renal failure.

- More recent studies have examined the role of fluid excess (primarily crystalloid) as a factor in outcome in high-risk surgical patients. Most of these studies have been performed on patients undergoing bowel surgery. This is discussed in Chapter 18.

- Harmful effects of the extra fluid may include:
  1. Increased lung H_2O, reduced pulmonary compliance and impaired gas exchange.
  2. Ileus may be promoted due to edema of the gut.
  3. Tissue oxygenation and, by association, wound healing may be impaired by the tissue edema associated with excessive crystalloid administration.

It has been suggested [61] that a more rational approach to perioperative fluid therapy would suggest that crystalloids should be limited in volume, blood loss replaced largely with colloid and red blood cells, and that balanced salt solutions such as Ringer's lactate should be preferred to 0.9% saline.

End points of fluid therapy

The end points of fluid therapy may need to be chosen with care in high-risk or critically ill patients. Reduction in tachycardia and improvement in blood pressure and urine volumes are important, albeit crude, signs of response to fluids. Both CVP and PCWP have limitations. More recent, dynamic approaches to assessing the circulation show promise.

- Central venous saturation. Saturation of the central venous blood ($ScvO_2$) has been shown to be a useful sign of tissue hypoxia and guide to early resuscitation in patients presenting to the ER with septic shock [62]. Preliminary work suggests that a low $ScvO_2$ perioperatively is associated with an increased risk of postoperative complications in high-risk surgery [63]. The use of $ScvO_2$ as a guide to fluid therapy warrants further study.

- Pulse pressure variation (PPV). Recent studies suggest that the presence of arterial PPV during the respiratory cycle indicates a relative hypovolemia and, indeed, predicts an increase in CO with fluid [64]. Most monitors can "freeze" the arterial trace and quantify this PPV or one can simply view the "swing" on the arterial trace.

- Additionally and importantly, it is suggested that if there is *no* PPV there will be no increase in CO no matter how much fluid is given [65]. This technique only seems to apply in the patient undergoing IPPV.

Permissive hypovolemia in trauma patients

- An important study in 1994 of penetrating trauma showed an improved survival in those patients with "delayed" fluid resuscitation, i.e. minimal IV fluids given prior to definitive operative intervention [66]. This has been called "permissive" hypovolemia.

- The rationale, borne out by previous animal studies, is that full resuscitation results in:
  - higher BP disrupting clot formation,
  - hemodilution and decreased viscosity disrupting clot formation, and
  - dilutional coagulopathy.
- The recommendation has, therefore, been made in penetrating injury to limit fluids to maintain a MAP not >50 until bleeding has been surgically controlled, *then* full resuscitation.
- The biggest problem is that this study was performed in *penetrating* injuries. Patients with blunt trauma are not so likely to have definitive surgical interventions.
- This approach is inapplicable in head-injured patients who require maintainence of cerebral perfusion pressure to reduce secondary brain injury.
- Further controlled trials are awaited, but it would be unfortunate if improvements in trauma management related to an understanding of the importance of rapid resuscitation with volume infusion as a cornerstone of that resuscitation were lost because fluid restriction was seen as appropriate in any but a few specific (and uncommon) circumstances.

Blood transfusion

From the perspective of the anesthetist certain points are worth emphasizing.

- The importance of communication with surgeon regarding bleeding. On occasion the surgeon may need to be told to stop dissecting and control active bleeding to allow one to "catch up".
- Similarly one must communicate early with the blood bank with regard to requirements, especially requirements for clotting factors.
- Many anesthetists only start to consider blood transfusion once approximately 10% of the patient's blood volume (based on 80 ml kg^{-1} body weight) has been lost. With ongoing brisk hemorrhage one should not wait until 10% has been lost!
- Maintaining body temperature will minimize coagulopathy and blood loss as previously described.
- Maintaining blood volume is probably more important in the short term than maintaining Hb. However, with major hemorrhage blood *will* be needed!
- Autologous transfusion systems, e.g. "cell savers", should be considered for appropriate "clean" operations.

Blood transfusion is further discussed in Chapter 9.

Inotropes and vasoactive drugs

In addition to the normal anesthetic goals that pertain to all patients, one must pay especial interest to the maintenance of organ blood flow and function in the critically ill patient. This is obviously the case for all our patients, but fortunately the vast majority of low-risk patients present few problems and rarely need any form of circulatory support. In septic or shocked patients this is the norm, and the choice of inotropes and vasopressors and monitoring of the circulation are discussed below.

- Adequate filling pressures and intravascular volume are crucial prior to anesthesia and also the use of inotropic agents. With hypovolemia the vasodilator effects of inotropic agents such as Dobutamine predominate leading to hypotension. The use of vasopressors in hypovolemia will reduce splanchnic and muscle blood flow.

- Cardiac function can be severely compromised in hemorrhagic shock so that an element of cardiogenic shock contributes to the shocked state. In such cases the response to resuscitation may be compromised and invasive monitoring and/or inotropes required as detailed below. As early as the 1950s the contribution of the heart to progressive, irreversible shock was recognized, and it was also demonstrated that the homeostatic mechanisms and vasoconstriction were not sufficient to maintain coronary perfusion in severe hemorrhage. Therefore, cardiac dysfunction needs to be detected and corrected as early after injury as possible.

- For myocardial support in the failing heart and low output states, Dobutamine is probably the agent of choice.

- For vascular support, e.g. with abnormal vasodilation, a vasopressor such as norepinephrine (noradrenaline) is probably the agent of choice.

- In view of concerns relating to gut blood flow and lactic acidosis, the role of epinephrine (adrenaline) infusions perioperatively is controversial.

Oxygen transport in the high-risk or critically ill surgical patient

Differences between hemorrhagic shock and traumatic shock

Hemorrhage results in well-known physiologic changes. Traumatic shock includes these responses, but they are modified by the tissue injury and its associated inflammatory response. This has several practical effects.

- HR responds to hemorrhage by an initial tachycardia followed eventually by a progressive bradycardia – the heart slowing in the absence of adequate venous return in an attempt to maintain stroke volume. With tissue injury there is no late slowing of the heart and tachycardia continues.

- Blood pressure is maintained by vasoconstriction until more than one-third of blood volume has been lost. With tissue injury, blood pressure is maintained to a greater degree by the surge in catecholamines and other nociceptive stimuli, but this is at the expense of tissue perfusion due to excessive vasoconstriction.

- Animal studies show that for an equivalent degree of blood loss, traumatic injury results in greater tissue hypoperfusion and a greater "injury" than simple hemorrhage.

- The wound and fracture sites are metabolically active with a resultant requirement for increased oxygen consumption and glucose oxidation – the concept of "the wound as an organ". In addition to the local reasons for increased metabolic demands, there are systemic inflammatory and catabolic causes of increased metabolic demand requiring an increased cardiac output compared to normal. This may imply a need for increased cardiac output and oxygen delivery in trauma and high-risk surgical patients as discussed in the chapter on perioperative optimization.

Oxygen debt and lactic acidosis in the high-risk surgical patient

Even when oxygen delivery is well maintained, oxygen consumption falls under anesthesia. Animal studies show that anesthesia reduces tissue oxygen extraction especially in septic models. This occurs with all agents, but is associated with lactic acidosis only with volatile agents.

Thus, although anesthesia reduces metabolic rate and oxygen demand, this may be countered in the critically ill patient by the reduction in the tissue's ability to extract oxygen. An oxygen debt may develop, especially if there are falls in cardiac output and/or oxygen delivery below a critical level [67]. Worryingly, the reduction of tissue oxygen extraction under anesthesia may increase the threshold for oxygen delivery to be "critical" [68], i.e. lesser degrees of fall in cardiac output and oxygen delivery may result in tissue hypoxia under anesthesia. This has obvious implications for anesthesia of the critically ill or shocked patient, in whom maintenance of cardiac output and oxygen delivery are crucial.

There are many studies demonstrating that high-risk surgical patients develop an intra-operative "oxygen debt", the magnitude and duration of which correlates with the development of lactic acidosis, organ failure and increased mortality [69, 70]. This oxygen debt is postulated to potentially arise from anesthetic cardiac depression, direct anesthetic reductions in tissue oxygen uptake as already described, failure to maintain adequate fluid intake during surgery and perhaps hypothermia.

The crucial message is that high-risk surgical patients may have reduced cardiac reserves, especially in the elderly, suffer occult tissue hypoperfusion with a developing oxygen debt postoperatively, proceed to multiple organ failure if there is no intervention to reverse the tissue hypoperfusion, and have a higher mortality than patients who *do* have sufficient reserves to reverse their oxygen debt and prevent serious tissue hypoxia. Appropriate interventions may include fluid therapy, oxygen, inotropes and vasopressors.

The role of the anesthetist in outcome of the critically ill patient

The anesthetist may influence overall outcome of the critically ill patient in the OR by several mechanisms, some more controversial than others.

- Obvious clinical errors. This will not be further discussed here.
- Choice of anesthetic agents. Some aspects of this have already been discussed in this chapter. Regional anesthesia is discussed in its own chapter.
- Poor hemodynamic control [71] or poor fluid balance – both of which may influence the development of ischemia or organ failure.
- Ischemia. Volatile agents (and probably opiates) seem to protect the heart from subsequent ischemia (preconditioning) similar to the preconditioning due to previous ischemia. The mechanisms seem similar, i.e. activation of the sarcolemmal and mitochondrial K(ATP) channels via stimulation of adenosine receptors and subsequent activation of protein kinase C. The opening of the K(ATP) channels causes cardioprotection by decreasing Ca^{2+}.
- Although individual studies of patients undergoing cardiac surgery have been underpowered to detect differences in mortality, volatile anesthetics, when compared to intravenous anesthetics, seem to result in better cardiac function, lower troponin concentrations, less requirement for inotropic support, reduced duration of mechanical ventilation, and reduced hospital length of stay [72].
- Myocardial preconditioning has been most studied, but similar ischemia protection effects may occur in other organs [73].
- Deep anesthesia (as reflected by a bispectral index score < 45) has been shown in a prospective observational study of adult patients undergoing major noncardiac

surgery to be associated with an increased risk of death during the first year after surgery [74]. This was a relatively minor factor compared with the presence of patient co-morbidities, but was an independent predictor of increased mortality. A mechanism is unclear (postoperative pulmonary complications from deep anesthesia would not be expected to have such long-term influences), but could involve postoperative cognitive dysfunction or exacerbated inflammatory response. This study has been hotly debated, but has been substantiated by another presented but, as yet, unpublished study.

- As regards the individual anesthetist, there have been few studies which have effectively come down to assessing the role of the *competence* of the anesthetist on risk and outcome. One study of patients undergoing coronary artery surgery found that the only nonpatient-related factors influencing outcome were cardiac bypass time and the anesthetist [75]. We can speculate on possible causes of this difference (poor hemodynamic control?), and can expect more such studies in the future.

Further reading

Recommendations for the safe transfer of patients with brain injury. Association of Anaesthetists of Great Britain and Ireland, 2006.

Schultz MJ, Haitsma JJ, Slutsky AS, Gajic O. What tidal volumes should be used in patients without acute lung injury? *Anesthesiology* 2007; **106**: 1226–31.

Wilson W, Grande CM, Hoyt DB, eds. *Trauma: Emergency Resuscitation, Perioperative Anesthesia, Surgical Management*, Volume I. London, Informa Health, 2007.

References

1. Brundage SI, McGhan R, Jurkovich GJ, *et al.* Timing of femur fracture fixation: Effect on outcome in patients with thoracic and head injuries. *J Trauma* 2002; **52**: 299–307.

2. Parr MJ, Alabdi T. Damage control surgery and intensive care. *Injury* 2004; **35**: 713–22.

3. Balogh Z, McKinley BA, Cocanour CS, *et al.* Supranormal trauma resuscitation causes more cases of abdominal compartment syndrome. *Arch Surg* 2003; **138**: 637–42.

4. Bercault N, Wolf M, Runge I, *et al.* Intrahospital transport of critically ill ventilated patients: A risk factor for ventilator-associated pneumonia – a matched cohort study. *Crit Care Med* 2005; **33**: 2471–8.

5. Schmied H, Kurz A, Sessler DI, *et al.* Mild hypothermia increases blood loss and transfusion requirements during total hip arthroplasty. *Lancet* 1996; **347**: 289–92.

6. Frank SM, Fleisher LA, Breslow MJ, *et al.* Perioperative maintenance of normothermia reduces the incidence of morbid cardiac events: A randomised clinical trial. *JAMA* 1997; **227**: 1127–43.

7. Berti M, Casati A, Torri G, *et al.* Active warming, not passive heat retention, maintains normothermia during combined epidural–general anesthesia for hip and knee arthroplasty. *J Clin Anesth* 1997; **9**: 482–6.

8. Aubier M, Vines N, Syllie G, *et al.* Respiratory muscle contribution to lactic acidosis in low cardiac output. *Am Rev Resp Dis* 1982; **126**: 648–52.

9. Neumann P, Rothen HU, Berglund JE, *et al.* Positive end-expiratory pressure prevents atelectasis during general anaesthesia even in the presence of a high inspired oxygen concentration. *Acta Anaesthesiol Scand* 1999; **43**: 295–301.

10. Wrigge H, Uhlig U, Zinserling J, *et al.* The effects of different ventilatory settings on pulmonary and systemic inflammatory responses during major surgery. *Anesth Analg* 2004; **98**: 775–81.

11. Benoît Z, Wicky S, Fischer JF, *et al.* The effect of increased FIO(2) before tracheal

extubation on postoperative atelectasis. *Anesth Analg* 2002; **95**: 1777–81.

12. Bitterman H, Reissman P, Bitterman N, *et al.* Oxygen therapy in hemorrhagic shock. *Circ Shock* 1991; **33**: 183–91.

13. Rosenberg-Adamsen S, Lie C, Bernhard A, *et al.* Effect of oxygen treatment on heart rate after abdominal surgery. *Anesthesiology* 1999; **90**: 380–4.

14. Anderson KJ, Harten JM, Booth MG, *et al.* The cardiovascular effects of inspired oxygen fraction in anaesthetized patients. *Eur J Anaesthesiol* 2005; **22**: 420–5.

15. Kotani N, Hashimoto H, Sessler DI, *et al.* Supplemental intraoperative oxygen augments antimicrobial and proinflammatory responses of alveolar macrophages. *Anesthesiology* 2000; **93**: 15–25.

16. Belda FJ, Aguilera L, García de la Asunción J, *et al.* Supplemental perioperative oxygen and the risk of surgical wound infection: A randomized controlled trial. *JAMA* 2005; **294**: 2035–42.

17. Jevtovic-Todorovic V, Wozniak DF, Benshoff ND, *et al.* A comparative evaluation of the neurotoxic properties of ketamine and nitrous oxide. *Brain Res* 2001; **895**: 264–7.

18. Willman EV, Andolfatto G. A prospective evaluation of "ketofol" (ketamine/propofol combination) for procedural sedation and analgesia in the emergency department. *Ann Emerg Med* 2007; **49**: 23–30.

19. McConachie I, Chandrasekar B. Tolerance following remifentanil infusion. *CPD Anaesthesia* 2006; **8**: 29–31.

20. Durieux ME, Sperry RJ, Longnecker DE. Effects of hypoxemia on regional blood flows during anesthesia with halothane, enflurane, or isoflurane. *Anesthesiology* 1992; **76**: 402–8.

21. Mayer N, Zimpler M, Kotai E, *et al.* Enflurane alters compensatory hemodynamic and humoral responses to hemorrhage. *Circ Shock* 1990; **30**: 165–70.

22. Bennetts FE. Thiopentone anaesthesia at Pearl Harbor. *Br J Anaesth* 1995; **75**: 366–8.

23. Bogetz MS, Katz JA. Recall of surgery for major trauma. *Anesthesiology* 1984; **61**: 6–9.

24. Longnecker DE, Sturgill BC. Influence of anesthetic agent on survival following

hemorrhage. *Anesthesiology* 1976; **45**: 516–21.

25. Idvall J. Influence of ketamine anesthesia on cardiac output and tissue perfusion in rats subjected to hemorrhage. *Anesthesiology* 1981; **55**: 297–304.

26. Johnson KB, Egan TD, Kern SE, *et al.* The influence of hemorrhagic shock on propofol: A pharmacokinetic and pharmacodynamic analysis. *Anesthesiology* 2003; **99**: 409–20.

27. Johnson KB, Egan TD, Layman J, *et al.* The influence of hemorrhagic shock on etomidate: A pharmacokinetic and pharmacodynamic analysis. *Anesth Analg* 2003; **96**: 1360–8.

28. Johnson KB, Kern SE, Hamber EA, *et al.* Influence of hemorrhagic shock on remifentanil: A pharmacokinetic and pharmacodynamic analysis. *Anesthesiology* 2001; **94**: 322–32.

29. Yli-Hankala A, Kirvela M, Randell T, *et al.* Ketamine anaesthesia in a patient with septic shock. *Acta Anaesthesiol Scand* 1992; **36**: 483–5.

30. Van der Linden P, Gilbart E, Engelman E, *et al.* Comparison of halothane, isoflurane, alfentanil and ketamine in experimental septic shock. *Anesth Analg* 1990; **70**: 608–17.

31. Flondor M, Hofstetter C, Boost KA, *et al.* Isoflurane inhalation after induction of endotoxemia in rats attenuates the systemic cytokine response. *Eur Surg Res* 2008; **40**: 1–6.

32. Kawasaki T, Ogata M, Kawasaki C, *et al.* Ketamine suppresses proinflammatory cytokine production in human whole blood in vitro. *Anesth Analg* 1999; **89**: 665–9.

33. Kawasaki C, Kawasaki T, Ogata M, *et al.* Ketamine isomers suppress superantigen-induced proinflammatory cytokine production in human whole blood. *Can J Anaesth* 2001; **48**: 819–23.

34. Beilin B, Rusabrov Y, Shapira Y, *et al.* Low-dose ketamine affects immune responses in humans during the early postoperative period. *Br J Anaesth* 2007; **99**: 522–7.

35. Taniguchi T, Yamamoto K, Ohmoto N, *et al.* Effects of propofol on hemodynamic and inflammatory responses to endotoxemia in rats. *Crit Care Med* 2000; **28**: 1101–6.

36. Yu HP, Lui PW, Hwang TL, *et al*. Propofol improves endothelial dysfunction and attenuates vascular superoxide production in septic rats. *Crit Care Med* 2006; **34**: 453–60.

37. Kidani Y, Taniguchi T, Kanakura H, *et al*. Sevoflurane pretreatment inhibits endotoxin-induced shock in rats. *Anesth Analg* 2005; **101**: 1152–6.

38. Gelissen HP, Epema AH, Henning RH, *et al*. Inotropic effects of propofol, thiopental, midazolam, etomidate, and ketamine on isolated human atrial muscle. *Anesthesiology* 1996; **84**: 397–403.

39. Paris A, Philipp M, Tonner PH, *et al*. Activation of alpha 2B-adrenoceptors mediates the cardiovascular effects of etomidate. *Anesthesiology* 2003: **99**; 889–95.

40. Bovill JG. Intravenous anesthesia for the patient with left ventricular dysfunction. *Semin Cardiothorac Vasc Anesth* 2006; **10**: 43–8.

41. Mackay CA, Terris J, Coats TJ. Prehospital rapid sequence induction by emergency physicians: Is it safe? *Emerg Med J* 2001; **18**: 20–24.

42. den Brinker M, Hokken-Koelega AC, Hazelzet JA, *et al*. One single dose of etomidate negatively influences adrenocortical performance for at least 24 hr in children with meningococcal sepsis. *Intensive Care Med* 2008; **34**: 163–8.

43. Jackson WL Jr. Should we use etomidate as an induction agent for endotracheal intubation in patients with septic shock? A critical appraisal. *Chest* 2005; **127**: 1031–8.

44. Morris C, McAllister C. Etomidate for emergency anaesthesia; mad, bad and dangerous to know? *Anaesthesia* 2005; **60**: 737–40.

45. Annane D. ICU physicians should abandon the use of etomidate! *Intensive Care Med* 2005; **31**: 325–6.

46. Stuttmann R, Allolio B, Becker A, *et al*. Etomidate versus etomidate and hydrocortisone for anaesthesia induction in abdominal surgical interventions. *Anaesthetist* 1988; **37**: 576–82.

47. McConachie I. Update on etomidate. *CPD Anaesthesia* 2007; **9**: 16–20.

48. Badner NH, Beattie WS, Freeman D, *et al*. Nitrous oxide-induced increased homocysteine concentrations are associated with increased postoperative myocardial ischemia in patients undergoing carotid endarterectomy. *Anesth Analg* 2000; **91**: 1073–9.

49. Myles PS, Leslie K, Chan MT, *et al*. Avoidance of nitrous oxide for patients undergoing major surgery: A randomized controlled trial. *Anesthesiology* 2007; **107**: 221–31.

50. Del Guercio LRN, Cohn JD. Monitoring operative risk in the elderly. *JAMA* 1980; **297**: 845–50.

51. Valentine RJ, Duke ML, Inman MH, *et al*. Effectiveness of pulmonary artery catheters in aortic surgery: A randomized trial. *J Vasc Surg* 1998; **27**: 203–11.

52. Tuman KJ, McCarthy RJ, Spiess BD, *et al*. Effect of pulmonary artery catheterization on outcome in patients undergoing coronary artery surgery. *Anesthesiology* 1989; **70**: 199–206.

53. Harvey S, Harrison DA, Singer M, *et al*. Assessment of the clinical effectiveness of pulmonary artery catheters in management of patients in intensive care (PAC-Man): A randomised controlled trial. *Lancet* 2005; **366**: 472–7.

54. American Society of Anesthesiologists Task Force on Pulmonary Artery Catheterization. Practice guidelines for pulmonary artery catheterization: an updated report by the American Society of Anesthesiologists Task Force on Pulmonary Artery Catheterization. *Anesthesiology* 2003; **99**: 988–1014.

55. Perel P, Roberts I. Colloids versus crystalloids for fluid resuscitation in critically ill patients. *Cochrane Database Syst Rev* 2007; **4**: CD000567.

56. Wilkes NJ, Woolf R, Mutch M, *et al*. The effects of balanced versus saline-based hetastarch and crystalloid solutions on acid–base and electrolyte status and gastric mucosal perfusion in elderly surgical patients. *Anesth Analg* 2001; **93**: 811–6.

57. Waters JH, Gottlieb A, Schoenwald P, *et al*. Normal saline versus lactated Ringer's solution for intraoperative fluid management in patients undergoing

abdominal aortic aneurysm repair: an outcome study. *Anesth Analg* 2001; **93**: 817–22.

58. Takil A, Eti Z, Irmak P, *et al.* Early postoperative respiratory acidosis after large intravascular volume infusion of lactated ringer's solution during major spine surgery. *Anesth Analg* 2002; **95**: 294–8.

59. Mythen MG, Webb AR. Perioperative plasma volume expansion reduces the incidence of gut mucosal hypoperfusion during cardiac surgery. *Arch Surg* 1995; **130**: 423–9.

60. Gan TJ, Soppitt A, Maroof M, *et al.* Goal-directed intraoperative fluid administration reduces length of hospital stay after major surgery. *Anesthesiology* 2002; **97**: 820–6.

61. Joshi GP. Intraoperative fluid restriction improves outcome after major elective gastrointestinal surgery. *Anesth Analg* 2005; **101**: 601–5.

62. Rivers E, Nguyen B, Havstad S, *et al.* Early goal-directed therapy in the treatment of severe sepsis and septic shock. *N Engl J Med* 2001; **345**: 1368–77.

63. Pearse R, Dawson D, Fawcett J, *et al.* Changes in central venous saturation after major surgery, and association with outcome. *Crit Care* 2005; **9**: R694–9.

64. Kramer A, Zygun D, Hawes H, *et al.* Pulse pressure variation predicts fluid responsiveness following coronary artery bypass surgery. *Chest* 2004; **126**: 1563–8.

65. Michard F, Teboul JL. Predicting fluid responsiveness in ICU patients: A critical analysis of the evidence. *Chest* 2002; **121**: 2000–8.

66. Bickell WH, Wall MJ Jr, Pepe PE, *et al.* Immediate versus delayed fluid resuscitation for hypotensive patients with penetrating torso injuries. *N Engl J Med* 1994; **331**: 1105–9.

67. Lugo G, Arizpe D, Dominguez G. Relationship between oxygen consumption and oxygen delivery during anesthesia in high-risk surgical patients. *Crit Care Med* 1993; **21**: 64–9.

68. Van der Linden P, Schmartz D, Gilbart E, *et al.* Effects of propofol, etomidate, and pentobarbital on critical oxygen delivery. *Crit Care Med* 2000; **28**: 2492–9.

69. Shoemaker WC, Appel PL, Kram HB. Role of oxygen debt in the development of organ failure sepsis, and death in high-risk surgical patients. *Chest* 1992; **102**: 208–15.

70. Hess W, Frank C, Hornburg B. Prolonged oxygen debt after abdominal aortic surgery. *J Cardiothorac Vasc Anesth* 1997; **11**: 149–54.

71. Reich DL, Bennett-Guerrero E, Bodian CA, *et al.* Intraoperative tachycardia and hypertension are independently associated with adverse outcome in noncardiac surgery of long duration. *Anesth Analg* 2002; **95**: 273–7.

72. Symons JA, Myles PS. Myocardial protection with volatile anaesthetic agents during coronary artery bypass surgery: A meta-analysis. *Br J Anaesth* 2006; **97**: 127–36.

73. Minguet G, Joris J, Lamy M. Preconditioning and protection against ischaemia-reperfusion in non-cardiac organs: A place for volatile anaesthetics? *Eur J Anaesthesiol* 2007; **24**: 733–45.

74. Monk TG, Saini V, Weldon BC, *et al.* Anesthetic management and one-year mortality after noncardiac surgery. *Anesth Analg* 2005; **100**: 4–10.

75. Merry AF, Ramage MC, Whitlock RM, *et al.* First-time coronary artery bypass grafting: the anaesthetist as a risk factor. *Br J Anaesth* 1992; **68**: 6–12.

Chapter 15

The elderly patient

S. Vaughan, I. McConachie and N. Imasogie

Throughout the developed world the population is aging. This, plus the advancement of anesthetic and surgical techniques, will result in more and more elderly (defined as aged 65 years and older) patients presenting for major elective and emergency surgery.

The risks of anesthesia, surgery and critical illness in the elderly, especially the very old, are increased compared to younger patients. Thus, the increase in geriatric surgery workload results in an increase in the proportion of surgical patients considered high risk [1].

It is vital, therefore, that the practising anesthetist is aware of the important differences that exist between the elderly patient and the young adult, and consider risk-reduction strategies outlined in this and other chapters.

Physiological changes associated with aging

After the age of 30 years, there is a gradual deterioration in organ function. The rate and extent of decline often determines those who are "physiologically young for their age" or those who are "physiologically old for their age". The following discussion apples to elderly patients in good health.

The aging cardiovascular system [2, 3]

- The arterial system becomes less compliant due to a loss in elastic tissue in the vessel wall. This results in an increased left ventricular afterload and systolic hypertension. The arteries also become less responsive to vasodilators such as nitric oxide, atrial naturetic peptide and β_2 adrenoceptor stimulation.

- The venous system also becomes less compliant, with a reduction in the strength of smooth muscle contraction within the vessel wall. Therefore the elderly have less blood in the capacitance vessels and less ability to squeeze this blood into the central circulation in the face of intravascular fluid depletion.

- Whether the changes in the vascular system lead to compensatory changes in the heart or whether both occur simultaneously and independently is a matter of debate.

- The ventricle hypertrophies with age. This may be as a response to the increased afterload and also due to a primary effect of aging. Ventricular hypertrophy reduces ventricular compliance, increases left ventricular end diastolic pressure (LVEDP) and reduces early diastolic filling of the ventricle. The elevated LVEDP increases the importance of atrial contraction (hence sinus rhythm) on late ventricular filling. Atrial hypertrophy develops to the increased impedance (LVEDP) to atrial emptying.

- The myocardium and pacemaker cells become less responsive to β_2 adrenoceptor stimulation. Therefore there is a reduction in both inotropic and chronotropic effects of β_2 stimulation.

Anesthesia for the High Risk Patient, ed. I. McConachie. Published by Cambridge University Press.
© Cambridge University Press 2009.

- At rest, cardiac index is unchanged or reduced in proportion to the reduction in basal metabolic rate. In the exercising young adult, cardiac output is increased by an increase heart rate and ejection fraction (i.e. a lower left ventricular end diastolic volume (LVEDV) and left ventricular end systolic volume (LVESV)). In the elderly, heart rate *falls* during exercise, LVEDV *increases* (by 20–30%) but LVESV decreases less, and therefore ejection fraction increases less, than in the young adult. It is apparent, then, that cardiac output in the elderly patient is more preload-dependant than in the young adult during times of cardiovascular stress.

- Pacemaker activity of the heart declines with age. The cells of the sino atrial node atrophy, conduction through the A-V node is increased, and conduction through the bundles is impaired. Heart block, bundle branch block and arrhythmias (both brady- and tachyarrythmias) become increasingly common with age.

- Coronary artery vascular resistance increases in the elderly because of the increased LVEDP and ventricular hypertrophy, but the reduced coronary flow is counterbalanced by a reduced myocardial oxygen consumption.

Aging of the respiratory system [4, 5]

- As one ages there are changes in the structure of the lung and airways along with changes in the thoracic wall.

- There is a loss in elastic tissue within the lung parenchyma as well as loss of alveolar surface area and therefore loss in surface tension forces. Both elastic tissue and surface tension contribute to the elastic recoil of the lung, hence the compliance of the aging lung is *increased* (compliance is the reciprocal of elastance). Calcification of the costal cartilage and the rib articulations reduce the thoracic compliance that counterbalances the increased lung compliance. There is some debate as to whether total compliance is unaltered or reduced because of the greater reduction in thoracic compliance over the increase in lung compliance.

- The losses in alveolar surface area results in V/Q mismatch, an increased physiological shunt (increased A-a gradient) and consequently a lower PaO_2.

- Changes in lung volumes also contribute to an increased physiological shunt. Throughout life, there is an increase in the volume of air required to prevent small airway collapse also known as closing volume (CV). At around 45 years of age, CV exceeds functional residual capacity (FRC) in the supine position, and in the seated position by 65 years of age. Once CV exceeds FRC, then airway closure occurs during tidal ventilation. The increase in closing volume can be explained by the loss in elastic tissue with age.

- Aside from an increase in CV with age there is an increase in residual volume. FRC, the point at which the outward pull of the thorax is balanced by the tendency for the lung to collapse, is unchanged at the expense of a reduced expiratory reserve volume (ERV). As ERV is reduced then it follows that vital capacity (VC) must be reduced. It is believed that total lung capacity is unchanged, or only reduced slightly (10%) with age.

- The large airways increase in size as one ages, resulting in an increased anatomical and physiological deadspace. Airway resistance is unchanged as the resistance (proximal) airways dilate and the smaller, distal, airways collapse, thus offsetting each other. Although total compliance is unchanged or marginally reduced, the loss in elasticity of the lungs and rigidity of the chest wall increases the work of breathing.

- The elderly have a diminished response to both hypercapnia and hypoxia. The elderly have blunted protective laryngeal reflexes and therefore are more at risk of pulmonary aspiration during anesthesia.
- Pulmonary vascular resistance increases with age, but it is doubtful if this is of any clinical significance.

Changes in renal function with age [6]

- Renal mass declines with age. After the third decade there is 1% loss per year. The reduction in mass is due to glomerular loss (up to 30% by the eighth decade) which is predominantly cortical. The exact cause of the glomerular atrophy is unknown, but it mirrors a reduction in renal blood and plasma flow (10% per decade).
- Loss of glomeruli has been implicated in the fall in glomerular filtration rate (GFR) with age. Absolute creatinine clearance falls approximately $1 \, \text{ml} \, \text{min}^{-1} \, 1.73 \, \text{m}^2$ per year or from $140 \, \text{ml} \, \text{min}^{-1} \, 1.73 \, \text{m}^2$ in the third decade to $97 \, \text{ml} \, \text{min}^{-1} \, 1.73 \, \text{m}^2$ in the eighth decade. However, plasma creatinine levels are unchanged in the elderly because a reduced muscle mass results in a reduced production of creatinine.
- Renal tubular function declines with age. Tubular dysfunction may be explained on the loss of glomerular units and a reduction in metabolically active tubular cells with age.
- The aged kidney is less effective at concentrating urine and conserving water in the face of water deprivation. This may result from a lowering in the medullary concentration gradient caused by disturbance of the counter-current mechanism by alterations in renal blood flow and a relative resistance to anti-diuretic hormone (ADH). Moreover, thirst perception during periods of dehydration is impaired. The nephron is also impaired in its ability to dilute the urine in the face of water overload. The elderly may be especially at risk of developing hyponatremia if excessive hypotonic intravenous solutions are given [7].
- The elderly face problems in salt conservation. Plasma renin and aldosterone levels are reduced in the elderly. This may be due to the relative unresponsiveness to β_2 receptor stimulation as renin is released in response to β_2 adrenoceptor stimulation. Moreover, changes in the heart with age lead to atrial distension and release of atrial naturetic factor (ANF), which also suppresses renin and aldosterone release. Not only does the relative deficiency of these two hormones lead to sodium loss, but it also places the elderly at risk of hyperkalemia.

The effect of age on hepatic function [8, 9]

- The liver, like most other organs, involutes with age, so by the eighth decade the liver has lost two-fifths of its mass. There is also a reduction in hepatic blood flow that not only represents the loss in hepatic cellular mass but also an absolute reduction in terms of percentage of cardiac output.
- Despite the reduction in mass and blood flow, it appears that hepatocellular enzyme function is preserved with advancing age. In vitro studies in patients with normal histology on liver biopsy failed to demonstrate any deterioration in hepatic microsomal oxygenase or hydrolase activity (phase I metabolic reactions) and also showed that reduced glutathione (phase II conjugation reactions and a major hepatic antioxidant) concentrations are maintained.

227

- In parallel with the apparent preservation of hepatocellular function, serum concentration of bilirubin, alkaline phosphatase, and transaminases are unaffected by age.
- Coagulation studies are also unchanged by age, but there is a gradual decline in serum albumin concentration.

Changes in the nervous system with age [10, 11]

- Memory loss, confusion and dementia are the clinical manifestations of aging of the brain.
- Normal pressure hydrocephalus results from global atrophy of the brain and an increase in CSF volume. The brain weighs 20% less by the eighth decade than in the second decade of life, and CSF volume increases by 10% in the same time period.
- Cerebral blood flow is reduced in line with brain volume, but autoregulation to carbon dioxide and mean arterial blood pressure is preserved.
- Within the brain the most metabolically active cells (gray matter of the cerebral and cerebellar cortices, basal ganglia, thalamus) atrophy more than the white matter. Regional blood flow reflects the neuronal loss with flow to the gray matter reduced more than that to the white.
- The levels of excitatory neurotransmitters (norepinephrine, serotonin, dopamine and tyrosine) are reduced.

The peripheral neurones like their counterparts in the brain undergo age-related degeneration. In particular there is:

- an increased threshold to stimulate sensory organs, such as pain corpuscles, and a reduced conduction velocity in afferent neurones and ascending spinocortical tracts. There is also a reduced conduction velocity in motor neurones and in the corticospinal tracts so that the reflex arc for painful stimuli is increased and righting reflexes are impaired; and
- skeletal muscle mass is reduced and extrajunctional acetylcholine receptors increased in response to degeneration of motor neurones. The reduction in muscle mass with aging is termed sarcopenia.

Neuroendocrine changes with age [12]

- Aging produces a state akin to a hyperadrenergic state. The impaired responses in the elderly to β_2 adrenoceptor stimulation lead to increased plasma norepinephrine and epinephrine concentrations despite atrophy of the adrenal medulla.
- Cardiovascular reflexes are also impaired in the elderly. Reduced responsiveness of the baroreceptors results in an underdamped cardiovascular system, and there is a reduced vasoconstrictor response to cold and less heart rate change in response to changes in posture. The elderly are therefore more vulnerable to cardiovascular instability, particularly during sympathetic blockade.

Changes in body fluids composition and metabolism with aging

The key changes that occur are summarized below.

- Basal metabolic rate falls as a consequence of a reduced skeletal mass and a reduction in the metabolically active areas of the brain, kidney and liver.
- Increased body fat results in a reduction in total body water.

- Testosterone and tri-iodothyronine levels are reduced.
- Glucose intolerance occurs.

Changes in pharmacokinetics and pharmacodynamics with age [13, 14]

In general, absorption of drugs from the gastrointestinal tract is unaffected by age. There are, however, important changes in distribution, metabolism and elimination of drugs because of age-related changes of the organs.

- A reduction in total body water means that the volume of distribution of water-soluble drugs (e.g. nondepolarizing muscle relaxants) is decreased, with an effective increase in the tissue concentration. Conversely, an increase in body fat results in an increased volume of distribution for lipid-soluble drugs.

- The reduction in albumin concentration in the elderly increases the free fraction of protein-bound (i.e. lipid-soluble) drugs and therefore increases the bioavailability at their effector sites.

- Hepatic clearance of a drug is dependent on three factors: the intrinsic clearance (CL_{int}), the free fraction of the drug (f) and the hepatic blood flow (Q_H). The hepatic clearance of drugs with a low CL_{int} is dependent on CL_{int} and f, and are said to be "capacity-limited". Examples of such drugs are barbiturates, benzodiazepines and theophyllines. If the free fraction of a highly protein-bound drug is increased, then the hepatic clearance becomes more dependent upon Q_H than CL_{int}. The elderly have a reduced Q_H, but CL_{int} is largely unchanged. Therefore, the hepatic clearance of capacity-limited drugs with low protein binding is unchanged with age. The reduction in serum albumin will increase the f of highly protein-bound drugs (e.g. thiopentone), and so their hepatic clearance will be reduced as a result of a reduced Q_H.

- Drugs with a high CL_{int} will be dependent on Q_H only for the hepatic clearance. They are said to be "flow-limited" and their clearance will be reduced as a result of the age-related fall in Q_H. Examples of flow-limited drugs are β-blockers, tricyclic antidepressants, opioid analgesics and amide local anesthetics.

- Biliary excretion of drug metabolites is unaffected by age, but renal excretion of water-soluble drugs and drug metabolites may be reduced by age-related reduction in GFR and tubular secretion.

- As well as changes in drug pharmacokinetics (e.g. increased free fraction of drugs, reduced volume of distribution, reduced clearance), the increased sensitivity to some drugs in the elderly is also due to pharmacodynamic changes.

- The reduction in excitatory neurotransmitters in the brain with gray matter atrophy is thought to be the basis for the enhanced sensitivity to intravenous induction agents and reduced MAC to volatile anesthetics. Changes in receptor sensitivity may also account for the enhanced analgesia seen with morphine, and altered sensitivity to benzodiazepines.

Co-existing disease and age-related organ dysfunction

- The deterioration in the various organ systems described above can be accelerated and worsened by co-existing disease.

- Pulmonary function is particularly affected by smoking and can result in emphysema or chronic bronchitis. Chronic asthma may also lead to fixed obstructive airways disease.
- It is important not to forget that drug therapy for medical conditions may adversely affect some organs. Examples would include renal damage from use of nonsteroidal anti-inflammatory agents and penicillamine used in the treatment of RA. The liver particularly can be adversely affected by a long list of drugs, and this should be borne in mind if faced with abnormal liver function tests or jaundice.
- Acute confusional states in the elderly may also be drug-induced and usually resolve once the drug is discontinued.

Organ reserve and risk

Invasive monitoring studies reveal that organ functional reserve in the elderly is reduced [15] by both the changes in organ function associated with aging and resulting from actual pathology. The increase in oxygen and metabolic demands imposed by major surgery may not be able to be supplied by these limitations in organ function. Occult organ ischemia may result. This is fully explored in Chapter 14. In addition, reduced functional organ reserve in, for example, the kidney results in an increased vulnerability during periods of physiological stress.

Anesthesia for the elderly patient

Increasing numbers of elderly patients present for surgery compared to previous decades and, in addition, the magnitude of the surgery thought suitable to be undertaken has also increased (although in many patients advances in minimally invasive techniques have reduced the surgical stress associated with certain procedures).

Preoperative preparation

- The preoperative visit for the elderly is often more taxing and takes longer than in the younger adult. Elderly patients may have cognitive impairment, memory loss and impaired hearing and vision. Extraction of information can be prolonged and difficult, so it is vital that the patient's chart be available for perusal.
- It is important to realize that the elderly often have different symptoms of a disease. For example, ischemic heart disease will often present as dyspnea rather than chest pain. This can be explained on the basis of the age-related cardiac changes, in that myocardial ischemia further elevates LVEDP and results in pulmonary edema. Internal Medicine and Cardiology consults may be required.
- Although clinical assessment of cardiac systolic function may be generally accurate, elderly patients with normal left ventricular (LV) ejection fraction often have isolated diastolic filling abnormalities that could not be predicted by clinical factors. LV diastolic dysfunction is almost certainly underestimated in the elderly surgical patient [16]. The significance of diastolic dysfunction in the elderly in terms of risk, complications and outcomes remains to be established.
- Assessment of hydration is important but also difficult. The signs of dehydration such as loss of skin turgor, dry eyes and mouth are common findings in the elderly, so one will

have to look for more subtle signs such as loss of jugular venous pulsation in the supine position, postural hypotension, and a raised urea.

- The presence of cardiac murmurs, particularly of the aortic valve, should be sought, especially if a regional anesthetic technique is being considered.

- It is a common assumption that all patients over 65 years of age should have hematology and biochemistry investigations and an ECG performed as part of a routine preoperative workup. However, a large study has shown that abnormal laboratory tests in elderly patients had low predictive values for complication rates and did not, in general, alter perioperative management [17]. The authors suggested that routine preoperative laboratory testing on the basis of age alone may not be indicated in elderly patients. Tests should be ordered as guided by the history and physical examination.

- Similarly abnormal resting preoperative ECGs are common but are of limited value in predicting postoperative cardiac complications in older patients undergoing noncardiac surgery. Studies suggest that ordering preoperative ECGs based on age criteria alone may not be indicated [18], because ECG abnormalities in older people are prevalent but nonspecific and less useful than the presence and severity of co-existing disease states in predicting postoperative cardiac complications.

- When ordering more advanced investigations, one should give thought to the accuracy of the results. For example, an exercise ECG may be of limited value when the patient is disabled by arthritis. Radionucleotide imaging or stress echocardiography of the heart may be a more appropriate test.

- The age, physical status of the patient, the degree of urgency of surgery and the type of surgery performed determine postoperative outcome. Therefore very careful consideration should be given to the risk–benefit when an elderly patient of poor physical status presents for major surgery. Where risks outweigh perceived benefit, surgery should be deferred.

Anesthetic technique

The usual principles of intraoperative management, e.g. avoidance of hypotension, hypovolemia and hypoxia, must be adhered to in the elderly patient along with the avoidance of hypothermia. In addition, oxygen delivery to the tissues must be maintained to avoid further reductions in organ function and reserve.

Specific problems that can be encountered during anesthesia for the elderly are as follows.

- The elderly often have fragile veins, making venous access difficult.

- Edentulous patients may present a difficult airway once anesthesia is induced as the face "collapses", making a seal with the facemask and therefore ventilation difficult. Cervical spondylosis may make intubation difficult as neck extension is reduced.

- Elderly patients have thin skin and arthritic joints. Special care should be taken when transferring and positioning on the operating table. All bony prominences should be well padded.

- Elderly patients are more at risk of hypothermia both during general anesthesia (GA) and regional anesthesia [19, 20]. Warming mattresses, warmed intravenous fluids and warm air blowers must be readily available and used for all but the shortest of cases.

- The 1999 UK CEPOD report [21] highlighted the high incidence of intraoperative hypotension and how this was largely inadequately treated. In major surgical cases or cases in which there is expected to be large fluid losses, invasive monitoring of blood pressure and central venous pressure should be instituted. There should be earlier use of inotropic cardiovascular support when hypotension fails to respond to fluid loading.

Choice of anesthetic technique

This depends on the type of surgery proposed, the physical status of the patient and patient preference. The regional anesthesia versus general anesthesia debate is discussed in Chapter 8. When choosing anesthetic agents in the elderly, the following should be considered.

- All elderly patients should be preoxygenated prior to induction of anesthesia. Intravenous induction agents should be given slowly. In general, the induction dose is lower and induction time prolonged. The MAC of inhalational agents is reduced, but the dose of both depolarizing and nondepolarizing muscle relaxants is the same as a younger adult.

- The elderly are more sensitive to opioid analgesics but have delayed elimination, and so doses should be reduced and dosing interval prolonged.

- Inhalational anesthetic agents all depress the ventilatory responses to hypoxia and hypercarbia, and this will be exacerbated in the elderly who already have blunted responses to changes in oxygen and carbon dioxide levels. All elderly patients should receive supplementary oxygen in the postanesthesia recovery unit (PACU).

- Central neural blockade may be more technically difficult [22] in the elderly due to osteoarthritis, kyphoscoliosis and osteoporotic collapse. Vertebral collapse means that the spinal cord ends at a lower vertebral level in the elderly and is at risk of damage if the L3/4 space is used. A study showed that there is a great variability between the surface localization of the L3/4 space and the true space [23].

- Sympathetic blockade from spinal anesthesia reduces cardiac preload and in the elderly may result in profound hypotension that must be treated promptly and aggressively with fluids and vasoconstrictors. Failure to appreciate the magnitude of cardiovascular changes associated with spinal anesthesia in the elderly may result in poor outcome [24].

Postoperative care

- Carefully selected, elderly patients may be eligible for "fast-tracking" through the PACU and hospital system following brief surgery and anesthesia. This is facilitated by the use of short-acting inhalational agents such as Desflurane [25]. However, despite concerns relating to possible complications related to excessive depth of anesthesia, the use of bispectral index monitoring does not improve early recovery from anesthesia [26].

- Fluid prescription postoperatively will depend upon the nature of the procedure performed, the expected ongoing losses and the expected period that oral intake will be limited. Any prescription must take into account the volume of ongoing loss as well as the daily maintenance requirements. A well-organized fluid balance chart is invaluable. Ongoing losses that are extracellular should be replaced with a balanced salt solution such as compound sodium lactate. Maintenance fluids can be roughly calculated from $60\,ml\,kg^{-1}$ for the first 30 kg body weight plus $1\,ml\,kg^{-1}$ for each kg thereafter and should total $1\,mmol\,kg^{-1}$ of Na^+ and K^+ every 24 h.

- Oxygen prescription also depends on the nature of the procedure and the pre-existing medical condition of the patient. Supplemental oxygen should be prescribed for those who have had thoracic or abdominal surgery, a history of ischemic heart disease or respiratory insufficiency. The duration of oxygen therapy is determined on an individual basis so that a patient with angina having had gastric surgery should receive oxygen for at least 72 h after surgery. Any elderly patient with a patient-controlled analgesia (PCA) device should receive oxygen for the duration of use of the PCA.

- Analgesic regimens should be tailored to the type of surgery and physical status of the patient. Analgesia is discussed in Chapter 7, but it should be emphasized that nonsteroidal anti-inflammatory agents should be used with particular care in the elderly, especially those with borderline renal function. If opioids are used then the dosing interval should be increased. Elderly patients can be safely given a PCA device on the ward, but should only receive one if they understand how, and have the dexterity, to use it.

- Age should not, in itself, be a discriminator to admission to ICU. Indeed, if it is felt that major surgery will be of benefit to the patient, then it seems perverse to deny them appropriate postoperative care. However, as discussed below, the very elderly patient probably has a worse outcome from critical illness.

Outcome

In any discussion of outcome in elderly patients it is crucial to examine functional outcomes, in particular the ability to return to independent activities of daily living, as well as mortality figures.

Anesthesia outcome in the elderly

- Complication rates and morbidity following anesthesia are increased in the elderly [27]. Not surprisingly, the occurrence of complications increases hospital stay.

- One of the key points in the UK CEPOD report [28] in 2000 was: "The profile of patients who die within 30 days of an operation has changed since the report of 1990. Patients are more likely to be older, have undergone an urgent operation, be of poorer physical status and have co-existing cardiovascular or neurological disorder". The 1999 UK CEPOD report [20] that looked specifically at patients over 90 years at the time of operation recognized that "elderly patients have a high incidence of coexisting disorders and a high risk of early postoperative death".

- The occurrence of postoperative complications, especially respiratory and renal complications, are independent predictors of reduced survival [29] and must be vigorously prevented and treated. High ASA score, emergency surgery, poor preoperative functional status and the presence of congestive cardiac failure are all predictors of postoperative complications.

- Pre-existing medical problems are probably more significant in predicting poor postoperative outcome than events during the anesthetic [30]. However, one study identified intraoperative tachycardia as a predictor of cardiac complications [31].

Trauma outcome

- Mortality and functional outcome are worse in elderly patients suffering major trauma – especially the very old [32].
- Fractured hip is a common injury in the elderly patient. Close attention to preoperative care, early surgery, management of medical problems, nutrition, early mobilization and early involvement of specialist Geriatricians are important in improving outcome in this challenging group of patients. With an active management program surprisingly good results can be obtained in these patients – even in the very old [33].

ICU outcome

- It is generally acknowledged that outcome from critical illness is worse in the very old [34]. However, there is controversy over admission criteria for elderly patients and duration of treatment – highlighted by the debate in the literature provoked by a case report [35] that documented the pre- and postoperative care of a 113-year-old on an ICU.
- Following ICU discharge, perceived quality of life (QAL) in elderly survivors of critical illness is not different from younger patients, but objective assessment of QAL variables shows worse outcome in the elderly with reduced activities of daily living and an increased incidence of discharge to a care facility [36].

Postoperative cognitive dysfunction

Definition

Postoperative cognitive dysfunction (POCD) can be defined as a new onset impairment of attention and memory in a fully conscious patient, associated with a decline in activities of daily living, not present before the operation. It must be distinguished from delirium, impairment of consciousness and dementia, a permanent impairment of memory. There is a continuum of POCD which is shown in Figure 15.1.

The earliest report of cognitive decline in the literature was that by Bedford [37] in 1955 reporting a 7% incidence of cognitive decline in elderly patients undergoing surgery. However, no neuropsychological testing was done, and hypoxia and hypotension were proposed to be the cause.

More recent studies investigating cognitive function have introduced neuropsychological tests aimed at detecting the subtle changes in the domains of cognitive function.

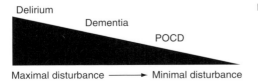

Figure 15.1 Continuum of cognitive dysfunction.

Incidence

- In the largest study of its kind to date, the International Study of Postoperative Cognitive Dysfunction group (ISPOCD1) recruited 1218 patients aged 60 years and above scheduled for major noncardiac surgery, and found the incidence of postoperative dysfunction was 25% at 1 week and 10% after 3 months [38].

- The incidence of postoperative cognitive dysfunction following cardiac surgery is 25–80% [39] measured at several months postoperatively.

- Canet *et al.* examined 372 patients aged 60 years and over [40] and found that the incidence of POCD after minor surgery at 1 week was much less than after major surgery. Three months following minor surgery, there was no significant POCD compared to controls.

- Studies, however, have shown that neuraxial anesthesia does not decrease the incidence of POCD compared to general anesthesia [41].

Risk factors for POCD

Preoperative factors:

- age (over 70 years),
- baseline cognitive impairment,
- poor baseline functional status (alcohol abuse).

Intraoperative factors:

- surgical procedures such as coronary artery bypass and aortic aneurysm repair,
- operative duration (duration of over 1 h) [38].

Postoperative factors:

- postoperative infection [38],
- postoperative pain and analgesics particularly in the first 24 h [40].

Clinical studies

The ISPOCD1 multi-center study [38] examined long-term POCD in patients 60 years and over scheduled for major abdominal and orthopedic surgery. The major findings were:

- anesthesia and surgery cause long-term postoperative decline with the risk increasing with age. Those over 70 years of age are most at risk;

- a definite correlation between a decline in activities of daily living and long-term postoperative cognitive dysfunction; and

- no correlation was found between hypoxemia and hypotension in the perioperative period and POCD.

A follow up study [42] by the same group examined cognitive function 1–2 years after noncardiac surgery.

- The results showed 10.4% of the patients had POCD after 1–2 years. However, 10.6% of the controls also had POCD after 1–2 years.

- They concluded that POCD is a reversible condition in a majority of cases, but may persist in 1% of patients.

- Logistic regression identified age, early POCD and infection within the first three months as significant risk factors for long-term POCD.

The ISPOCD2 study [43] examined middle-aged patients (aged 40–60 years), scheduled for major or orthopedic surgery.

- Their findings were 19.25% POCD at 7 days and 6.2% at 3 months. At 3 months, there was no difference between the study group and the control group.

Pathophysiology of POCD

More research has been performed on the causes of delirium than for postoperative cognitive dysfunction. Although both are forms of cognitive dysfunction, their features are distinct from one another. The ISPOCD1 found that the patients that developed delirium were not the ones that developed POCD.

The etiology of POCD is unknown, but is thought to be multi-factorial.

- Perioperative imbalance of neurotransmitter systems, especially acetylcholine and serotonin have been postulated [41].
- Central cholinergic deficiency or inhibition is thought to be associated with POCD [44]. Central nervous system inflammatory mediators have also been implicated.
- Cytokines such as interleukins are released in stressful conditions. Infusions of interleukin 2 have been associated with cognitive dysfunction and delirium [11].

Postoperative pain and analgesics have also been implicated in the increased rate of POCD seen following major surgery as compared to minor surgery [40].

- In one study, poorly controlled pain was associated with delirium [45].
- Duggleby and Lander found that pain, not analgesic intake, predicted cognitive decline after surgery [46].
- Hypoxia, hypothermia, and depression were not found to be risk factors in the development of POCD in the ISPOCD group studies.

How does anesthesia contribute to POCD?

It is known that drug interaction with central nicotinic acetylcholine receptors (nAcHRs) modulates cognitive function [47]. Many drugs used in anesthesia are known to interact with these receptors: atracurium metabolite laudanosine activates these receptors, while inhalational anesthetics and ketamine are potent inhibitors. Whereas activation of these receptors may elicit improvement in cognitive function, inhibition may cause varied clinical syndromes, delirium being one of them [48].

- Belluardo et al. suggest that activation of nAcHRs is associated with neuroprotection [49].
- Furthermore, Perry et al. have discovered that loss of nAcHRs occurs in early stages of histopathological changes associated with neurodegenerative disease before neuronal loss takes place [50].
- Central nAcHRs may therefore be the key to POCD, and their protection from drugs that interact with them may be the way to reduce POCD in the elderly.

Testing for POCD

The domains of cognitive function investigated are:

1. memory and learning;
2. attention, concentration and perception;
3. visual and spatial skills;
4. visuomotor and manual skills;
5. numerical;
6. executive functions;
7. verbal and language skills.

The battery of tests used by ISPOCD1 in testing the above domains is as follows.

1. The visual verbal learning test – a list of 15 words has to be learned in three consecutive presentations at a fixed rate on a computer screen. Patients are asked to recall as many as possible.
2. The concept shifting test. It is a test of cognitive speed, visual motor tracking and cognitive flexibility. Subjects are asked to identify letters and numbers as fast as possible in ascending order, e.g. 1-A, 2-B, 3-C, etc. Time taken and number of errors is used to score the patient.
3. The Stroop color word interference test. The ability to distinguish the written name of a color from the color it is printed in. This is a test of attention.
4. The paper and pencil memory scanning test – the subject has to identify a target letter among 20 distracting letters. This is a test of sensorimotor speed and speed of memory.
5. The letter-digit coding – tests several areas of cognitive function: visual memory, visuo-constructive, perception, visual scanning and motor skills. The subject is asked to fill in digits near letters according to a key presented at the top of the test sheet.
6. The four boxes test. This test is administered on a computer. When a black circle appears in one of the four fields on the screen, the patient presses the corresponding key on the keyboard as quickly as possible. Correct responses and errors are recorded.
7. The Mini Mental State exam. This test is not adequate for predicting POCD, but is included in the battery for screening purposes.

Consequences of POCD

The consequences of POCD when viewed from the perspective of an aging population requiring increasing numbers of surgical treatment are spiralling health costs. Patients who suffer long-term POCD become dependent on others for daily care whereas they had been independent before surgery. They also have longer hospital stays and higher rates of discharge to rehabilitative facilities.

Further reading

Dodds C, Kumar C, Servin F, eds. *Anaesthesia for the Elderly Patient*. Oxford, Oxford University Press, 2007.

Sieber FE, ed. *Geriatric Anaesthesia*. New York, McGraw Hill, 2006.

References

1. Klopfenstein CE, Herrmann FR, Michel JP, Clergue F, Forster A. The influence of an aging surgical population on the anaesthesia workload: A ten-year survey. *Anesth Analg* 1998; **86**: 1165–70.

2. Folkow B, Svanborg A. Physiology of cardiovascular aging. *Physiol Rev* 1993; **73**: 725–64.

3. Priebe H-J. The aged cardiovascular risk patient. *Br J Anaesth* 2000; **85**: 763–78.

4. Wahba WM. Influence of aging on lung function – Clinical significance of changes from age twenty. *Anesth Analg* 1983; **62**: 764–76.

5. Crapo RO, Campbell EJ. Aging of the respiratory system. In: Fishman AP, ed. *Pulmonary Diseases and Disorders*. New York, McGraw-Hill. 1998; 251–64.

6. Lindeman RD. Renal physiology and pathophysiology of aging. *Contrib Nephrol* 1993; **105**: 1–12.

7. Lane N, Allen K. Hyponatraemia after orthopaedic surgery. *Br Med J* 1999; **318**: 1363–4.

8. Kampmann JP, Sinding J, Moller-Jorgensen I. Effect of age on liver function. *Geriatrics* 1975; **30**: 91–5.

9. Woodhouse KW, Mutch E, Williams FM, *et al.* The effect of age on pathways of drug metabolism in human liver. *Age Ageing* 1984; **13**: 328–34.

10. Creasy H, Rapoport SI. The ageing human brain. *Ann Neurol* 1985; **17**: 2–10.

11. Dorfman LJ, Bosley TM. Age-related changes in peripheral and central nerve conduction in man. *Neurology* 1979; **29**: 38–44.

12. Collins KJ, Exton-Smith AN, James MH. Functional changes in autonomic nervous responses with ageing. *Age Ageing* 1980; **9**: 17–24.

13. Montamat SC, Cusack BJ, Vestal RE. Management of drug therapy in the elderly. *N Engl J Med* 1989; **231**: 303–09.

14. Calvey TN, Williams NE, eds. Variability in drug response. In: *Principles and Practice of Pharmacology for Anaesthetists*. Oxford, Blackwell Scientific Publications. 1991; 133–5.

15. DelGuercio LR, Cohn JD. Monitoring operative risk in the elderly. *JAMA* 1980; **243**: 1350–5.

16. Phillip B, Pastor D, Bellows W, Leung JM. The prevalence of preoperative diastolic filling abnormalities in geriatric surgical patients. *Anesth Analg* 2003; **97**: 1214–21.

17. Dzankic S, Pastor D, Gonzalez C, Leung JM. The prevalence and predictive value of abnormal preoperative laboratory tests in elderly surgical patients. *Anesth Analg* 2001; **93**: 301–8.

18. Liu LL, Dzankic S, Leung JM. Preoperative electrocardiogram abnormalities do not predict postoperative cardiac complications in geriatric surgical patients. *J Am Geriatr Soc* 2002; **50**: 1186–91.

19. Kurz A, Plattner O, Sessler DI, Huemer G, Redl G, Lackner F. The threshold for thermoregulatory vasoconstriction during nitrous oxide/isoflurane anaesthesia is lower in elderly than in young patients. *Anesthesiology* 1993; **79**: 465–9.

20. Frank SM, Shir Y, Raja SN, Fleisher LA, Beattie C. Core hypothermia and skin-surface temperature gradients. Epidural versus general anaesthesia and the effects of age. *Anesthesiology* 1994; **80**: 502–08.

21. Extremes of age. The 1999 Report of the National Confidential Enquiry into Perioperative Deaths. National CEPOD. ISBN 0 95222069 6 X.

22. Tessler MJ, Kardash K, Wahba RM, Kleiman SJ, Trihas ST, Rossignol M. The performance of spinal anaesthesia is marginally more difficult in the elderly. *Reg Anesth Pain Med* 1999; **24**: 126–30.

23. Broadbent CR, Maxwell WB, Ferrie R, Wilson DJ, Gawne-Cain M, Russell R. Ability of anaesthetists to identify a marked lumbar interspace. *Anaesthesia* 2000; **55**: 1122–6.

24. Holland R. Trends recognised in cases reported to the New South Wales Special Committee Investigating Deaths under

Anaesthesia. *Anaesth Intens Care* 1987; **15**: 97–8.

25. Fredman B, Sheffer O, Zohar E, *et al.* Fast-track eligibility of geriatric patients undergoing short urologic surgery procedures. *Anesth Analg* 2002; **94**: 560–4.

26. Zohar E, Luban I, White PF, Ramati E, Shabat S, Fredman B. Bispectral index monitoring does not improve early recovery of geriatric outpatients undergoing brief surgical procedures. *Can J Anaesth* 2006; **53**: 20–5.

27. Tiret L, Desmonts JM, Hatton F, Vourc'h G. Complications associated with anaesthesia – A prospective survey in France. *Can Anaesth Soc J* 1986; **33**: 336–44.

28. Then and Now. The 2000 Report of the National Confidential Enquiry into Perioperative Deaths. National CEPOD ISBN 0 9522069 7 8.

29. Manku K, Bacchetti P, Leung JM. Prognostic significance of postoperative in-hospital complications in elderly patients. I. Long-term survival. *Anesth Analg* 2003; **96**: 583–9.

30. Liu LL, Leung JM. Predicting adverse postoperative outcomes in patients aged 80 years or older. *J Am Geriatr Soc* 2000; **48**: 405–12.

31. Leung JM, Dzankic S. Relative importance of preoperative health status versus intraoperative factors in predicting postoperative adverse outcomes in geriatric surgical patients. *J Am Geriatr Soc* 2001; **49**: 1080–5.

32. Grossman M, Scaff DW, Miller D, Reed J, Hoey B, Anderson HL. Functional outcomes in octogenarian trauma. *J Trauma* 2003; **55**: 26–32.

33. Shah MR, Aharonoff GB, Wolinsky P, Zuckerman JD, Koval KJ. Outcome after hip fracture in individuals ninety years of age and older. *J Orthop Trauma* 2001; **15**: 34–9.

34. Boumendil A, Somme D, Garrouste-Orgeas M, Guidet B. Should elderly patients be admitted to the intensive care unit? *Intens Care Med* 2007; **33**: 1252–62.

35. Oliver CD, White SA, Platt MW. Surgery for fractured femur and elective ICU admission at 113 yr of age. *Br J Anaesth* 2000; **84**: 260–2.

36. Rady MY, Johnson DJ. Hospital discharge to care facility: A patient-centered outcome for the evaluation of intensive care for octogenarians. *Chest* 2004; **126**: 1583–91.

37. Bedford PD. Adverse cerebral effects of anaesthesia on old people. *Lancet* 1955; **2**: 259–63.

38. Moller JT, Cluitmans P, Rasmussen LS, *et al.* Long term postoperative cognitive dysfunction in the elderly: ISPOCD1 study. *Lancet* 1998; **351**: 857–61.

39. Borowicz LM, Goldsborough MA, Selnes OA, *et al.* Neuropsychologic change after cardiac surgery: A critical review. *J Cardiothorac Vasc Anesth* 1996; **10**: 105–12.

40. Canet J, Raeder J, Rasmussen LR, *et al.* Cognitive function after minor surgery in the elderly. *Acta Anaesth Scand* 2003; **47**: 1204–10.

41. Wu CL, Hsu WBS, Richman JM, Raja SN. Postoperative cognitive dysfunction as an outcome of regional anesthesia and analgesia. *Reg Anesth Pain Med* 2004; **29**: 257–68.

42. Abildstrom H, Rasmussen LS, Rentowl P, *et al.* Cognitive function 1–2 years after non-cardiac surgery in the elderly. *Acta Anaesthesiol Scand* 2000; **44**: 1246–51.

43. Johnson T, Monk T, Rasmussen LS, *et al.* ISPOCD2 Investigators. Postoperative cognitive dysfunction in middle-aged patients. *Anesthesiology* 2002; **96**: 1351–7.

44. Flacker JM, Lipsitz LA. Serum anticholinergic activity changes with acute illness in the elderly medical patient. *J Gerontol Med Sci* 1999; **54A**: M12–16.

45. Schor JD, Levkoff SE, Lipsitz LA, *et al.* Risk factors for delirium in hospitalized elderly. *JAMA* 1992; **267**: 827–31.

46. Duggleby and Lander J. Cognitive status and postoperative pain: Older adults. *J Pain Symptom Mgmt* 1994; **9**: 19–27.

47. Fovale V. Drugs of anesthesia, central nicotinic receptors and post-operative cognitive dysfunction. *Acta Anaesth Scand* 2003; **47**: 1180.

48. Tunn LE, Damlouji NF, Holland A, *et al.* Association of postoperative delirium with

raised levels of anticholinergic drugs. *Lancet* 1981; **8248**: 651–3.

49. Belluardo N, Mudo G, Blum M, *et al.* Neurotrophic effects of central nicotinic receptor activation. *J Neural Transm Suppl* 2000; **60**: 227–45.

50. Perry EK, Morris CM, Court JA, *et al.* Alteration in nicotinic binding sites in Parkinson's disease, Lewy body dementia and Alzheimer's disease: Possible index of early neuropathology. *Neuroscience* 1995; **64**: 385–95.

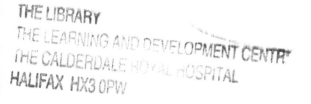

chapter 16

The patient with cardiac disease undergoing noncardiac surgery

C. Harle

Cardiac disease is common and represents a significant source of risk in patients presenting for noncardiac surgery. An understanding of the principles of anesthesia for patients with cardiac disease and approaches to reducing this risk is essential for all anesthesiologists. Patients with coronary artery disease, valvular heart disease and pulmonary artery hypertension are discussed in this chapter. This chapter will not address the management of patients with dysrhythmia or congenital cardiac disease

Coronary artery disease

It is essential that anesthesiologists have a sound understanding of the pathophysiology of coronary artery disease (CAD), the preparation of at risk patients and the perioperative management of myocardial ischemia.

- Effective treatment of and reduction of risk factors for CAD have resulted in a significant reduction in death rates from CAD over the last two decades. Nevertheless, CAD remains the leading cause of mortality in Western adults – CAD causes 1 of every 5 deaths in the USA.
- Furthermore, the prevalence in the general public is high – between 6% and 7% of *all* adults over 18 years have CAD [1], and someone will die from a coronary event approximately once every minute in the USA in 2008. The prevalence of CAD increases with age.
- Thus many patients undergoing noncardiac surgery have CAD, diagnosed or otherwise.
- Cardiovascular disease remains a leading cause of morbidity and 30-day mortality following surgery, particularly in patients older than 70 years of age undergoing major thoracic, abdominal or vascular surgery [2].
- Patients who suffer postoperative myocardial infarction (MI) following noncardiac surgery have in-hospital mortality rates between 15 and 25%, and nonfatal perioperative MI is an independent predictor of subsequent cardiovascular death within 6 months [3].

Pathophysiology

- Intraluminal occlusion of the epicardial coronary arteries arises from the progressive growth of atherosclerotic plaques. It is believed that these plaques are the consequence of an attempt at healing an endothelial injury mediated by a complex inflammatory process.
- Genetic predisposition, cigarette smoking, diabetes, hyperlipidemia, sedentary lifestyle and obesity are all associated with increased risk of CAD.
- Reduced coronary blood flow results in an imbalance between delivery and demand for myocardial oxygen, with myocardial ischemia resulting. This typically manifests as stable angina. Coronary arterial spasm can exacerbate this imbalance.

Anesthesia for the High Risk Patient, ed. I. McConachie. Published by Cambridge University Press.
© Cambridge University Press 2009.

- Acute coronary syndromes are usually the consequence of plaque rupture with intra-luminal thrombosis and near or complete occlusion of the vessel, which results in unstable angina, MI, and may cause sudden cardiac death.
- Patients with CAD who are subjected to surgical stress, inflammation and increased platelet activation are at risk of suffering perioperative myocardial injury. Significantly, postmortem studies in patients who died from MI following noncardiac surgery suggest that the patho-physiological mechanism of MI following noncardiac surgery involves disruption of vulner-able coronary artery plaque, followed by thrombosis of the diseased coronary artery [4].

Preoperative assessment

Identification of patients at risk of CAD is the first step in reducing the perioperative risk. The various methods of identifying and predicting cardiac risk are discussed in Chapter 3.

Having identified patients at risk, the next step is to decide whether any intervention or therapies are required, which may reduce the risk.

Preoperative revascularization

Revascularization is probably only indicated for those in whom revascularization would be beneficial independent of noncardiac surgery.

- The CARP trial [5] suggests that pre-emptive revascularization per se is of no benefit prior to major vascular surgery. Limitations to this study are significant, and the authors do not distinguish between outcomes following percutaneous coronary intervention (PCI) and those following CABG.
- Historical data suggest that pre-emptive CABG is indicated in patients undergoing major elective vascular surgery by virtue of improved long-term outcomes [6], specifically in patients with multi-vessel CAD and impaired ventricular function. However, CABG confers procedure-related morbidity and mortality and may delay the proposed non-cardiac surgery, with significant implications [7].
- More recently, CABG has been suggested to confer significant survival benefit to patients with CAD amenable to surgical revascularization undergoing nonvascular abdominal surgery [8].
- CABG has also recently been found superior to PCI in the prevention of perioperative MI in patients undergoing subsequent vascular surgery [9], probably due to more complete revascularization in the CABG group.

The choice of revascularization technique should be carefully considered.

- Coronary artery bypass grafting (CABG) should be offered to those patients in whom it would be indicated in concordance with the updated AHA/ACC guidelines from 2004 [10].
- It seems that PCI before noncardiac surgery will not prevent perioperative cardiac events, and it should be reserved only for patients in whom PCI is indicated for an acute preoperative coronary syndrome [2].

Patients who have recently undergone PCI pose significant perioperative challenges.

- Dual anti-platelet therapy is standard practice in these patients, and effective platelet inhibition will increase the risks of bleeding and requirements for transfusion of blood and blood products.

- Abrupt cessation of anti-platelet therapy is associated with increased incidence of stent thrombosis, and MI in this setting has a mortality rate of up to 45% due to the interruption of blood flow in a high-flow vessel supplying a myocardial territory with poor collateral blood flow, which has not had the opportunity to have been preconditioned by previous ischemia [11].

Medical optimization

Optimization of medical therapy is important in these patients, and should be an integral part of the perioperative management, as mentioned above. This should begin in the preoperative stage. An understanding of the pharmacological basis for these therapies as well as their limitations will aid decision making for the physician.

Beta-blocker therapy

Beta-blockers have long been considered an important weapon in the battle against perioperative MI. Proposed mechanisms by which they are cardioprotective include an improvement in the ratio of myocardial oxygen supply to demand, by a reduction in heart rate and contractility, a well as anti-arrhythmic and anti-inflammatory effects and anti-renin–angiotensin properties. The role of beta-blockers is discussed in Chapters 4 and 5.

Nitrates

Nitrates have long been the mainstay treatment for angina. Nitrates facilitate coronary vasodilation and improve coronary blood flow. They are effective anti-anginal and anti-ischemic agents. They *may*, however, cause coronary steal and myocardial ischemia, and they frequently cause hypotension [12]. There is a small association with perioperative nitrate administration and adverse cardiac outcomes following noncardiac surgery [13]. Indeed, long-term nitrate therapy following MI is associated with increased cardiac death [14].

Calcium channel blockers (CCB)

CCB improve the balance between myocardial oxygen supply and demand by a combination of a reduction in inotropy, a reduction in chronotropy, coronary vasodilatation and afterload reduction. CCB, in particular diltiazem, appears to reduce death rates and the incidence of MI in a meta-analysis [15]. There is, however, counterintuitive evidence of an increase in postoperative silent myocardial ischemia in patients receiving CCB [13].

Angiotensin converting enzyme inhibitors (ACE-I) and angiotensin receptor antagonist (ARA)

These drugs are indicated in the management of patients with CAD and left ventricular dysfunction, where they have a survival benefit for patients who have had an MI [16]. Their role in the perioperative management of patients with CAD undergoing either cardiac or noncardiac surgery remains controversial and is fully discussed in Chapter 4.

Statins

There is evidence that statin therapy improves endothelial function, reduces vascular inflammation and stabilizes atherosclerotic plaque [2]. The cardioprotective mechanisms of statins include scavenging of oxygen radicals, antithrombotic effects, anti-inflammatory effects and a reduction in endothelial cell apoptosis [17]. Statins are discussed further in Chapter 4.

Alpha-2 agonists

The alpha-2 agonists clonidine and mivazerol generate a Class IIb recommendation from the ACC/AHA guidelines for perioperative control of hypertension in patients with known CAD or at least one risk factor. A meta-analysis of 23 trials with 3395 patients showed that alpha-2 agonists are associated with significant reduction in death and MI during vascular surgery [18]. Pre-emptive Clonidine therapy has also been shown to reduce perioperative myocardial mortality and improved survival two years after noncardiac surgery in patients at risk of CAD [19]. Clonidine decreases central sympathetic activity, and enhances adenosine induced coronary vasodilatation [20], both of which mechanisms may explain its beneficial effects on myocardial ischemia.

Aspirin and anti-platelet therapy

Aspirin (ASA) has an established role in the prevention and treatment of myocardial infarction [21]. It can be reasonably expected to confer benefits in the perioperative period when platelet reactivity is increased. Abrupt cessation of anti-platelet medication is undesirable, increasing the risk of acute coronary thrombosis. Both patients with intracoronary stents and those with untreated CAD are at risk.

- This risk is now believed to be significantly greater than the risk of surgical bleeding if these drugs are continued [11].
- The risk of stroke is also increased if aspirin is withdrawn [22].

The risk of surgical bleeding *is* increased with anti-platelet therapy; however, low-dose ASA therapy per se is not associated with significant bleeding complications, nor with increased perioperative mortality, with the notable exceptions of intracranial surgery and prostatectomy [23].

However, patients who have recently undergone PCI and those who have drug eluting stents require *dual* anti-platelet therapy with ASA and the irreversible adenosine diphosphate receptor antagonist clopidogrel.

- Unlike ASA, clopidogrel is a significant risk factor for perioperative bleeding, blood and blood product requirement, morbidity [24] and possibly mortality in cardiac surgery [25]. Less is known about bleeding complications in noncardiac surgery; however, it is reasonable to assume an increased risk for bleeding, and it has been recommended that clopidogrel be held for 5 days prior to surgery in patients on dual antiplatelet therapy [26].
- Abrupt cessation of clopidogrel is associated with death and MI following both PCI and acute coronary syndrome, suggesting a possible clopidogrel rebound effect [27].

Dipyridamole has similar effects on platelet function to those of clopidogrel, and is sometimes used as an alternative to ASA.

Abciximab, integrilin, tirofiban and ticlodipine all antagonize the binding of fibrinogen with the glycoprotein IIb/IIIa fibrinogen receptor on the platelet surface membrane. These agents are mostly used in the management of patients undergoing PCI and in those with unstable angina, or acute MI. Ticlodipine has a proven role in the prevention and treatment of transient ischemic attacks. The exact role of these agents in the management of stable patients with CAD is unclear; however, several patients have been treated with these agents, and will likely continue to be. Little other than anecdote is known about the effects of these agents on blood loss in the perioperative period; however, these are potent anti-platelet agents, and are undoubtedly associated with increased bleeding. Similarly, abrupt cessation of these agents may be associated with significant increased thrombotic risk. Knowledge of the pharmacology of these agents, their respective half-lives and estimation of relative risk of continuing therapy versus cessation in the perioperative period is an important aspect of providing anesthesia to patients with CAD.

The patient with a coronary stent, or a recent PCI

These patients present significant clinical challenges in the perioperative period. Firstly, one has to appreciate the type of stent and the implications thereof. Broadly speaking, there are two types of stent:

- bare metal stents (BMS), and
- drug-eluting stents (DES).

A feared complication of any stent procedure is thrombosis. Postmortem examination of thrombosed stents reveals that the pathology is a combination of neointimal hyperplasia and subsequent thrombosis. Neointimal hyperplasia results from a healing process, related to proliferation and migration of smooth muscle cells [28].

DES elute either paclitaxel or sirolimus. Sirolimus is a macrolide which is immunosuppressive and anti-mitotic, and paclitaxel is primarily an anti-cancer cytotoxic chemotherapeutic agent with potent anti-mitotic properties. The rationale for having these agents eluted is to suppress endothelial growth and prevent neointimal hyperplasia.

- It was thought that, particularly when combined with dual anti-platelet therapy, the DES would remain patent longer than the BMS.
- Recently, however, we have been able to appreciate that this is not necessarily the case, and DES have been associated with much higher rates of late stent thrombosis and related MI and death than BMS [29].
- Further preliminary evidence that DES confer no benefit over BMS, and that sirolimus stents may in fact increase noncardiac mortality [30], has provoked discussion and controversy.
- A meta-analysis of 9 trials including more than 5000 patients concludes that stent thrombosis is more common 1 year after DES than with BMS [31].
- It is clear that patients who have DES in particular require dual anti-platelet therapy, usually with ASA and clopidogrel, for at least a year, and possibly longer. The premature cessation of dual anti-platelet therapy is undesirable, with stent thrombosis being the undesirable outcome. Even a year after cessation of clopidogrel, patients with DES appear at greater risk of late complications in stent stenosis than patients with BMS [29].

It is therefore important to consider the merits of cases on an individual basis, and a multidisciplinary discussion including the anesthesiologist, surgeon and cardiologist should take place to plan the perioperative management of high-risk patients on dual anti-platelet therapy who are scheduled for elective surgery [26]. This planning must consider the patient's ischemic risk, the risk of withholding antiplatelet therapy, and the risk of bleeding. Table 16.1 proposes an approach to facilitate planning in these patients, which takes into account the nature of the surgery, the risk of bleeding and the risk of stopping anti-platelet therapy.

It is recommended, where possible, that surgery be delayed 2–4 weeks following PCI without stenting, 4–6 weeks after stenting with BMS, and for 12 months following PCI with DES [11].

Table 16.1 An approach to surgery and antiplatelet therapy (modified from [11, 26])

Surgical hemorrhagic risk	Cerebro- and cardiovascular risk		
	Low	**Intermediate**	**High**
	>6 months after MI, PCI, BMS, CABG, stroke. >12 months if complications	6–24 weeks after MI, PCI +BMS, CABG, or stroke (Ø complication): >12 months after DES; high-risk stents (long, proximal, multiple, overlapping, small vessels, bifurcation); low EF, diabetes	<6 weeks after MI, PCI, BMS, CABG; <6 months after same if complications; <12 months after high-risk DES; <2 weeks after stroke
Low risk			
Transfusion normally not required: peripheral, plastic and general surgery, biopsies: minor orthopedic, ENT, and general surgery; endoscopy; eye anterior chamber, dental extraction and surgery	Elective surgery OK; maintain ASA	Elective surgery OK; maintain ASA and clopidogrel if prescribed	Elective surgery: postpone; vital or emergency surgery OK; maintain ASA and clopidogrel
Intermediate risk			
Transfusions frequently required; visceral surgery; cardiovascular surgery; major orthopedic, ENT, reconstructive surgery; endoscopic urology	Elective surgery OK; maintain ASA	Elective surgery: postpone; surgery absolutely required: OK; maintain ASA (clopidogrel if prescribed)	Elective surgery: postpone; vital or emergency surgery: OK; maintain ASA and clopidogrel
High risk			
Possible bleeding in a closed space; intracranial neurosurgery: spinal canal surgery; eye posterior chamber surgery	Elective surgery: OK; maintain statin; withdraw ASA (maximum 7 days)	Elective surgery: postpone; surgery absolutely required: OK; maintain ASA, clopidogrel (if prescribed)	OK only for vital surgery; maintain ASA. Bridge with tirofiban/ eptifibatide and heparin

Summary:

Bleeding risk:

Major: Intervention cannot proceed on antiplatelet agents

Moderate: Intervention can proceed on ASA alone

Minor: Intervention can proceed on ASA and clopidogrel

Risk of stent thrombosis:

Major: DES in place less than 6 months, patient requires ASA and clopidogrel

Moderate: DES in place more than 6 months to a year

Whichever anti-anginal, anti-platelet or anti-ischemic therapy is contemplated, the peri-operative physician has to balance the risks of hypotension and reflex tachycardia with the associated reduction in coronary perfusion pressure and coronary perfusion time against the coronary vasodilation and reduction in myocardial oxygen consumption these agents confer.

Anesthetic management

Anesthesia for patients with CAD must be planned and executed with the goals of optimizing myocardial oxygen delivery and minimizing myocardial oxygen demand.

Coronary blood flow and arterial oxygen content are the major determinants of myocardial oxygen delivery.

Coronary blood flow depends on:

1. coronary perfusion pressure, which is the aortic diastolic pressure minus left ventricular end diastolic pressure;
2. resistance to flow within the coronary artery, influenced by coronary smooth muscle tone, obstruction to flow as caused by atheromatous plaques and blood viscosity; and
3. diastolic time, which is the phase of the cardiac cycle when coronary blood flow takes place.

Myocardial oxygen demand is predominantly influenced by:

1. heart rate;
2. left ventricular afterload; and
3. myocardial contractility.

Consequently the following clinical parameters are undesirable:

⇑ heart rate   ⇓ diastolic pressure,

⇑ afterload   ⇓ arterial oxygen content

⇑ left ventricular end diastolic pressure

⇑ contractility

No single technique can guarantee these conditions; however, by paying attention to these physiological goals, and with appropriate monitoring to detect myocardial ischemia, the outcome of these patients may be significantly influenced by the choice of anesthetic technique. Particular attention should be given to avoiding the stressors associated with intense stimulation, such as that associated with laryngoscopy, intense surgical stimulus and tracheal extubation, as tachycardia and hypertension are undesirable.

Monitoring

Selection of monitors should be guided by availability, practicality and expertise of the attending anesthesiologist at interpreting the information the monitors provide.

Most national anesthesia societies have similar minimum standards for monitoring. Additional monitoring may include, but is not limited to 5-lead ECG monitoring with ST segment analysis, continuous temperature measurement, urine output, direct arterial pressure monitoring, central venous pressure monitoring, trans esophageal echo (TEE), pulmonary artery flotation catheters (PAFC), and other less-invasive monitors, such as those which use pulse wave form analysis or aortic Doppler signals to estimate cardiac output. Monitoring should aid the diagnosis and quantification of ischemia, as well as the hemodynamic consequences of ischemia, and the response to intervention.

Volatile agents

Volatile inhalational anesthetic agents have beneficial effects on vulnerable myocardium through the phenomenon of ischemic preconditioning. Furthermore, these agents may also modify the effect of ischemia during the ischemic insult and following reperfusion (post-conditioning). Animal studies have consistently demonstrated a myocardial protective effect mediated by ischemic preconditioning associated with the use of volatile anesthetic agents. Studies are now beginning to support this in the clinical context with reduced troponin release, reduced ICU length of stay and reduced in-hospital stay being credited to volatile mediated ischemic preconditioning [32]. There are data to support the use of Isoflurane, Sevoflurane and Desflurane for the purpose of ischemic preconditioning.

Opioid agents

There are opioid receptors in the myocardium, and animal experiments have shown that selective δ and κ opioid receptor agonists confer significant myocardial protection in induced ischemic models. μ receptor agonists appear to have no benefit, and myocardial opioid antagonist pretreatment is associated with a reduction in function and metabolic integrity in these models [33]. The clinical relevance of these findings remains to be elucidated.

Analgesia

Pain is associated with tachycardia, hypertension and exacerbation of myocardial ischemia. Opioid analgesia is effective in the treatment of severe angina, and has beneficial effects on the pulmonary vasculature, and it is logical that effective analgesia is an important component of the anesthetic for the patient with CAD. Provided they are not used excessively, opioids are useful in pain management for these patients

Multi-modal analgesia (MMA) using opioids, local anesthetics, nonsteroidal anti-inflammatory drugs (NSAIDs) and other "co-analgesics" is now an established practice.

- Caution should be exercised, however, when prescribing NSAIDs to patients with cardiovascular disease due to the risks of exacerbation of hypertension, fluid and electrolyte shifts, congestive heart failure and acute renal failure [34].

- The role of the selective cyclo-oxygenase-2 (COX-2) inhibitors is not absolutely clear. Rofecoxib was withdrawn from world markets in 2004 due to an increase in adverse cardiac events.

- The European regulatory authorities and the FDA appear to have inconsistent conclusions regarding the safety of NSAIDs in patients with cardiovascular disease [35].

- It is possible that the short-term benefits in the perioperative period outweigh the risks; however, a careful risk–benefit assessment is important before using either NSAIDs or COX-2 inhibitors [36].

- Acetaminophen appears safe in patients at risk and is a reliable component of MMA in patients at risk for cardiac events [34].

- Gabapentin appears to be generally safe, although caution should again be exercised in prescribing this class of drug to patients with chronic heart failure, as there have been case reports of exacerbation of heart failure associated with Pregabalin [37].

Central neuraxial analgesia (CNA)

These techniques are popular and effective analgesic options for an array of surgical procedures. Thoracic epidural analgesia (TEA) in particular confers significant benefits in the setting of CAD, by virtue of vasodilation of diseased coronaries [38], improved coronary blood flow, reduced afterload and reduced heart rate with the associated "sympathectomy". Furthermore, there is evidence that epidural analgesia reduces postoperative cardiovascular complications following major vascular surgery, and in high-risk patients [39].

The risk of conducting CNA has to be balanced against the risk of hematoma formation, given the possible concomitant use of anti-platelet agents, and other anti-coagulants. The American Society of Regional Anesthesia and Pain Medicine (ASRA) have issued extensive guidelines regarding the timing of regional anesthetic techniques and anticoagulation. In essence, clopidogrel should be stopped 7 days before the planned intervention [40], which may be impossible or impractical depending on the patient's circumstances. Nevertheless, where reasonable and safe, these techniques can be very important in reducing cardiac risk.

Mechanical support systems

Severe and refractory myocardial ischemia may be reversed, or at least temporized, with an intra-aortic balloon pump (IABP). This device has an established role in patients with severe CAD undergoing CABG. There are several case reports and small case series which support the use of an IABP in noncardiac surgery; however, there is probably insufficient evidence at present to adequately assess the risk–benefit ratio of this intervention as prophylaxis against ischemia [2]. It should, however, be considered in high-risk and unstable patients.

Postoperative disposition

The level of postoperative care will depend on the patient's condition, the facilities available, the patient's pre-existing risk and the extent of the procedure undertaken. The intensive care, high dependency or coronary care units are suitable places for high-risk patients to be monitored and cared for following surgery. It is important to recall that postoperative ischemia commonly occurs on the second and third postoperative days. Postoperative goals include preservation of oxygen delivery, hemoglobin and oxygenation, maintenance of the hemodynamic goals balancing myocardial oxygen supply and demand, restoration of normal fluid and electrolyte balance, normothermia, hemodynamic stability and re-introduction anti-ischemic therapies.

Valvular heart disease and pulmonary hypertension

This second half of this chapter aims to provide an outline of the management of patients with valvular heart disease with or without pulmonary hypertension, who are undergoing noncardiac surgery.

- There are few data regarding valvular heart disease and perioperative risk analysis.
- However, the presence of ventricular dysfunction, arrhythmia, pulmonary hypertension and co-existing coronary artery disease all increase cardiac risk when patients with valvular disease undergo noncardiac surgery.
- There is good evidence that aortic stenosis (AS) is a strong independent predictor of perioperative risk, and that the severity of AS is predictive of the risk [41].

- Aortic incompetence (AI) has also been associated with increased perioperative mortality.
- Less is known about the risk conferred by mitral stenosis (MS) and mitral regurgitation (MR).
- It appears that in the absence of heart failure or recent myocardial infarction, lesions of the mitral valve do not contribute significantly to perioperative mortality.
- It is, however, very important to note that all of these four valve lesions are associated with an increased incidence of postoperative congestive heart failure.

Preoperative assessment

As for the patient with CAD, the ACC/AHA have issued comprehensive guidelines on perioperative evaluation of these patients [2]. Investigation should focus on identification and quantification of valvular disease. Echocardiography remains the most effective means of assessing valvular structure and function. Furthermore, it is useful in estimating ventricular function, chamber dimensions, ventricular hypertrophy, detecting intracardiac thrombus and the anatomical and pathological consequences of valvular disease, including pulmonary hypertension and diastolic dysfunction. Estimation of the severity of valvular disease is imperative in planning and executing safe anesthesia and surgery in these patients.

The evaluation of patients with valvular heart disease should include an analysis of the need for endocarditis prophylaxis. Historically, antibiotic prophylaxis was routinely prescribed for allcomers with valvular heart disease. There is increasing evidence that for dental procedures, routine prophylaxis is likely to prevent only an exceedingly small number of cases of infective endocarditis (IE).

Cardiac conditions associated with the highest risk of adverse outcomes from endocarditis, for which prophylaxis with dental procedures is reasonable:

- prosthetic cardiac valve or prosthetic material used for cardiac valve repair;
- previous IE;
- congenital heart disease (CHD)*;
- unrepaired cyanotic CHD, including palliative shunts and conduits;
- completely repaired congenital heart defect with prosthetic material or device, whether placed by surgery or by catheter intervention, during the first 6 months after the procedure†;
- repaired CHD with residual defects at the site or adjacent to the site of a prosthetic patch or prosthetic device (which inhibit endothelialization); and
- cardiac transplantation recipients who develop cardiac valvulopathy.

*Except for the conditions listed above, antibiotic prophylaxis is no longer recommended for any other form of CHD.

†Prophylaxis is reasonable because endothelialization of prosthetic material occurs within 6 months after the procedure [42].

Similarly for nondental surgery, the prescribing of antibiotic prophylaxis should take into account the risk of IE, as well as the risk for adverse outcomes from IE. Advancing age, diabetes mellitus, impaired immunity and dialysis each increase the risk of adverse outcomes from IE, and they frequently co-exist. Fleisher *et al.* recommend that physicians review all available data, and use clinical judgment before prescribing prophylaxis [2].

Conduct of anesthesia

- Awareness of the pathophysiological processes involved in valvular heart disease and pulmonary hypertension is essential to the successful anesthetic management of patients presenting for noncardiac surgery.

- Anticipation of the effects of surgical stresses including blood loss and other interventions such as the introduction of pneumoperitoneum during laparoscopy, alterations in position, application of tourniquets to limbs or cross-clamps to large blood vessels and the reperfusion associated with their release will surely facilitate reducing morbidity and mortality in these high-risk surgical patients.

- Anesthetic planning should include appropriate investigations, premedication and plans for the conduct of anesthesia, including monitoring techniques, analgesic strategies and plans for the postoperative management of these patients.

Monitoring

It is essential that appropriate monitoring be instituted before the induction of any form of anesthesia in these high-risk patients. In addition to routine standard monitoring, anesthesiologists should have a very low threshold for using direct arterial blood pressure monitoring. Central venous pressure (CVP) monitoring and the use of a pulmonary artery flotation catheter (PAFC) in particular may assist in monitoring fluid therapy. It must be borne in mind, however, that arrhythmias can be induced by the insertion of guide wires and catheters into the heart. Ventricular arrhythmias in particular are sometimes difficult to treat in patients with severe ventricular hypertrophy, and a defibrillator should be present whenever such procedures are being undertaken. Where the expertise is available, transesophageal echocardiography (TEE) can be a very useful adjunct to monitoring, and can be used to guide volume replacement, as well as to monitor ventricular performance. Institutional facilities and expertise will inevitably vary, and monitoring should be appropriate to the ability to interpret the information obtained. Other monitoring should be employed as discussed above in relation to CAD, and in compliance with national guidelines and standards.

Aortic stenosis

AS is a significantly underappreciated risk factor and accounts for substantial perioperative morbidity and mortality. Targeted intraoperative monitoring and prompt correction of hemodynamic abnormalities can allow for safe anesthesia in patients with severe, symptomatic AS undergoing noncardiac surgery [43].

Definitions

The severity of AS is traditionally estimated at cardiac catheterization, and expressed as the peak-to-peak pressure gradient (PG) between the left ventricle (LV) and the aorta:

$$PG = P(LV) - P(aorta)$$

- A PG greater than 50 mmHg is defined as critical AS. It is important to remember that this value is true for patients with normal cardiac output, and smaller gradients may occur in those who have LV failure, and worse degrees of AS. It is possible to quantify PGs

251

using Doppler echocardiography; however, patients older than 50 should have coronary angiography to exclude concomitant coronary artery disease.

- Valve surface area (the area of the orifice of the open valve) is also an important measurement in AS. The normal valve surface area is 2.6–3.5 cm^2. A valve surface area of 1 cm^2 or less is likely to cause clinically significant aortic valve obstruction.

Etiology and risk

Isolated AS is usually an acquired disease. Degeneration and/or calcification may occur on a previously normal valve, or on a congenitally bicuspid valve. The end result is obstruction of the aortic outflow. Isolated rheumatic disease of the aortic valve is not common.

- Presenting symptoms include angina, syncope and heart failure.
- Onset of symptoms from AS is usually followed by death within 2–5 years if the diseased valve is not replaced.
- The optimal timing for valve replacement in patients with significant AS without symptoms is less clear [44].

Decisions to proceed with anesthesia and surgery in these patients need to be made with due consideration of severity of AS, and relative urgency of proposed surgery. Certainly, patients with New York Heart Association (NYHA) class 4 symptoms, i.e. breathless at rest, ought to have valvular surgery before elective noncardiac surgery. Patients needing urgent or emergency surgery present a major challenge. Balloon aortic valvuloplasty has unfavorable outcomes, and is not recommended as a temporizing measure. The advances in percutaneous valve implantation technology will likely render balloon valvuloplasty completely obsolete, and this procedure may be an option to consider when patient condition or urgency of imminent surgery preclude surgical valve replacement [45].

Pathophysiology

- Obstruction of the outflow of blood from the left ventricle (LV) causes an increase in LV wall tension, with compensatory and characteristic concentric hypertrophy of the LV.
- This LV pressure overload-induced hypertrophy results in reduced ventricular compliance, and higher end diastolic pressures are needed to fill the "stiff" LV.
- Patients with AS are particularly dependent on the contribution of atrial contraction to ventricular filling, hence atrial arrhythmias can produce critical loss of cardiac output and should be avoided at all costs.
- End-stage AS is associated with severe loss of compliance and the inability of the LV to sustain cardiac output, with loss of stroke volume as well as a reduced ejection fraction. This leads to a state known as afterload mismatch, with the heart failing because of excessive afterload rather than contractility failure. Surgical correction of the high afterload by valve replacement should restore ejection fraction; however, in severe cases, decompensated heart failure is a poor prognostic sign.
- The hypertrophied myocardium associated with AS is vulnerable to ischemia, because of increased oxygen demand and high wall tension. Even with normal coronary arteries, subendocardial ischemia can occur, as coronary blood flow cannot keep pace with the ventricular hypertrophy. Tachycardia should be avoided as it aggravates ischemia.

- Pharmacological afterload reduction does *not* alleviate the mechanical afterload to the LV, and should be avoided as the associated reduction in diastolic blood pressure may cause myocardial ischemia.

Conduct of anesthesia

It may be reasonable to consider regional anesthetic techniques, including epidural [46, 47] and even spinal anesthesia [48], for selected patients with AS. However, the fall in diastolic blood pressure, and the potential bradycardia that may occur, make these anesthetic techniques potentially hazardous. Judicious use of regional anesthetic techniques appear warranted in selected cases [49].

The choice of anesthetic agents should be aimed at avoiding myocardial depression, and avoiding peripheral arteriolar vasodilation.

Certain hemodynamic objectives need to be met or maintained.

- The patient with AS should be kept "well filled", with high normal ventricular filling pressures.
- The afterload should be maintained with judicious use of vasopressor agents.
- Tachycardia should be avoided.
- In particular, diastolic hypotension should be avoided, and falls in blood pressure should be corrected with volume replacement and alpha-agonist drugs.
- Arrhythmias should be treated promptly by cardioversion in the event of hemodynamic compromise.
- Appropriate observation and monitoring should be continued into the postoperative period.
- Vasodilating and myocardial depressant induction agents (propofol and thiopentone) should best be avoided or used with great caution. Opiates are generally well tolerated, and may allow for reduced concentrations of inhalational anesthetic agents. Vecuronium, cisatracurium, and rocuronium are all suitable muscle relaxants; however, histamine release is undesirable.

Aortic incompetence (AI)

Definitions

Incompetence of the aortic valve results in regurgitation of a portion of the stroke volume back into the LV during diastole. The severity of AI is quantified by the volume of regurgitant blood as estimated during angiography, or by color flow Doppler echocardiography. It may be mild, moderate or severe.

- Regurgitant volumes under $3\,l\,min^{-1}$ are deemed mild, while more than $6\,l\,min^{-1}$ is classed as severe AI.
- It is possible to have regurgitant volumes in excess of $20\,l\,min^{-1}$.

Etiology

Disease of the valve leaflets, or the wall of the aortic root, or both can cause AI. Causes include: rheumatic fever, infective endocarditis, trauma, a congenitally bicuspid valve, failure of a bioprosthetic valve and myxomatous disease of the aortic valve. AI can occur in the presence of ventricular septal defect, and as a consequence of aortic dissection. More rare causes include connective tissue diseases and congenital defects as well as treatment with the appetite suppressant phentermine-fenfluramine.

Pathophysiology

- The regurgitant volume in chronic AI causes increased diastolic volume in the LV, which in turn provides a degree of hemodynamic compensation for the loss of forward stroke volume by the process of preload augmentation.
- Progression of the disease results in increased wall tension and eccentric hypertrophy of the LV.
- The heart can be grossly enlarged.
- The competent mitral valve protects the left atrium (LA) and pulmonary vasculature from the volume overload of AI. In severe AI, the regurgitant jet impinges on the anterior leaflet of the mitral valve and produces the presystolic mitral murmur of Austin Flint.
- The LV is initially very compliant, and unlikely to become ischemic until late in the disease process, when LV failure occurs. LV failure occurs when the chronically increased wall tension and muscle mass result in loss of compliance and contractility.
- The onset of LV failure is followed by rapid deterioration. Reduced afterload and moderate tachycardia are the chief mechanisms to offset the effects of AI.
- A reduction in afterload as achieved by the lower diastolic aortic pressure augments forward flow.
- A faster heart rate ($>90 \, \text{min}^{-1}$) reduces diastolic time and hence the regurgitant fraction.
- Acute AI is poorly tolerated and patients rapidly develop heart failure with distension of the LV and increased LA and pulmonary artery occlusion pressure (PAOP), as the mitral valve is unable to contain the regurgitant volume.

Conduct of anesthesia

To minimize the effects of an incompetent aortic valve, the anesthetic should aim to reduce or maintain a low afterload, and to keep a heart rate of about 90 beats per minute. Regional anesthesia is a logical choice where patients do not have any other contraindications to its use, and epidural anesthesia has been successfully employed in patients with severe AI [50]. Bradycardia should be treated aggressively, and in low cardiac output states dobutamine or milrinone are both reasonable choices if inotropic drugs are needed. Moderate vasodilation from both induction and inhalational anesthetic agents may be beneficial to patients with AI.

Mitral stenosis

Definitions

The normal mitral valve orifice in adults is between 4 and 6 cm^2.

- Clinically significant mitral stenosis (MS) occurs when the valve orifice is less than 2 cm^2.
- When the mitral valve opening is reduced to 1 cm^2, the MS is said to be critical.

The diastolic transmitral pressure gradient can be accurately estimated by Doppler echocardiography.

- A gradient of less than 5 mmHg is consistent with mild MS;
- 5–12 mmHg is consistent with moderate MS;
- a gradient of greater than 12 mmHg is severe MS.

Etiology

Rheumatic heart disease is the most common cause of MS. Women are four times more likely to be affected than men. Congenital MS is rarely seen in infants and children. Malignant carcinoid, amyloid deposits, systemic lupus erythematosus, rheumatoid arthritis and the Hunter Hurler mucopolysaccharidososes are other rare causes. Large vegetations from infective endocarditis of the mitral valve, as well as left atrial tumors (usually myxomas) and congenital membranes in the left atrium (cor triatriatum) may all mimic MS.

Pathophysiology

- MS causes chronic underfilling of the LV, and results in increased pressure and volume upstream of the mitral valve.
- In order to generate adequate flow through a valve with a $1 \, cm^2$ orifice to maintain a normal cardiac output, the left atrial pressure has to be approximately 25 mmHg.
- This increased LA pressure causes dilation of the LA and with disease progression the pulmonary venous and capillary pressure increases. The pressure in the pulmonary arteries (PA) also increases and medial hypertrophy occurs in these vessels.
- The right ventricle (RV) has to work harder and RV hypertrophy occurs. RV dysfunction and failure is a poor prognostic sign, and secondary dysfunction of the right-sided valves (tricuspid and pulmonic regurgitation) occurs in severe MS.
- For a given orifice size, the transvalvular pressure gradient is proportional to the square of the transvalvular flow rate. Therefore a doubling of flow rate will quadruple the pressure gradient. Exercise, pregnancy, hypervolemia, and hyperthyroidism or any other cause of increased cardiac output will significantly increase the transvalvular pressure gradient.
- Atrial contraction contributes approximately 30% of ventricular filling in patients with MS. Atrial fibrillation (a common feature in MS with left atrial enlargement) therefore significantly decreases cardiac output. Tachycardia reduces diastolic time more than systolic time, thereby reducing the time available for flow across the mitral valve. This increases the transvalvular gradient and LA pressures further. Thus atrial fibrillation should be aggressively managed and, when it does occur, it is very important to control ventricular rate.

Conduct of anesthesia

- The single most important aspect of the anesthetic plan in patients with MS is to avoid tachycardia.
- Atrial fibrillation or tachycardia should be treated promptly by cardioversion or β blockade.

Filling pressures should be kept fairly high, but pulmonary edema should be avoided. Pulmonary artery pressure monitoring may be desirable, as it can help to maintain optimal LA pressure; however, there is increased risk of PA rupture during balloon inflation, and the wedge pressure trace may not be attainable.

Afterload reduction should be avoided, as hypotension ensues with the stenotic mitral valve precluding compensatory increase in cardiac output to maintain blood pressure. LV function is usually normal, although it will be relatively small and noncompliant.

As with AS, it is advisable to avoid vasodilating induction agents, and volatile agents should be used with caution and titrated carefully.

Mitral regurgitation

Definitions

Mitral regurgitation (MR) may be acute or chronic. Acute MR is usually a result of infection (endocarditis) or ischemia with papillary muscle or chordal dysfunction. This usually requires urgent cardiac surgical intervention, and anesthesia for these patients is beyond the scope of this chapter. Chronic MR is described as mild, moderate or severe. The quantification of MR is made by cine-angiography, and/or color flow Doppler and pulsed wave Doppler echocardiography.

- The volume of MR can be estimated from the difference between left ventricular stroke volumes, measured during angiography, and the effective forward stroke volumes measured indirectly using the Fick method.

- In severe MR, the regurgitant stroke volume approaches or even exceeds forward stroke volume.

- Echocardiographic quantification of severity of MR is made using Doppler color flow mapping to estimate the size and volume of the regurgitant jet, and pulsed wave Doppler to observe flow reversal in the pulmonary veins as occurs in severe MR. Echocardiography also provides useful information regarding the cause of MR and the dimensions of the left atrium.

Etiology

Abnormalities of any of the components of the mitral valve apparatus can cause MR. This includes the mitral valve leaflets, the chordae tendineae, the papillary muscles, and the mitral annulus. Mitral leaflet pathology is usually of rheumatic origin, although endocarditis is also implicated. The mitral valve prolapse syndrome is another important cause. Rarely, blunt or penetrating trauma may cause destruction of the mitral leaflets.

Chordal dysfunction may follow acute MI or endocarditis. Ischemia or infarction commonly causes posterior papillary muscle dysfunction.

Degenerative disease of the mitral annulus is common and is an important cause of MR, particularly in female patients. Dilation of the annulus occurs in any cardiac disease associated with left ventricular dilatation. It is particularly associated with ischemic cardiomyopathy.

Pathophysiology

- The pathophysiology of MR is best thought of in terms of chronic LV overload.

- The incompetent valve allows a proportion of the LV stroke volume back into the LA.

- The LA is highly compliant and may dilate to massive proportions. A significant proportion of the stroke volume will flow retrograde through the mitral valve before the aortic valve opens.
- The LV ejection fraction should therefore be increased (>80%). A normal ejection fraction (50–60%) may indicate depressed myocardial contractility.
- With large regurgitant volumes in the LA, pulmonary venous congestion ensues, and pulmonary arterial hypertension is a feature of chronic volume overload.
- The regurgitant fraction is influenced by LV afterload, the size of the regurgitant defect, the pressure gradient between the LA and LV, as well as the heart rate.
- Moderate tachycardia reduces systole and the time for regurgitant blood flow, as well as reducing diastole and the time for diastolic filling of the LV.
- The absence of a competent mitral valve means that there is no isovolemic contraction phase during systole.

Conduct of anesthesia

Anesthetic goals include:

- avoid increases in afterload,
- maintain a relative tachycardia (about 90 beats min^{-1}); and
- maintain relatively high filling pressures.

As with mitral stenosis, excessive filling is bad, and hypotension is best treated with inotropes rather than with vasopressors. Pulmonary artery catheters provide useful information, both in terms of pulmonary hypertension and the severity of MR, which may be seen as a "v" wave on the pulmonary artery wedge trace. Where inotropes are needed both milrinone and dobutamine are logical choices, as the reduction in afterload is augmented by the reduction in pulmonary artery pressure. In the event of excessive loss of systemic vascular tone, judicious vasopressor (norepinephrine) infusion is appropriate to allow continued use of inotropes. Regional anesthetic techniques are desirable, as the reduction in afterload, and the avoidance of the sympathetic surges associated with laryngoscopy, are beneficial to the patient. Regional anesthetic techniques can never replace monitoring and vigilance. In severe MR, the use of an IABP may be beneficial, as it has significant effects on afterload reduction, and reduces myocardial work, while augmenting diastolic coronary perfusion.

In circumstances of cardiogenic shock, the IABP should be considered, as it may be a life-saving, or at least a temporizing, intervention [51]. The IABP should not be used against an incompetent aortic valve.

Pulmonary hypertension

Definitions

Pulmonary hypertension is defined as pulmonary artery (PA) systolic pressure greater than 30 mmHg and mean pressure greater than 20 mmHg. Pulmonary hypertension may be primary (idiopathic) or secondary.

Etiology

Primary pulmonary hypertension is a rare but progressive and fatal disease. Secondary causes of pulmonary hypertension include mitral regurgitation, mitral stenosis, left ventricular diseases, pericardial diseases, left atrial myxomas, congenital cardiac defects, pulmonary embolism or thrombosis, pulmonary parenchymal disease and chronic hypoxemic states, as well as some collagen vascular diseases.

Pathophysiology

- Chronic resistance to pulmonary blood flow may cause secondary pulmonary hypertension.
- Reactive processes can also result in pulmonary hypertension – increased resistance to flow often results in an additive reactive component.
- The effects of pulmonary hypertension and increased resistance to flow on the right ventricle (RV) are complex. The RV is a thin-walled structure whose function is highly influenced by its geometry. Chronically elevated PA pressures cause RV hypertrophy, which in turn results in loss of compliance and poor performance. Right ventricular failure is notoriously difficult to manage.
- Apart from the deleterious effects on RV function, the hydrostatic effects of pulmonary hypertension predispose to the development of pulmonary edema and hypoxemia from ventilation perfusion mismatch.
- The loss of RV compliance means that filling pressure in the RV is difficult to optimize – underfilling leads to underperformance, while the overfilled ventricle rapidly fails.
- Excessive distension of the RV also results in leftward displacement of the interventricular septum, causing a form of "internal tamponade."
- Pulmonary vascular resistance (PVR) is the standard for measuring pulmonary vascular reactivity. PVR measures the mean component of RV afterload, and does not account for pulsatile effects.
- Pulmonary vascular impedance may be a more valid measure than PVR, as impedance calculations allow for the effects of blood viscosity, pulsatile flow, reflected waves, and arterial compliance [52]. Thus the dynamic relationship between flow and pressure can be more comprehensively understood. Unfortunately, it remains difficult to obtain all the data required for this calculation, and the simpler calculations of vascular resistance are used. None the less, a very important factor in calculating impedance in the pulmonary circulation is the heart rate, and for a given cardiac output, impedance is lowest at a faster heart rate, typically greater than 90 beats per minute.

Conduct of anesthesia

Severe pulmonary hypertension and incipient RV failure present some of the most challenging problems to the anesthesiologist.

As with all anesthetic plans, the nature of the planned surgery will influence the choice of technique. Where appropriate, RA may be the option of choice.

- Increases in pulmonary vascular resistance/impedance are poorly tolerated by the compromised RV, and hypertensive surges should be avoided.
- Hypoxemia will worsen existing pulmonary hypertension.
- Correct fluid loading is critical, and monitoring strategies should include means to estimate both RV and LV filling pressures.

There are many therapeutic options to reduce PA pressure and support the failing or vulnerable RV:

- Increasing the inspired oxygen concentration.
- Speeding up the heart rate to relative tachycardia ($90-120\,min^{-1}$).
- Vasodilators have a role to play, and nitroglycerine can reduce PA pressure, although often at the expense of systemic blood pressure.
- Inhaled agents such as nitric oxide (NO), milrinone and prostacycline reduce PA pressure.
- Inhaled NO rapidly improves pulmonary hemodynamic function in the context of pulmonary embolism, cardiac surgery, lung transplantation and acute lung injury [53].
- Abrupt cessation of NO can precipitate circulatory collapse.
- It is difficult to show a significant survival benefit for inhaled NO in adults, but it should be kept in mind as an option in patients with severe pulmonary hypertension and RV failure. Dipyridamole combined with inhaled NO may enhance the vasodilatory effects of NO in select circumstances [54].
- Inhaled milrinone has been shown to be a potentially useful agent to reduce pulmonary arterial pressure in cardiac surgery patients with pulmonary hypertension [55], and should also be considered in managing the patient with severe pulmonary hypertension and heart failure.
- Calcium channel blockers are useful in the management of pulmonary hypertension with a vasoreactive component. Sildenafil and iloprost are used in the management of chronic pulmonary hypertension [56] and could be considered when patients with pulmonary hypertension present for surgery.
- Systemic milrinone has significant beneficial effects on reducing PVR, and is inotropic with significant scope to improve RV function [57].
- Dobutamine also has the potential to improve RV hemodynamics and reduce PA pressure, particularly where LV failure is a feature.
- Isoprenaline has also been used extensively in the cardiac surgical patient population to treat RV failure and pulmonary hypertension.
- Even though no major study has been conducted to estimate the impact of RV failure and pulmonary hypertension on outcome, there is consensus that these patients are at high risk of perioperative mortality [2].
- Patients who have pulmonary hypertension and intracardiac shunts are at risk of increased right to left shunting when they develop systemic hypotension. A vicious cycle of acidosis and further reduction in systemic vascular resistance can ensue, and this cycle should be arrested at the earliest possible time.

References

1. Rosamond W, Flegal K, Furie K, *et al.* Heart disease and stroke statistics 2008 update. A report from the American Heart Association Statistics Committee and Stroke Statistics Subcommittee. *Circulation* 2008; **117**: e25–146.

2. Fleisher LA, Beckman JA, Brown KA, *et al.* ACC/AHA 2007 guidelines on perioperative cardiovascular evaluation and care for noncardiac surgery: A report of the American College of Cardiology/American Heart Association Task Force on Practice Guidelines (Writing Committee to Revise the 2002 Guidelines on Perioperative Cardiovascular Evaluation for Noncardiac Surgery). *J Am Coll Cardiol* 2007; **50**: e159–241.

3. Devereaux PJ, Goldman L, Cook DJ, *et al.* Perioperative cardiac events in patients undergoing noncardiac surgery: A review of the magnitude of the problem, the pathophysiology of the events and methods to estimate and communicate risk. *CMAJ* 2005; **173**: 627–34.

4. Dawood MM, Gutpa DK, Southern J, *et al.* Pathology of fatal perioperative myocardial infarction: Implications regarding pathophysiology and prevention. *Int J Cardiol* 1996; **57**: 37–44.

5. McFalls EO, Ward HB, Moritz TE, *et al.* Coronary-artery revascularization before elective major vascular surgery. *N Engl J Med* 2004; **351**: 2795–804.

6. Rihal CS, Eagle KA, Mickel MC, Foster ED, Sopko G, Gersh BJ. Surgical therapy for coronary artery disease among patients with combined coronary artery and peripheral vascular disease. *Circulation* 1995; **91**: 46–53.

7. Mesh CL, Cmolik BL, Van Heekeren DW, *et al.* Coronary bypass in vascular patients: A relatively high-risk procedure. *Ann Vasc Surg* 1997; **11**: 612–9.

8. Karapandzic VM, Vujisic-Tesic BD, Colovic RB, Masirevic VP, Babic DD. Coronary artery revascularization prior to abdominal nonvascular surgery. *Cardiovasc Revasc Med* 2008; **9**: 18–23.

9. Ward HB, Kelly RF, Thottapurathu L, *et al.* Coronary artery bypass grafting is superior to percutaneous coronary intervention in prevention of perioperative myocardial infarctions during subsequent vascular surgery. *Ann Thorac Surg* 2006; **82**: 795–800; discussion 800–1.

10. Eagle KA, Guyton RA, Davidoff R, *et al.* ACC/AHA 2004 guideline update for coronary artery bypass graft surgery–Summary article: A report of the American College of Cardiology/American Heart Association Task Force on Practice Guidelines (Committee to Update the 1999 Guidelines for Coronary Artery Bypass Graft Surgery). *Circulation* 2004; **110**: 1168–76.

11. Chassot PG, Delabays A, Spahn DR. Perioperative antiplatelet therapy: The case for continuing therapy in patients at risk of myocardial infarction. *Br J Anaesthesia* 2007; **99**: 316–28.

12. Thadani U, Rodgers T. Side effects of using nitrates to treat angina. *Expert Opin Drug Saf* 2006; **5**: 667–74.

13. Sear JW, Foex P, Howell SJ. Effect of chronic intercurrent medication with beta-adrenoceptor blockade or calcium channel entry blockade on postoperative silent myocardial ischaemia. *Br J Anaesthesia* 2000; **84**: 311–5.

14. Ishikawa K, Kanamasa K, Ogawa I, *et al.* Long-term nitrate treatment increases cardiac events in patients with healed myocardial infarction. Secondary Prevention Group. *Jpn Circ J* 1996; **60**: 779–88.

15. Wijeysundera DN, Beattie WS. Calcium channel blockers for reducing cardiac morbidity after noncardiac surgery: A meta-analysis. *Anesth Analg* 2003; **97**: 634–41.

16. Pfeffer MA, Braunwald E, Moye LA, *et al.* Effect of captopril on mortality and morbidity in patients with left ventricular dysfunction after myocardial infarction. Results of the survival and ventricular enlargement trial. The SAVE Investigators. *N Engl J Med* 1992; **327**: 669–77.

17. Kersten JR, Fleisher LA. Statins: The next advance in cardioprotection? *Anesthesiology* 2006; **105**: 1079–80.

18. Wijeysundera DN, Naik JS, Beattie WS. Alpha-2 adrenergic agonists to prevent perioperative cardiovascular complications: A meta-analysis. *Am J Med* 2003; **114**: 742–52.

19. Wallace AW, Galindez D, Salahieh A, *et al*. Effect of clonidine on cardiovascular morbidity and mortality after noncardiac surgery. *Anesthesiology* 2004; **101**: 284–93.

20. Kitakaze M, Hori M, Gotoh K, *et al*. Beneficial effects of alpha 2-adrenoceptor activity on ischemic myocardium during coronary hypoperfusion in dogs. *Circ Res* 1989; **65**: 1632–45.

21. Collaborative overview of randomised trials of antiplatelet therapy – II: Maintenance of vascular graft or arterial patency by antiplatelet therapy. Antiplatelet Trialists' Collaboration. *Br Med J* 1994; **308**: 159–68.

22. Maulaz AB, Bezerra DC, Michel P, Bogousslavsky J. Effect of discontinuing aspirin therapy on the risk of brain ischemic stroke. *Arch Neurol* 2005; **62**: 1217–20.

23. Burger W, Chemnitius JM, Kneissl GD, *et al*. Low-dose aspirin for secondary cardiovascular prevention – cardiovascular risks after its perioperative withdrawal versus bleeding risks with its continuation – review and meta-analysis. *J Intern Med* 2005; **257**: 399–414.

24. Purkayastha S, Athanasiou T, Malinovski V, *et al*. Does clopidogrel affect outcome after coronary artery bypass grafting? A meta-analysis. *Heart* 2006; **92**: 531–2.

25. Filsoufi F, Rahmanian PB, Castillo JG, *et al*. Clopidogrel treatment before coronary artery bypass graft surgery increases postoperative morbidity and blood product requirements. *J Cardiothorac Vasc Anesth* 2008; **22**: 60–6.

26. Albaladejo P, Marret E, Piriou V, *et al*. Perioperative management of antiplatelet agents in patients with coronary stents: Recommendations of a French Task Force. *Br J Anaesthesia* 2006; **97**: 580–2.

27. Ho PM, Peterson ED, Wang L, *et al*. Incidence of death and acute myocardial infarction associated with stopping clopidogrel after acute coronary syndrome. *JAMA* 2008; **299**: 532–9.

28. Guerin P, Rondeau F, Grimandi G, *et al*. Neointimal hyperplasia after stenting in a human mammary artery organ culture. *J Vasc Res* 2004; **41**: 46–53.

29. Pfisterer M, Brunner-La Rocca HP, Buser PT, *et al*. Late clinical events after clopidogrel discontinuation may limit the benefit of drug-eluting stents: An observational study of drug-eluting versus bare-metal stents. *J Am Coll Cardiol* 2006; **48**: 2584–91.

30. Nordmann AJ, Briel M, Bucher HC. Mortality in randomized controlled trials comparing drug-eluting vs. bare metal stents in coronary artery disease: A meta-analysis. *Eur Heart J* 2006; **27**: 2784–814.

31. Stone GW, Moses JW, Ellis SG, *et al*. Safety and efficacy of sirolimus- and paclitaxel-eluting coronary stents. *N Engl J Med* 2007; **356**: 998–1008.

32. Weber NC, Schlack W. Inhalational anaesthetics and cardioprotection. *Handb Exp Pharmacol* 2008; 187–207.

33. Romano MA, McNish R, Seymour EM, *et al*. Differential effects of opioid peptides on myocardial ischemic tolerance. *J Surg Res* 2004; **119**: 46–50.

34. Whelton A. Clinical implications of nonopioid analgesia for relief of mild-to-moderate pain in patients with or at risk for cardiovascular disease. *Am J Cardiol* 2006; **97**: 3–9.

35. Furberg CD. Decisions by regulatory agencies: Are they evidence-based? *Trials* 2007; **8**: 13.

36. Joshi GP, Gertler R, Fricker R. Cardiovascular thromboembolic adverse effects associated with cyclooxygenase-2 selective inhibitors and nonselective antiinflammatory drugs. *Anesth Analg* 2007; **105**: 1793–804.

37. Murphy N, Mockler M, Ryder M, *et al*. Decompensation of chronic heart failure associated with pregabalin in patients with neuropathic pain. *J Card Fail* 2007; **13**: 227–9.

38. Blomberg S, Emanuelsson H, Kvist H, *et al*. Effects of thoracic epidural anesthesia on coronary arteries and arterioles in patients with coronary artery disease. *Anesthesiology* 1990; **73**: 840–7.

39. Liu SS, Wu CL. Effect of postoperative analgesia on major postoperative complications: A systematic update of the evidence. *Anesth Analg* 2007; **104**: 689–702.

40. Horlocker TT, Wedel DJ, Benzon H, *et al*. Regional anesthesia in the anticoagulated

261

patient: Defining the risks (the second ASRA Consensus Conference on Neuraxial Anesthesia and Anticoagulation). *Reg Anesth Pain Med* 2003; **28**: 172–97.

41. Kertai MD, Bountioukos M, Boersma E, *et al.* Aortic stenosis: An underestimated risk factor for perioperative complications in patients undergoing noncardiac surgery. *Am J Med* 2004; **116**: 8–13.

42. Wilson W, Taubert KA, Gewitz M, *et al.* Prevention of infective endocarditis: guidelines from the American Heart Association: A guideline from the American Heart Association Rheumatic Fever, Endocarditis, and Kawasaki Disease Committee, Council on Cardiovascular Disease in the Young, and the Council on Clinical Cardiology, Council on Cardiovascular Surgery and Anesthesia, and the Quality of Care and Outcomes Research Interdisciplinary Working Group. *Circulation* 2007; **116**: 1736–54.

43. O'Keefe JHJ, Shub C, Rettke SR. Risk of noncardiac surgical procedures in patients with aortic stenosis. *Mayo Clin Proc* 1989; **64**: 400–5.

44. Otto CM. Valvular aortic stenosis: Disease severity and timing of intervention. *J Am Coll Cardiol* 2006; **47**: 2141–51.

45. Conradi L, Reichenspurner H. Review on balloon aortic valvuloplasty: A surgeon's perspective in 2008. *Clin Res Cardiol* 2008; **97**: 285–7.

46. Brighouse D. Anaesthesia for caesarean section in patients with aortic stenosis: the case for regional anaesthesia. *Anaesthesia* 1998; **53**: 107–9.

47. Colclough GW, Ackerman WE, Walmsley PM, *et al.* Epidural anaesthesia for a parturient with critical aortic stenosis. *J Clin Anesth* 1995; **7**: 264–5.

48. Collard CD, Eappen S, Lynch EP, *et al.* Continuous spinal anaesthesia with invasive hemodynamic monitoring for surgical repair of the hip in two patients with severe aortic stenosis. *Anesth Analg* 1995; **81**: 195–8.

49. McDonald SB. Is neuraxial blockade contraindicated in the patient with aortic stenosis? *Reg Anesth Pain Med* 2004; **29**: 496–502.

50. Zangrillo A, Landoni G, Pappalardo F, *et al.* Different anesthesiological management in two high risk pregnant women with heart failure undergoing emergency cesarean section. *Minerva Anestesiol* 2005; **71**: 227–36.

51. Sanborn TA, Feldman T. Management strategies for cardiogenic shock. *Curr Opin Cardiol* 2004; **19**: 608–12.

52. Hunter KS, Lee PF, Lanning CJ, *et al.* Pulmonary vascular input impedance is a combined measure of pulmonary vascular resistance and stiffness and predicts clinical outcomes better than pulmonary vascular resistance alone in pediatric patients with pulmonary hypertension. *Am Heart J* 2008; **155**: 166–74.

53. Steiner MK, Preston IR, Klinger JR, *et al.* Pulmonary hypertension: Inhaled nitric oxide, sildenafil and natriuretic peptides. *Curr Opin Pharmacol* 2005; **5**: 245–50.

54. Jiang ZY, Costachescu T, Derouin M, *et al.* Treatment of pulmonary hypertension during surgery with nitric oxide and vasodilators. *Can J Anaesth* 2000; **47**: 552–5.

55. Lamarche Y, Perrault LP, Maltais S, *et al.* Preliminary experience with inhaled milrinone in cardiac surgery. *Eur J Cardiothorac Surg* 2007; **31**: 1081–7.

56. Benedict N, Seybert A, Mathier MA. Evidence-based pharmacologic management of pulmonary arterial hypertension. *Clin Ther* 2007; **29**: 2134–53.

57. Chen EP, Bittner HB, Davis RDJ, *et al.* Milrinone improves pulmonary hemodynamics and right ventricular function in chronic pulmonary hypertension. *Ann Thorac Surg* 1997; **63**: 814–21.

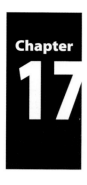

Chapter 17

Vascular surgery

D. Sebastian and I. McConachie

The provision of anesthesia for surgery on the aorta and its major branches is challenging in that it is associated with high morbidity and mortality.

This chapter will focus on:

1. principles of the management for carotid endarterectomy;
2. the anesthetic management of a ruptured abdominal aortic aneurysm; and
3. peripheral vascular surgery.

This will encompass most of the challenges of vascular surgery.

The key problems encountered in vascular anesthesia are as follows.

1. The impairment of vital organ perfusion by pre-existing vascular disease or the consequence of intraoperative cross-clamping.
2. Potential of perioperative hemorrhage.
3. Consequences of massive blood transfusion (discussed in Chapter 9).
4. Consequences of changes in left ventricular afterload produced by clamping and unclamping of the abdominal and thoracic aorta.
5. Effects of exteriorization of bowel and retroperitoneal dissection.
6. Effects of dissection around the thoracic aorta and use of one lung ventilation for thoracolumbar aortic surgery. This is outside the scope of this text.

Carotid endarterectomy

- Carotid artery endarterectomy (CAE) has been established as a safe and effective procedure for the treatment of patients with transient ischemic attacks associated with atherosclerosis or severe stenosis of the bifurcation of the common carotid artery or proximal portion of the internal carotid artery in the neck.
- Evidence suggests that with symptomatic carotid stenosis of <50%, medical therapy is preferable to surgical intervention. There is an increased 5-year stroke risk with surgery.
- With tighter stenoses, surgery is increasingly beneficial over best medical therapy unless the artery is nearly occluded [1].
- The perioperative mortality rate following carotid endarterectomy is 1.6% with a risk of stroke and death of 5.6% in symptomatic carotid stenosis [2].
- Coronary artery disease is prevalent (40–75%) amongst patients presenting for carotid endarterectomy [3]. In contrast to a decline in neurologic morbidity and mortality rates, cardiac complications have not declined.

Anesthesia for the High Risk Patient, ed. I. McConachie. Published by Cambridge University Press.
© Cambridge University Press 2009.

Appropriate selection of patients, advanced surgical techniques, increasingly effective cerebral monitoring procedures, introduction of intraoperative quality controls for vascular reconstruction, and improved anesthetic techniques have reduced some perioperative complications among patients undergoing carotid endarterectomy.

Recent evidence according to the pooled data from the MRC European Carotid Surgery Trial (ECST) and the North American Symptomatic Carotid Endarterectomy Trial (NASCET) has shown that maximum benefit in stroke reduction is achieved if surgery is performed within 2 weeks of the patient's last symptoms. Thus, preoperative management should be expedited to achieve as short a "symptom to surgery" time as possible but should include:

- blood pressure optimization based on readings taken from both arms and decisions made on the higher reading arm;

- continue regular cardiac medications including aspirin, ACE inhibitors, statin, and beta blockers unless there are definite contraindications.

- preoperative evaluation of myocardial function and ischemic potential are not required unless patients have unstable angina, recent MI with evidence of ongoing ischemia, decompensated congestive cardiac failure or significant valvular heart disease.

Intraoperative management for carotid endarterectomy

The procedure can be done under either general or regional anesthesia.

There are no definite data to indicate that one of the above methods is better than the other with regards to the perioperative stroke rate or death rate. Hence the technique chosen is often based on the anesthetist, surgeon and patient preference.

The main principles of anesthetic management should be:

- the protection of the heart and brain from ischemia,

- control of the heart rate,

- avoidance of surgical pain and stress responses, and

- the final goal is having an awake patient at the end of surgery to assess neurological status.

Regional or local anesthesia

Blocking the C2–C4 dermatomes provides regional or local anesthesia. This is done by the use of a superficial and deep cervical plexus block or only a superficial plexus block with local anesthetic infiltration of the surgical field as necessary (especially the lower border and ramus of the mandible). A systematic review concluded that superficial/intermediate block is safer than any method that employs a deep injection [4]. There is a higher rate of conversion to general anesthesia with the deep/combined block which may have been influenced by the higher incidence of direct complications, but which may also suggest that the superficial/combined block provides better analgesia during surgery. Cervical epidural anesthesia has also been used, but may have a lower success rate and increased complications compared to cervical plexus block [5].

- Regional anesthesia provides for the most sensitive and cheapest method of monitoring for cerebral hypoperfusion. If sedation is used this must be kept to a minimum with the ability to maintain continuous verbal contact with the patient.

- The other advantages with regional anesthesia are claimed to be better cardiovascular stability, lower requirement for vascular shunts, and a smoother, shorter recovery phase with lower overall costs.

- The disadvantages of regional anesthesia are that there should be significant patient understanding and cooperation from the patient. Failure requires rapid conversion to general anesthesia in a less than ideal situation!

- The rates of conversion from regional to general anesthesia are reported to be between 2% and 6%.

- A large multi-center trial comparing general anesthesia and local anesthesia (the GALA trial) has finished recruiting and may answer some of the questions regarding outcomes from both techniques.

General anesthesia

Any form of general anesthesia can be used as long as the main principles mentioned above are maintained. The advantages of general anesthesia are the ability to have a secure airway and to maintain a normal arterial carbon dioxide tension. The other advantages are the cerebral protective effects of the anesthetic drugs and a more controlled environment for the surgeon.

The disadvantage of general anesthesia is that ideally some form of cerebral perfusion monitoring has to be used, although most available methods are either difficult to interpret or expensive.

Potential methods of cerebral perfusion monitoring are:

1. direct observation in an awake patient,
2. internal carotid artery stump pressure (SP) measurement,
3. EEG and somatosensory-evoked potential (SEP) measurement,
4. regional cerebral blood flow (rCBF) using injection of xenon-133,
5. jugular venous oxygen saturation,
6. cerebral oximetry,
7. transcranial Doppler monitoring (TCD), and
8. near infrared spectroscopy (NIRS).

TCD, NIRS, SP and SEP were compared in one of the few (admittedly small) studies comparing different cerebral monitoring methods for the detection of cerebral ischemia during carotid endarterectomy. TCD, NIRS, and SP measurements provided similar accuracy, while lower accuracy was found for SEP monitoring [6]. TCD was not useful due to a high rate of technical difficulties preventing measurement.

Full discussion of all these techniques is beyond the scope of this text.

The other disadvantages of general anesthesia are the higher incidence of temporary shunting with the risks associated with it, such as difficulty with insertion, air or atheroma embolization, intimal dissection, malfunction due to kinking and potential for thrombus formation.

Postoperative management

Hemodynamic instability is the most common complication that occurs in the postoperative period.

- Hypertension is common (30–50%) after carotid endarterectomy, especially in patients with poorly controlled preoperative hypertension.

- Neurologic and cardiac complications are associated with postoperative hypertension, hence hypertension should be treated aggressively with short-acting drugs such as sodium nitroprusside or nitroglycerin. Beta-blockers help reduce systolic hypertension.

- Postoperative hypotension is seen as commonly as hypertension but may be more common after regional anesthesia. To avoid cerebral or cardiac injury this should also be treated aggressively with short-acting agents such as phenylephrine or metaraminol. Cardiac complications causing hypotension should be excluded or treated.

- Cerebral hyperperfusion syndrome. This was first reported as a syndrome including ipsilateral, frontal headache, transient seizures, and intracerebral hemorrhage after carotid endarterectomy. This is thought to result from restoration of normal pressure and flow through the carotid and an initial inability to regain autoregulation leading to hyperperfusion in the previously hypoperfused brain.

- Other complications that can occur are myocardial infarction, seizures, cranial nerve injury and wound hematoma with potential airway compromise.

Considering the potential for the above complications to occur, it is recommended that these patients be monitored closely for the first 12–24 h.

Anesthesia for abdominal aortic surgery (AAA)

The vast majority of abdominal aortic aneurysms are related to atherosclerotic disease (90% of infrarenal aneurysms). Some of the other causes include infection, cystic medial necrosis, arteritis, trauma, and inherited connective tissue disorders.

The signs and symptoms that present as ruptured aortic aneurysm surgery are usually dramatic. Sudden abdominal pain radiating to the back presents in 70% according to the literature, and is associated with a throbbing abdominal pulsatile mass in 80% of patients.

In some cases of a "leaking" (i.e. a contained bleed) or painful, rapidly expanding aneurysm, an operation better described as "urgent" may be possible, but in general patients present shocked and often moribund, and anesthesia, operation and resuscitation are simultaneous and interrelated.

Incidence and prognosis

- Of people over 60, 5–7% have abdominal aortic aneurysms in the US.
- The frequency rate of asymptomatic AAA is 8.2% in the UK.
- The frequency of rupture is 13 cases per 100 000 persons in the UK.
- The peak incidence of AAA occurs in people above 70 years of age.
- The male-to-female incidence ratio in people younger than 80 years is 2:1.
- When older than 80 years, the ratio changes to 1:1.
- Increasing incidence occurs with male sex, smoking, age, diabetes and hypertension.
- A family history of AAA is a risk factor (25% of cases in persons with first-degree relatives with AAA).
- Mortality in the elective setting is around 6–7%.
- Mortality in the emergency setting varies between 29 and 40%.

- Approximately 30–50% of patients with a ruptured AAA die before they ever reach a hospital.
- Rupture of an abdominal aortic aneurysm usually occurs in men over the age of 60, with most of them occurring below the origin of the renal arteries.
- Without surgery, a ruptured aneurysm is fatal.

Aneurysm size is classically related to aneurysm rupture. However, there is no scientific evidence that aneurysm size has any correlation with a better or worse prognosis after rupture.

The Cochrane database reviewers [7] have cautiously supported routine ultrasound screening (and by implication elective intervention) to reduce the mortality from rupture of undetected abdominal aortic aneurysms – at least in men aged 65–79.

Assessment

It is important that a brief history is sought particularly with relevance to general health and co-morbidity. Two scoring systems for aortic aneurysm repair have been proposed: the Hardman index and the Glasgow aneurysm score. The literature is conflicting as to their ability to accurately predict outcome. Poor prognostic signs include:

- females;
- age > 75;
- actual aortic rupture;
- cardiopulmonary resuscitation prior to surgery;
- hypotension (despite fluid resuscitation);
- transfusion requirements in excess of 3000 ml;
- raised serum creatinine;
- obtunded consciousness and preoperative HB <10 g%;
- pre-existing medical problems such as:
  - ischemic heart disease,
  - cardiac failure,
  - chronic lung disease,
  - renal impairment, and
  - hypertension.

In addition, the current use of medications such as anti-coagulants and anti-hypertensives can complicate the management of the patient.

For elective aortic aneurysm surgery issues around cardiac assessment and cardiac optimization become important and are extensively discussed in other chapters of this text.

Decision to proceed with surgery

Considering that the decision to take the patient for a laparotomy and repair has to be made in a short span of time, the management of the patient should continue on the assumption that the patient will be taken to the operating room (OR) for surgery. Resuscitation and preparation for surgery are done simultaneously – preferably in the OR.

Ideally, the decision to proceed to surgery should be an active one, taken jointly by a senior surgeon and anesthetist, with the accent on a possible survivor rather than a last desperate throw of the die.

In practice, there is often very little time for consideration or discussion, and the anesthetist may well be presented with a "fait accomplis" in that the patient and relatives are expecting an operation, and are aware that survival is unlikely without. In any case, there is a large element of judgment involved, and it is natural to "give the patient a chance" unless it is obvious (usually only in hindsight) that the patient has no realistic prospect of survival.

Centralization of vascular surgery services has resulted in patients being transferred longer distances for treatment of ruptured aortic aneurysms. It seems that the transfer of these patients may not worsen the already high mortality from this condition, despite delays in treatment [8]. However, this may be partly due to preselection – only the less shocked patients being considered suitable for transfer or tolerating the journey.

Preparation

Appropriate preparation for a procedure that has high morbidity and mortality may improve the outcome. However, it is important that time is not spent on obtaining unnecessary investigations prior to taking the patient to the OR. Various procedures and investigations, however, are essential.

- Two 14G intravenous cannulae.
- Full blood count, serum biochemistry, coagulation profile.
- Blood for cross-match – at least 10–12 units.
- Request type-specific or O-negative blood sent immediately to the OR.
- Assume a massive blood transfusion will happen and a coagulopathy would develop – request for fresh frozen plasma and platelets.
- Organizing the availability of cell saver in the operating theater, ready to be applied at the start of the surgical procedure.
- 12-lead ECG if possible.
- Arterial cannula and arterial blood gas preinduction if time and patient condition permits.

The patient is often hypotensive secondary to bleeding into the retroperitoneal space. The formation of a clot and retroperitoneal tamponade usually slows the hemorrhage. Hence it is important that intravenous fluids and vasopressors are used very judiciously [9]. The increase of aortic blood pressure with fluid resuscitation could dislodge the clot or overcome the tamponade and make matters worse! Large volumes of intravenous fluids should only be given if there is an acute threat to life such as compromised cerebral perfusion causing confusion or coma, myocardial ischemia or imminent cardiac arrest.

Analgesia should be dealt with as in any other similar circumstances: in small increments to relieve pain. There is considerable danger that usual doses of fentanyl or other opiates can result in vasodilation, producing catastrophic falls in blood pressure as well as decreased conscious state, especially in the elderly.

Anesthetic management

As indicated earlier, it is important that the urgency of the situation is realized and the patient is appropriately resuscitated in the OR. The eventual mortality is directly proportional to the amount of time taken to achieve proximal control of the aorta.

Any procedure likely to provoke a valsalva maneuver such as placement of a nasogastric tube or insertion of a urinary catheter may also induce further bleeding, and is best left for after the patient is anesthetized or after proximal control of aorta is obtained.

- The necessary equipment to give the patient warm fluids rapidly should be available and primed.
- It is an advantage to have two anesthetists, at least one of whom should have the experience and competence to deal with an acute emergency of a leaking or ruptured abdominal aortic aneurysm.
- Experienced and competent surgeon and assistants [10].
- The surgeon and assistants should be scrubbed and ready with the patient's abdomen prepared and draped while the patient is still awake and being preoxygenated for induction of anesthesia.
- Monitoring with ECG, SpO_2, NIBP, $ETCO_2$ is the mandatory minimum prior to induction.
- Inserting an intra-arterial cannula into one of the peripheral arteries in the upper limb for monitoring of blood pressure can be done at this stage or before if it is an easy cannulation, but time should not be wasted in trying repeatedly to obtain arterial access.
- Rapid sequence induction with an appropriate induction agent that would maintain cardiovascular stability. The patient should be considered to have a "full stomach" and the precautions appropriate to the institution should be employed to prevent aspiration of gastric contents.
- Various combinations of drugs can be used with drugs such as midazolam, ketamine, thiopentone, fentanyl, alfentanil or remifentanil.
- This is followed by an intubating dose of suxamethonium (succinylcholine) or rocuronium.
- Surgery usually commences as soon as intubation is achieved. Clearly, communication between anesthetist and surgeon is essential throughout the operation, but never more so than at this point.

Induction of anesthesia may cause the loss of sympathetic tone, causing hypotension. It is important to be able to treat this with a combination of rapid infusion of fluids and vaso-constrictors such as ephedrine, phenylephrine or metaraminol. Tilting the operating table head-down might aid in correcting the hypotension along with the other measures mentioned. It is important to remember that correction of hypotension should be done to prevent cardiac arrest or myocardial or cerebral ischemia, and is not to achieve normotension until surgical control of the proximal aorta is obtained, i.e. cross-clamping of the aorta.

Maintenance of anesthesia

- If suxamethonium has been used, it is important to follow it by the use of a nondepolarizing muscle relaxant so as to avoid the possibility of coughing and increasing the bleeding around the leaking aneurysm or causing an acute rupture when the suxamethonium has worn off.

- The access to the aneurysm is via laparotomy performed as midline, paramedian or a transverse incision, depending on the surgeon's choice.
- Anesthesia is maintained using volatile agents or propofol infusion and opiates with an aim to maintain cardiac stability and provide an adequate anesthetic for the patient.
- Ventilation with oxygen/air mixtures avoids the possibility of nitrous oxide causing bowel distension which could contribute to postoperative raised intra-abdominal pressure. Air is added as opposed to using 100% oxygen in order to limit the development of pulmonary atelectasis.
- Insertion of central venous catheters can be done at this stage after the aorta has been cross-clamped.
- Insertion of a 8.5 fr central venous catheter (pulmonary artery or Swan Ganz introducer catheter) allows for rapid infusion of fluids when needed.
- Methods for monitoring the cardiac output either with a pulmonary artery catheter, transesophageal Doppler or pulse contour analysis methods can be considered. These may be especially useful for managing the hemodynamic responses to clamping and unclamping the aorta and also for postoperative management. However, it is important that control of hemorrhage has occurred and the patient is relatively stable before time is spent on additional methods of monitoring.
- Nasogastric tube/temperature probe can be inserted at this stage.
- Epidural anesthesia plays a major role in the management of the elective aortic surgery patient. However, given the unpredictability of the coagulation process perioperatively, and the destabilization of the cardiovascular picture likely to be caused, the use of epidural regional blockade in the emergency context is not wise.

Anesthetic techniques for the shocked patient are discussed in greater detail in Chapter 14.

Cross-clamping of the aorta
Cross-clamping of the aorta causes significant stress on the cardiovascular system of the patient (and sometimes the anesthetist!). Clamping decreases the blood flow to tissues supplied below the clamp causing ischemia of the kidneys, abdominal organs and the spinal cord, and also the accumulation of acid metabolites in tissues below the clamp.

- Aortic cross-clamping simultaneously causes an increase in blood pressure and left ventricular afterload, and hence causes a decrease in cardiac output, stroke volume and ejection fraction.
- The left ventricular afterload is determined by the end diastolic myocardial tension and systolic intraventricular pressure.
- Because the left ventricle is functionally coupled to the systemic arterial circuit, its intracavity pressure varies directly with the input impedance of the arterial circuit into which it ejects.
- Because of these opposing forces in the cardiac output and the SVR, the resultant rise in arterial blood pressure may not be as great as expected.
- There is an increase in myocardial oxygen demand. Myocardial ischemia is common, which may respond to nitroglycerin.
- Venous return is decreased as the venous system distal to the clamp is devoid of effective perfusion pressure distal to the clamp.

- On cross-clamping as the systolic load increases, myocardial contractility decreases, resulting in reduced stroke volume, ejection fraction and cardiac output.
- Infrarenal aortic cross-clamping increases the systemic vascular resistance (SVR) by about 40%.

In emergency aortic surgery, the hemodynamic effects of cross-clamping may not be as pronounced as in elective aortic surgery due to the presence of hypovolemia.

The acute changes in the hemodynamics detailed above are determined and modified by the:

- intravascular volume status,
- presence of myocardial failure or ischemia, and
- the anesthetic technique employed.

Patients with ischemic heart disease and with limited myocardial reserve from previous myocardial infarction frequently develop signs of acute left ventricular decompensation and cardiac failure soon after aortic cross-clamping. It is therefore important to be clinically aware of and to plan meticulously for the high-risk patient.

Management of the cardiovascular changes associated with cross-clamping is usually dependent on the presentation of the cardiovascular changes. See the following.

Hypertension. This can be managed by a combination of:

- deepening anesthesia or the use of opiates,
- nitroglycerin, nitroprusside or esmolol infusion. Boluses of labetalol may also be useful.

Acute left ventricular strain or failure. This can be managed by a combination of:

- infusion of vasodilators, such as nitroglycerin, or combined inotropes and vasodilators (inodilators), such as dobutamine or epinephrine;
- diuretics are not useful for left ventricular failure from this cause.

Acute myocardial ischemia

- Nitroglycerin infusion may be useful.
- Occasionally, if hypotension and reduced coronary perfusion is contributing to myocardial ischemia, vasopressors may be required to restore myocardial (and other vital organ) perfusion.

Hypotension

- Rarely, a combination of severe hypovolemia and severe myocardial depression may produce hypotension on cross-clamping the aorta. It may seem illogical in the face of increased SVR and afterload to administer vasopressors, but occasionally these drugs are needed to maintain some vital organ perfusion and to keep the patient alive. The use of vasopressors in this situation is controversial and should, preferably, be guided by full invasive monitoring and cardiac studies.

Unclamping of aorta

Release of the aortic cross-clamp opens the distal vasculature for reperfusion. Unclamping should be done cautiously, with the anesthetist and surgeon working together to minimize the effects that will follow. The cross-clamp may have to be released in stages by the surgeon so as to allow time for the anesthetist to administer appropriate fluids and maintain the hemodynamic condition of the patient.

- The vascular resistance and arterial blood pressure are reduced. Ischemic vasodilation and vasomotor paralysis develop in the region below the cross-clamp as lactic acid and other anerobic metabolites accumulate in these tissues – hence the reduction of vascular resistance and arterial blood pressure. This could result in significant hypotension and could cause acute cardiac arrest and death.

- Washout of vasodilators and cardiodepressant mediators from ischemic tissues may also contribute to the hypotension.

- These include lactic acid, oxygen free radicals, prostaglandins, neutrophils, activated complement, cytokines and myocardial depressant factors [11]. These humoral mediators and factors may play a role in organ dysfunction in the postoperative period.

- It is important to appreciate this phenomenon and that its effects may be limited by appropriate fluid loading.

- Some clinicians administer calcium chloride and/or sodium bicarbonate prior to unclamping of the aorta, but this is poorly evidence-based.

- Stroke volume and cardiac output depend on the left ventricular filling pressures and this must be maintained above normal baseline values prior to release of the aortic clamp.

- Stop nitroglycerin infusion before the release of clamps. An increase in inspired oxygen concentration may also be appropriate.

- Monitoring of central venous pressure with or without pulmonary artery pressure should be utilized to achieve the highest cardiac output (flatter portion of the Frank Starling curve) by infusing fluids, blood or blood products.

- Inotropic support may be required to achieve optimum cardiac output.

When the above measures are employed the fall in cardiac output and drop in blood pressure may not be as pronounced.

Organ dysfunction following cross-clamping of the aorta

The basic pathological model involves:

- hemorrhagic shock – first ischemic insult primes the inflammatory response;
- resuscitation – first reperfusion insult;
- aortic clamping – second ischemic insult;
- aortic unclamping – second reperfusion insult.

There is some evidence for improved organ function following cross-clamping of the aorta as a result of treatment with mannitol or antioxidants.

- An early study showed that mannitol administered before aortic clamping reduced the rise in thromboxane, pulmonary artery pressure, reduced the fall in leukocytes and prevented the development of noncardiogenic pulmonary edema when compared with control patients [12].

- In another study, multi-antioxidant supplementation was associated with a reduction in serum CK and aspartate aminotransferase after aneurysm repair. This may have been due to a reduction in oxidative stress and decreased leukocyte sequestration and activation, but clinical differences were not identified [13].

- Another study of antioxidant administration for aortic surgery demonstrated an improved creatinine clearance on the second postoperative day [14].

Larger studies with more convincing outcome measures would be welcomed before these therapies can be recommended confidently.

Complications of abdominal aneurysm repair

Hypovolemia can be caused by inadequate fluid resuscitation, or because of sequestration of blood in the dilated vascular tree (i.e. central hypovolemia syndrome) or the persistence of bleeding.

Hypotension can be caused due to myocardial ischemia and failure, or by the temporary ischemic vasodilatation or vasomotor paralysis in the lower extremities after the release of the cross-clamp.

Hypovolemia and hypotension are corrected by the use of appropriate fluids and inotropes with the aim of achieving a near normal CVP and PAOP and a SVR on the low side of normal.

Anemia. Transfusion of blood should be given to achieve a hemoglobin concentration above 8 g% and in the presence of heart disease above 9 g%. This is discussed further in Chapter 9.

Coagulopathy occurs as with any other operation with severe blood loss because of the consumption of clotting factors. This situation is further worsened by the dilution of the clotting factors with intravenous fluids, transfusion of large volumes of blood, prolonged organ ischemia and the presence of hypothermia causing disseminated intravascular coagulation (DIC). Bleeding may be difficult to control at the operative site as well as the sites of vascular access. Correction is usually achieved by using fresh frozen plasma and platelets. In persistent bleeding there might be a role to use cryoprecipitate or recombinant factor VIIa (rVIIa).

Renal damage is caused by the reduced renal blood flow. The renal medulla is extremely sensitive to hypoperfusion. Ischemia results in cell membrane and microsomal disruption causing a rise in intracellular calcium, which is made worse during reperfusion. This can occur with both suprarenal and infrarenal clamping of the aorta. Embolization of atheromatous material and direct mechanical trauma to the kidneys may also be involved in causing renal damage.

- Renal failure occurs in approximately 20% of patients in the postoperative period with a mortality rate of 50–70%.

Renoprotective strategies that can be tried include:

- maintenance of intravascular volume,
- surgeon giving careful consideration of the proximal aortic cross-clamp time,
- minimizing the aortic cross-clamp time,
- avoiding high sodium loads,
- mannitol as an osmotic diuretic and a free radical scavenger,
- the role of dopamine and furosemide is controversial.

273

The controversies around renal protection strategies are fully discussed in Chapter 13.

Systemic inflammatory response syndrome (SIRS) is caused by a variety of factors including organ ischemia, reperfusion injury, release of cytokines and other inflammatory mediators, massive blood transfusion, and sepsis. Liver and renal dysfunction is common, and multiple organ failure may develop with a high mortality. Mannitol and antioxidants have already been briefly discussed. Further discussion on its prevention and management is beyond the scope of this chapter.

Spinal cord damage is seen rarely in about 0.2–2% of patients postoperatively. It may be apparent immediately after surgery, although it can occur up to 3 weeks into the post-operative period [15]. A review of the relevant anatomy is helpful in understanding this complication

- The arterial supply of the spinal cord is maintained by one anterior and two posterior spinal arteries.
- The anterior spinal artery is a midline structure formed by the branches of each vertebral artery. This supplies the whole of the spinal cord anterior to the posterior gray columns. The posterior spinal arteries are smaller and derived from the inferior cerebellar arteries.
- Spinal branches of the vertebral, deep cervical, intercostal, lumbar, iliolumbar, and lateral sacral arteries support the spinal arteries throughout its course.
- The lower two-thirds of the spinal cord are dependent on the spinal branches to "augment" their blood supply. This is particularly relevant to the anterior spinal artery because of its single vessel supply.
- The anterior radicular arteries vary in size and number. Around the region of T9–T12 is a larger artery – the "artery of Adamkiewicz". This has a characteristic hairpin bend and perfuses the spinal cord distal to its junction with the anterior spinal artery. The artery may arise anywhere from T5 to L1. This portion of the spinal cord has minimal collateral blood supply and is at greatest risk of ischemia from prolonged cross-clamping or hypotension, causing spinal cord damage.

Various strategies to prevent spinal cord damage are available but outwith the scope of this book. In general, prevention of this disastrous complication is helped by fast surgery and maintaining best possible cardiac function.

Other complications that may occur after the repair of an abdominal aortic aneurysm repair include:

- intraoperative cerebral ischemia leading to stroke;
- intra-abdominal hypertension. If severe, this may lead to abdominal compartment syndrome compromising renal and other splanchnic organ function;
- embolic occlusion of the distal arteries;
- gut ischemia, sometimes leading to perforation; and
- prolonged paralytic ileus.

Postoperative care

The majority of survivors of emergency aortic surgery will require support in the post-operative period in an intensive care unit (ICU). The management of the various complications that can occur as mentioned previously are best managed in a sedated and ventilated patient until normality of most of the correctible parameters is achieved.

Endovascular repair (EVAR) of ruptured aneurysm

Endovascular repair of AAA is a minimally invasive procedure with the potential for reduced mortality and morbidity.

This can be performed under general anesthesia, epidural anesthesia or local anesthesia with sedation [16]. These procedures can sometimes be of a long duration. Approximately 60% of abdominal aneurysm repairs can potentially be done using the EVAR technique [17]. This procedure requires accurate determination of the aneurysm morphology using contrast-enhanced CT scans or angiography. Hence it is a procedure usually restricted to an elective setting.

Advantages include avoiding the need for surgical exposure of the aorta and the cross-clamping of the aorta. However, up to 25% of patients undergoing EVAR may still require open surgical access to the aorta.

This is a technique that is gaining acceptance, especially in the high-risk patient with significant co-morbidities. However, in a large UK multi-center study of patients judged unfit for open repair, EVAR had a considerable 30-day operative mortality and was associated with a need for continued surveillance and reintervention, at substantially increased cost [18].

Full evaluation of the indications for EVAR remains incomplete, but to supplant open repair in elective aneurysms the mortality must improve on open surgical mortality. Some large studies have failed to show this [19]. Many centers now have extremely low mortalities for elective aortic surgery.

In a situation with a ruptured AAA but with a hemodynamically stable patient, there has been some use of this technique with good results. It has been recommended by some that appropriate patients with ruptured abdominal aortic aneurysms who are undergoing treatment in experienced vascular centers should be offered EVAR as the treatment of choice [20]. In those centers unstable patients may especially benefit from EVAR and should not be excluded from repair.

Peripheral revascularization surgery

- Peripheral arterial disease is a common condition in individuals over 55 years of age. This is seen at an earlier age in individuals with the risk factors for atherosclerosis as discussed earlier for incidence of AAA.

- The presence of peripheral arterial disease is a strong indicator for generalized atherosclerosis and should be kept in mind when assessing these patients. Ischemic heart disease, cerebrovascular disease and aneurysmal disease are common.

- These patients may have a prothrombotic state predisposing them to hypercoagulable conditions such as spontaneous thrombosis of vessels and deep vein thrombosis.

- Peripheral arterial disease can present as an acute arterial occlusion or chronic occlusive disease.

- Acute occlusion is more commonly due to thrombus formation rather than embolic disease.

- In the case of embolic disease, the emboli usually originate from the heart following atrial fibrillation or acute myocardial infarction. Other causes of emboli could be due to vegetations from rheumatic heart disease, prosthetic valves, bacterial endocarditis or paradoxical venous embolism.

- Acute thrombotic disease usually occurs in someone with previous long-standing atherosclerosis. This is a sudden event and is symptomatic with pain, pallor, pulselessness, parasthesia and paralysis (5 Ps).

- Chronic arterial occlusion is also seen with long-standing atherosclerosis with progressive stenosis of the vessel lumen leading onto complete occlusion. This can sometimes be asymptomatic as there has been time for the development of collateral circulation.

- In lower limb arterial insufficiency calculating the ankle brachial index (ABI) by dividing the ankle systolic pressure with the brachial systolic pressure is a useful noninvasive test to approximate the degree of arterial insufficiency.
  - 0.3–0.9 – claudication.
  - <0.5 – disabling claudication or rest pain.
  - <0.2 – gangrenous extremities.

Management

Peripheral arterial disease is more commonly managed now with nonoperative options such as:

- modification of risk factors,
- exercise programs,
- intra-arterial thrombolytic therapy, and
- angioplasty and stent placement.

The surgical options available are balloon catheter embolectomy, endarterectomy, bypass grafting and amputation.

- As these patients have significant co-morbidity it is important to optimize the medical management and for the patient to be appropriately investigated in the nonacute situation.

- Arterial bypass grafting can be a prolonged procedure with minimal blood loss or fluid shifts. It is important to maintain hemodynamic stability to perfuse other organs such as the heart, brain and kidney. Invasive arterial blood pressure monitoring to allow continuous monitoring and the use of central venous catheters are important in these patients who require meticulous attention to intravascular fluid status.

- The debate of regional versus general anesthesia for this type of surgery continues as there is still no conclusive evidence to show that one technique is better than the other. The important message to take from all the studies done is that meticulous attention to detail is required in this group of patients in the perioperative setting, with the same care continuing into the postoperative period.

- Cardiac morbidity is the most common cause of death in this group of patients (10 times greater than nonvascular surgery patients), and there may be a role for epidural analgesia to improve outcome in these patients.

Further reading

Kaplan JA, Lake CL, Murray MJ, eds. *Vascular Anesthesia*. London, Churchill Livingstone, 2004.

Murray MJ. Vascular anesthesia. *Anesthesiol Clin N Am* 2004; **22**: 183–356.

References

1. Endarterectomy for Moderate Symptomatic Carotid Stenosis: Interim Results from the MRC European Carotid Surgery Trial. *Lancet* 1996; **3447**: 1591–3.

2. Rothwell PM, Slattery J, Warlow CP. A systematic review of the risks of stroke and death due to endarterectomy for symptomatic carotid stenosis. *Stroke* 1996; **27**: 260–5.

3. Kawahito S, Kitahata H, Tanaka K, *et al*. Risk factors for perioperative myocardial ischemia in carotid artery endarterectomy. *J Cardiothor Vasc Anesthesia* 2004; **18**: 288–92.

4. Pandit JJ, Satya-Krishna R, Gration P. Superficial or deep cervical plexus block for carotid endarterectomy: A systematic review of complications. *Br J Anaesth* 2007; **99**: 159–69.

5. Hakl M, Michalek P, Sevcík P, *et al*. Regional anaesthesia for carotid endarterectomy: An audit over 10 years. *Br J Anaesth* 2007; **99**: 415–20.

6. Moritz S, Kasprzak P, Arlt M, *et al*. Accuracy of cerebral monitoring in detecting cerebral ischemia during carotid endarterectomy: A comparison of transcranial Doppler sonography, near-infrared spectroscopy, stump pressure, and somatosensory evoked potentials. *Anesthesiology* 2007; **107**: 563–9.

7. Cosford PA, Leng GC. Screening for abdominal aortic aneurysm. *Cochrane Database Syst Rev* 2007; **2**: CD002945.

8. Hames H, Forbes TL, Harris JR, *et al*. The effect of patient transfer on outcomes after rupture of an abdominal aortic aneurysm. *Can J Surg* 2007; **50**: 43–7.

9. Bickell WH, Wall MJ, Pepe PE, *et al*. Immediate versus delayed fluid resuscitation for hypotensive patients with penetrating torso injuries. *N Engl J Med* 1994; **331**: 1105–9.

10. Dueck AD, Kucey DS, Johnston KW, *et al*. Survival after ruptured abdominal aortic aneurysm: Effect of patient, surgeon, and hospital factors. *J Vasc Surg* 2004; **39**: 1253–60.

11. Gelman S. The pathophysiology of aortic cross-clamping and unclamping. *Anaesthesiology* 1995; **82**: 1026–60.

12. Paterson IS, Klausner JM, Goldman G, *et al*. Pulmonary edema after aneurysm surgery is modified by mannitol. *Ann Surg* 1989; **210**: 796–801.

13. Wijnen MH, Roumen RM, Vader HL, *et al*. A multiantioxidant supplementation reduces damage from ischemia reperfusion in patients after lower torso ischemia. A randomised trial. *Eur J Vasc Endovasc Surg* 2002; **23**: 486–90.

14. Wijnen MH, Vader HL, Van Den Wall Bake AW, *et al*. Can renal dysfunction after infra-renal aortic aneurysm repair be modified by multi-antioxidant supplementation? *J Cardiovasc Surg* 2002; **43**: 483–8.

15. Rosenthal D. Spinal cord ischemia after abdominal aortic operation: Is it preventable? *J Vasc Surg* 1999; **30**: 391–9.

16. Aadahl P, Lundbom J, Hatlinghus S. Regional anaesthesia for endovascular treatment of abdominal aortic aneurysms. *J Endovasc Surg* 1997; **4**: 56–61.

17. Schumacher H, Eckstein H, Kallinowski F, *et al*. Morphometry and classification in abdominal aortic aneurysms: Patient selection for endovascular and open surgery. *J Endovasc Surg* 1997; **4**: 39–44.

18. EVAR trial participants. Endovascular aneurysm repair and outcome in patients unfit for open repair of abdominal aortic aneurysm (EVAR trial 2): Randomized controlled trial. *Lancet* 2005; **365**: 2187–92.

19. EVAR trial participants. Endovascular aneurysm repair versus open repair in patients with abdominal aortic aneurysm (EVAR trial 1): randomized controlled trial. *Lancet* 2005; **365**: 2179–86.

20. Moore R, Nutley M, Cina CS, *et al*. Improved survival after introduction of an emergency endovascular therapy protocol for ruptured abdominal aortic aneurysms. *J Vasc Surg* 2007; **45**: 443–50.

Gastrointestinal surgery

P. Jones and T. Turkstra

Gastrointestinal surgery is often high-risk surgery. Yet, despite the high risk, it is not given a position of prominence in many anesthesia textbooks. It seems to be assumed that knowledge of providing anesthesia care for the high-risk gastrointestinal surgical patient will be gleaned purely from experience gained in managing other patients. In other words, anesthesia for gastrointestinal surgery is just "general anesthesia".

- Paradoxically, certain rare conditions encountered in surgery in the abdomen (such as carcinoid or pheochromocytoma) are well covered in standard textbooks.

- Similarly, management of conditions such as acute pancreatitis, although surgical, are not commonly operated upon in most centers and are well covered in intensive care unit (ICU) textbooks.

These conditions will not be discussed in this chapter.

Gastrointestinal surgery – very high-risk surgery

The general public (and many physicians) would undoubtedly consider surgery such as open heart surgery as being amongst the riskiest of surgical procedures in terms of 30-day operative mortality. In fact, certain relatively common gastrointestinal operations are arguably amongst the highest-risk procedures performed.

Operation	30-day operative mortality (%)
Colon cancer resection	4 [1]
Small bowel obstruction	8 [2]
Pancreaticoduodenectomy	6–12 [1]
Esophagectomy	10–20 [1]
Major lung resection for lung cancer	3–5 [1]
Coronary artery bypass grafting	2–5 [3]

Many of these expected mortality rates will be increased if the operations are performed on an emergency basis.

The lessons to be learned are:

- gastrointestinal surgery is high-risk surgery and warrants careful consideration of the patient's preoperative status and pre-existing medical conditions, the surgical procedure proposed, and the postoperative disposition;

- with the expected mortality, palliation may be better for some patients than attempting a cure;

- patients and their families need to be aware of the high-risk nature of the surgery.

Anesthesia for the High Risk Patient, ed. I. McConachie. Published by Cambridge University Press.
© Cambridge University Press 2009.

Reasons for being high-risk

- Co-existing medical diseases. Many of the patients are elderly with significant medical problems.
- Type of surgery. Often long procedures with significant blood loss, fluid shifts, electrolyte imbalances, nutritional problems, and significant postoperative pain.
- Abdominal surgery is associated with a profound physiologic stress response.
- Emergency or elective. Many of these patients will present as urgent or emergent cases. This is well recognized to be associated with a worse outcome. Less time is available for a complete assessment of the patient, investigation of possible medical problems, and for treatment.
- Hypovolemia is very common.
- Abdominal surgery is associated with significant respiratory compromise (with upper abdominal incisions being worse than lower abdominal incisions).
- Many patients will suffer from pre-, peri-, or postoperative sepsis.

General principles of intraoperative management

- To avoid sudden, life-threatening hypotension upon anesthesia induction in hypovolemic patients, it is often useful to give a pre-induction bolus of warm IV fluids that will stay in the intravascular space and result in more predictable hemodynamic stability (e.g. 500–1000 ml of low- to medium-molecular weight hydroxyethyl starch).
- Pre-induction nasogastric tube decompression of the stomach contents is often useful in emergency cases such as bowel obstruction. The nasogastric tube should be kept in for induction and left to drain freely to the atmosphere.
- Patient positioning is important for surgical access for certain incisions. One should be guided by the surgeon, but we should not forget our responsibilities for protecting skin, joints, and major nerves. It is often useful to have access to one or both arms extended to the side on arm boards.
- Temperature monitoring is critical since significant heat can be lost from exposure and evaporation with the abdomen open [4]. Further information on perioperative hypothermia is given in Chapter 14.
- Respiratory function is at risk both from potential aspiration on induction and impaired ventilation and splinting postoperatively. While open abdominal surgery results in a 21–38% decrease in FRC, FEV_1, and FVC values, even laparoscopic surgery results in decreases of 7–22% [5, 6].
- Intraoperatively, laparoscopic surgery results both in a restrictive lung defect secondary to the increased abdominal pressure and an increased CO_2 load. The patient is also at risk for trocar injuries, pneumothorax, subcutaneous emphysema, tracheal tube migration, venous gas embolism, and is often positioned at extreme angles (steep Trendelenburg or reverse Trendelenburg). Extreme angles can have an adverse impact on cerebral blood flow due either to low cerebral arterial perfusion pressure or cerebral venous hypertension.
- Fluid status should be carefully monitored using a patient-appropriate combination of arterial blood pressure, urinary output, central venous pressure (CVP), or pulmonary artery catheterization (in rare cases). There is the potential for significant blood loss as well as fluid shifts. An arterial line for blood pressure monitoring and sampling is routine

for high-risk cases. CVP monitoring may also be useful in the postoperative period for monitoring of fluid status and/or administration of parenteral nutrition.

Aspiration risk and cricoid force

Patients having a high inherent risk of regurgitated stomach contents often present for gastrointestinal surgery – the prototypical problem being small bowel obstruction. In 1961, Sellick described a maneuver [7] by which the lumen of the esophagus is temporarily obliterated by pressing the circumferential cricoid cartilage against the vertebral column, thereby preventing the stomach contents from ever reaching the pharynx if they were to ascend within the esophagus. Since his original report in 1961, the application of cricoid pressure (or, more appropriately, *cricoid force*, since the area over which the force is applied is usually not known) has become the standard of care for any patient in whom the risk of regurgitation/aspiration is deemed to be increased, and has anecdotally proved to be useful [8]. None the less, considerable controversy exists about the efficacy of cricoid force (CF).

- Sellick's maneuver went from "the bench to the bedside" in very little time. The maneuver was never subject to a study in living humans before being accepted clinically, indeed, Sellick's original description was of a latex tube filled with contrast that was placed into the esophagus of a cadaver and pressurized. Cricoid force was then applied, and an X-ray was taken showing obliteration of the lumen of the tube. In addition, Sellick filled the stomachs of cadavers with water, placed the patient in steep head-down position, and saw no regurgitated water in the pharynx. These two observations were deemed to be sufficient evidence of efficacy, and the practice very quickly became incorporated into clinical practice without prospective human data showing proof of effectiveness.

- However, in 2007, an evidence-based review of the efficacy of rapid sequence induction (in which cricoid force usage is explicitly required) to prevent aspiration concluded that "an absence of evidence from randomized clinical trials suggests that the decision to use rapid sequence induction during management can neither be supported nor discouraged on the basis of quality evidence" [9]. This neutral conclusion reflects the poor quality clinical evidence base that exists to support the usage of CF.

How much force?

The amount of CF required has been studied, and most authors agree that about 40 N of force are required to increase the pressure at the upper esophageal sphincter to the amount observed when patients are awake (approximately 38 mmHg) [10, 11]. However, the timing of the application of CF is problematic.

- The upper esophageal sphincter pressure decreases before loss of consciousness – implying that CF should be applied *before* the patient undergoes the induction of anesthesia.

- However, half of awake volunteers have difficulty breathing when 40 N of force is applied to their cricoid cartilage, and about 10% have complete airway obstruction [12]. Therefore, the recommendations are that 20 N of CF are applied while conscious, increasing the amount to 40 N after loss of consciousness [12].

- Another problem with timing is that, in awake patients, the lower esophageal sphincter pressure (LESP) *decreases* when CF is applied, thereby lowering barrier pressure (LESP – gastric pressure) and increasing the chances of passive regurgitation of stomach contents.

Therefore, applying CF before unconsciousness may increase the chances of passive regurgitation and make breathing more difficult for the patient.

Therefore, if used, CF should probably be applied just *after* loss of consciousness.

How does cricoid force work?

The theory as to why CF works to prevent aspiration hinges on the axial alignment of the cricoid cartilage, the esophagus, and the vertebral column.

- Concerningly, two imaging studies [13, 14] showed that the esophagus often does not lie directly between the cricoid cartilage and the vertebral column when CF is applied.
- In fact, when CF was applied, the esophagus was displaced laterally relative to the cricoid cartilage in over 90% of patients, and an unopposed esophagus was observed in 71% of patients.

These findings cast serious doubt on the anatomic rationale of the Sellick maneuver.

Is aspiration common?

Another important concept to consider is that, in order to develop the life-threatening complication of aspiration pneumonitis, a patient must first regurgitate gastric contents, subsequently aspirate the stomach contents into the pulmonary tree, and then develop inflammatory and/or infectious responses to the aspirated material. The chances of all three of these discrete events happening in one patient are very low, as noted by a retrospective analysis of aspiration occurring at a single center [15] which found that:

- aspiration is an uncommon event, occurring with an overall frequency of approximately 1:3200 anesthetics in adults;
- even patients having emergency surgery aspirate infrequently, with an approximate incidence of 1:900 anesthetics; and
- the actual *mortality* of a documented aspiration episode is extremely low (about 1:71 000).

It is important to note that, in this study, CF usage was not tracked, and therefore it is not possible to know what proportion of patients had CF applied and yet still aspirated. However, 45 out of 67 aspirations occurred at a time when CF would not normally have been applied (i.e. before induction of anesthesia, during tracheal extubation, or greater than 5 min after extubation), calling into question the traditional view of tracheal intubation being the time of greatest risk for aspiration.

How does cricoid force affect airway instrumentation?

- Cricoid force makes the insertion of the laryngeal mask airway [16], the ProSeal laryngeal mask airway [17] and the laryngeal tube [18] more difficult.
- Cricoid force also causes airway obstruction when patients are ventilated by mask with CF applied at 44 N [19].
- For tracheal intubation, a CF of 30 N causes the laryngoscopic exposure to deteriorate in approximately half of subjects [20], and causes sufficient tracheal deformation to potentially prevent the passage of a tracheal tube [21].
- Cricoid force also makes intubation using a lighted stylet more difficult [22].

How consistently is the force applied?

Even if it assumed that 44 N of CF is clinically effective to prevent regurgitation, is the average person assisting with the intubation procedure and applying CF capable of consistently delivering the proper amount of CF? Several studies have examined this question, and the results have been startling. Without training immediately before the application of CF, most practitioners apply less or more than the recommended force of 30–44 N [23]. Furthermore, even when reminded with a simple training aid as to the correct amount of force, relatively few assistants can apply the correct amount of force within a week of the training [24]. Therefore, it has been recommended that assistants responsible for applying CF train with a simple device before each patient in whom CF is going to be used [25].

In summary:

- cricoid force is an anecdotally successful but clinically unproven method that attempts to reduce the frequency of regurgitation of stomach contents into the pharynx;
- it is associated with significant adverse effects with respect to airway management and mask ventilation, and is hampered by the fact that it is not likely to be applied to the right patient, in the right anatomical location, at the right time;
- despite these problems, it is likely that CF will continue to be the standard of care for patients at high risk of aspiration;
- in an effort to increase the consistency, assistants should train on a simple device before every patient for whom CF is planned.

Anesthetic factors

There are several areas of controversy concerning anesthesia for gastrointestinal surgery.

Nitrous oxide

Nitrous oxide is highly soluble – 34 times as soluble as nitrogen. Thus, during anesthesia, nitrous oxide rapidly enters gas-filled spaces, including the bowel.

- This may cause problems with bowel distension and potentially restrict abdominal closure and contribute to intra-abdominal hypertension. In obstruction, the increase in intraluminal pressure could precipitate perforation.
- A study in 1994 [26] claimed that nitrous oxide did not influence operating conditions or the postoperative course in patients undergoing colonic surgery.
- These results were refuted by a large study in 2004 that demonstrated higher pain scores, a greater severity of nausea, and a higher proportion of moderate-severe bowel distension in the nitrous oxide group [27].

Nitrous oxide also effectively causes an acquired vitamin B_{12} deficiency. Because vitamin B_{12} is a bound co-enzyme for methionine synthase, the activity of methionine synthase is inhibited in the presence of nitrous oxide. Since the normal metabolic function of methionine synthase is to convert homocysteine into methionine as well as regenerating folate, nitrous oxide can result in megaloblastic anemia, neurologic toxicity, altered DNA synthesis, accelerated atherosclerosis, and myocardial ischemia [28].

A very large randomized, blinded, multi-center trial (2050 patients) published in 2007 reported on the effects of nitrous oxide-free (80% oxygen, 20% nitrogen) or nitrous oxide-based (70% nitrous oxide, 30% oxygen) anesthesia on duration of hospital stay, duration of ICU stay, and postoperative complications [29].

- In the nitrous oxide-free group, there was a significant decrease in major postoperative complications and severe nausea and vomiting, but the hospital length of stay did not differ between groups.

- Although this trial introduced a major confounding variable (was it the high oxygen concentration that was beneficial, or the high nitrous oxide concentration that was detrimental?), it still demonstrated that, at the very least, there is no reasonable indication for using nitrous oxide in major abdominal surgery.

The nitrous oxide controversy is also discussed in Chapter 14.

Perioperative oxygen supplementation

Surgical site infections (SSIs) are a common problem that increase patient morbidity and mortality as well as increasing the cost of patient care. Anesthetists are able to modulate the incidence of SSIs by several means, including avoiding hypothermia, limiting allogeneic blood transfusions, treating hyperglycemia, and ensuring that patients receive prophylactic antibiotics before the time of incision [30].

One of the body's key defenses against pathogenic microorganisms is the bactericidal activity of neutrophils, which is mediated by oxidative killing. Not surprisingly, research has been conducted that aims to improve oxidative killing by enhancing the tissue partial pressure of oxygen. Three studies in patients undergoing abdominal surgery have been carried out, using high and low fractional inspired concentrations of oxygen (F_IO_2) as treatment and control groups. The results of these trials are summarized below.

- In 2000, Greif et al. performed a randomized, double-blind trial in 500 patients undergoing elective open colorectal resection. Treatment with oxygen within the study protocol was continued from the time of induction until 2 h postoperatively. A standardized anesthetic protocol and aggressive intraoperative fluid resuscitation were used, and the SSIs were evaluated prospectively using standard scoring systems. The authors found a 5.2% incidence of SSI in the 80% oxygen group versus 11.2% in the 30% oxygen group. There were no differences in the duration of hospitalization, the time until solid food was eaten, or the time until the surgical staples were removed. They concluded that 80% oxygen during the operation and for the first 2 h afterwards reduced the incidence of SSIs significantly [31].

- In 2004, Pryor et al. conducted a randomized, double-blind trial in 165 patients undergoing a variety of major intra-abdominal surgeries. Treatment with oxygen (80% or 35%) was started at the time of induction of nonstandardized general anesthesia, and continued for 2 h postoperatively. Surgical site infections were evaluated retrospectively using prospectively defined criteria. They found a significantly higher incidence of SSIs in the 80% oxygen group than in the 35% oxygen group (25.0% versus 11.3%). They also found a longer hospital stay in the 80% oxygen group (13.3 days versus 6.0 days). They concluded that the use of high F_IO_2 in the perioperative period may have deleterious effects [32].

- In 2005, Belda et al. performed a randomized, double-blind trial in 300 patients undergoing elective colorectal surgery. Oxygen therapy (80% or 30%) occurred intraoperatively and for 6 h postoperatively. Anesthesia was standardized. The authors found a 14.9% incidence of SSI in the 80% oxygen group, and a 24.4% incidence in the 30% oxygen group, and they concluded that 80% oxygen supplementation in the perioperative period significantly reduced SSIs [33].

Thus, out of three trials, two support the use of high concentration perioperative oxygen, and one does not. Why did the study by Pryor *et al.* differ so markedly from the other two trials? Some possible explanations are that it:

- had a smaller number of patients enrolled;
- had an uneven distribution of baseline co-morbid conditions (patients in the 80% oxygen group were more likely to be obese, had longer operations, and lost more blood – all of which can contribute to SSIs);
- assessed SSIs retrospectively via a chart review (which may have missed SSIs);
- had no information about the quality of glycemic control (a variable associated with infectious complications).

Although there remains some uncertainty, there is good quality evidence that providing the patient with 80% oxygen intraoperatively and for at least 2 h postoperatively reduces the chances of having an SSI.

Perioperative fluid management

It used to be common practice to administer large amounts of crystalloid perioperatively to patients undergoing major abdominal surgery [34] – hoping that euvolemia or even slight hypervolemia would improve organ oxygen delivery and improve hemodynamics. Specifically, there has traditionally been a fear that a contracted plasma volume leaves the patient at risk of renal dysfunction. Clearly, a patient who is hypovolemic will encounter more episodes of hypotension; however, none of the major trials examining restricted fluid therapy (discussed below) encountered hemodynamic compromise intraoperatively because of adequate (if judicious) volume replacement. In addition, there is no evidence that a low intraoperative urine output (in the absence of hypovolemia) is associated with postoperative renal dysfunction [35, 36].

In contrast, fluid overload increases the demand placed on both the cardiovascular and respiratory systems, and can lead to significant morbidity or mortality. Excess fluids also contribute to gut edema, resulting in decreased gut motility, a longer period of postoperative ileus, and poor absorption of enteral alimentation [34]. Therefore, it is crucial to know whether fluid restriction or liberal fluid administration is optimal for our patients. Much of this research has been carried out in patients undergoing major gastrointestinal surgery.

Further confounding the issue is that the clinical trials in this area have failed to standardize the definitions of a "wet", "dry", or "neutral balance" strategy as far as the volume infused is concerned. In addition, many of the trials have examined a fixed volume administration protocol $(ml\,kg^{-1})$ instead of a goal-directed protocol (CVP greater than 8 mmHg). Finally, not all studies have used the same intravenous fluids, and it is likely that the type of fluid administered affects clinical outcomes. In this context, the data on fluid administration can be examined.

Fluid restriction is beneficial

Three clinical trials in patients undergoing abdominal surgery have demonstrated a positive impact of perioperative fluid restriction.

- Brandstrup *et al.* performed a randomized, blinded, clinical trial in 172 patients examining the impact of a restricted or standard perioperative intravenous fluid regimen. Fewer complications were observed in the restricted group, with numbers needed to treat of 7, 4, and 6, for major, minor, and cardiopulmonary complications, respectively. No changes in serum creatinine were observed between groups [36].

- Lobo *et al.* demonstrated in a small study of 20 patients that postoperative administration of a smaller amount of fluid and sodium resulted in quicker return of bowel function, a shorter hospital stay, and less complications than a regimen including larger amounts of fluids and sodium [37].

- Nisanevich *et al.* examined the effect of two intraoperative fluid regimens on postoperative outcomes in a prospective randomized, blinded clinical trial of 152 patients. The restrictive group received $4\,\mathrm{ml\,kg^{-1}\,h^{-1}}$ of lactated Ringer's solution while the liberal group received a bolus of $10\,\mathrm{ml\,kg^{-1}}$ of lactated Ringer's solution followed by $12\,\mathrm{ml\,kg^{-1}\,h^{-1}}$, resulting in a large difference in intraoperative fluid administration (1.2 l in the restrictive group versus 3.7 l in the liberal group). Patients in the restrictive group had a significantly earlier return of bowel function, a lower incidence of complications, and a shorter hospital stay [38].

Then again, maybe fluid restriction is not beneficial!

In contrast to the above studies, two studies have shown detrimental effects of a restrictive fluid regimen during the perioperative period.

- Holte *et al.* [39] demonstrated significant improvements in pulmonary function, exercise capacity, neuroendocrine response to surgery, and hospital stay in the liberal group compared to a restrictive fluid strategy in 48 patients undergoing laparoscopic cholecystectomy.

- Arkilic *et al.* [40] showed that an aggressive intraoperative fluid management protocol ($16-18\,\mathrm{ml\,kg^{-1}\,h^{-1}}$) significantly increases tissue perfusion and tissue oxygen partial pressure when compared to a conservative regimen ($8\,\mathrm{ml\,kg^{-1}\,h^{-1}}$) in 56 patients. However, clinical outcomes such as major or minor complications, return of bowel function, and length of hospital stay were not examined.

How can the above data be reconciled?
- The two studies above that showed a benefit of a liberal fluid strategy either were not in high-risk patients (Holte *et al.*) or did not examine clinical outcomes (Arkilic *et al.*), rather a surrogate outcome which may or may not be associated with a clinical difference.

- The three trials demonstrating a beneficial effect of a restrictive fluid strategy, however, were larger trials done in higher-risk patients that looked at clinically important outcomes.

In summary, the current evidence in GI surgery patients points toward a benefit of restricting perioperative fluid administration – resulting in shorter hospital stays, a lower incidence of complications, and a quicker return of bowel function.

Does the type of fluid administered matter?

The full volume of intravenous crystalloid solutions remains in the intravascular space only transiently. Shortly after administration, only 9–18% of the crystalloid volume will remain in the intravascular space [41]. Therefore, intravascular volume deficits corrected with crystalloids will require 3–4-times as much volume compared with deficits corrected by colloid administration. This "excess" crystalloid volume is a major source of postoperative interstitial and intestinal edema [34].

Colloid administration minimizes increases in volume in the interstitial fluid compartment and hence decreases intestinal fluid accumulation [42]. Therefore, a colloid-only transfusion regimen may offer the combined benefit of adequate volume resuscitation and minimal edema formation. However, there are not yet any studies performing a head-to-head comparison of crystalloids and colloids in high-risk patients having abdominal surgery. Time will tell whether a perioperative fluid strategy centered around hydroxyethyl starches instead of crystalloids results in improved outcomes.

Some aspects of blood transfusion are presented in Chapter 9.

Goal-directed volume replacement therapy

Newer technologies such as esophageal Doppler analysis [43, 44] and direct tissue oxygen tension monitoring [40] may allow the anesthetist to guide fluid therapy more accurately in a "personalized" fashion.

- Instead of following a regimen of fluids indexed to body weight, these technologies permit optimization of maximal stroke volume or of tissue oxygen tension without relying on a simple all-inclusive formula.

- It is important to note that these newer monitoring technologies may in fact result in *more* fluids being administered, but the fluids will be given because of patient need, not because of a prescribed formula.

- One limitation of these studies is that most have investigated only the usage of colloid intraoperatively – it is therefore unknown whether the patients would have had similar clinical outcomes if volume augmentation was provided by crystalloid instead of colloid.

In summary, both the amount and type of intravenous fluid administered during the perioperative period are important. Newer monitoring may allow the anesthetist to tailor the volume of fluids to what the patient actually needs, instead of guessing or relying on protocols designed for groups, not individuals.

Neostigmine and the anastomosis

Routine reversal of nondepolarizing neuromuscular blockade has been identified as one of the most valuable maneuvers that an anesthetist can perform to improve patient safety [45]. However, anticholinesterase drugs such as neostigmine have been implicated in the past (mainly by surgeons) as a cause of anastomotic breakdown. Animal studies do not support this assumption. A large study in humans found no difference in the rate of anastomotic leakage with or without neostigmine [46]. Undoubtedly, surgical factors are the most important influence on the integrity of the anastomosis. Reversal of neuromuscular blockade should be the rule, not the exception.

Epidural analgesia

Major gastrointestinal surgery often involves a significant incision, with the potential for substantial postoperative pain. This pain may interfere with postoperative respiratory function, especially coughing, which may be further compromised by respiratory depression secondary to narcotic administration [5]. As a result, epidural pain control has been advocated and shown to be superior for pain control and patient satisfaction [5].

Concerns have been raised with respect to the potential for increased gastrointestinal complications associated with epidural use, the most important of which is anastomotic leakage – could the more rapid recovery of bowel function associated with epidural use increase anastomotic leakage [47]?

- A 2007 review limited to colorectal surgery showed no increase in anastomotic complications associated with epidural use [48].

- Additionally, a systematic review of epidural use during gastrointestinal surgery [49] found improved pain control, earlier return of bowel function, but no change in the length of stay; the only increased complication was pruritis.

- Thus, an epidural should be considered for major gastrointestinal surgery if there are no contraindications [49]. Unfortunately, patients presenting for urgent gastrointestinal surgery often have contraindications to the placement of an epidural catheter such as coagulopathy, inability to tolerate positioning because of pain, inability to give consent, or symptoms and laboratory values suggestive of infection or sepsis.

Perioperative nutrition

Nutrition is extremely important in the high-risk surgical patient. It is important to note that it is not just postoperative nutrition that is important – preoperative nutritional state is a powerful determinant of prognosis following surgery (see Chapter 10).

Parenteral nutrition
- Only indicated if unable to feed the patient via the enteral route.
- More expensive.
- Infectious complications.
- Normally requires central venous access (with all of its attendant complications).
- Associated with many problems such as acalculous cholecystitis, electrolyte abnormalities, trace element deficiency, volume overload, overfeeding, hyperglycemia, refeeding syndrome, and more.

Short-term parenteral nutrition should not be used because the complications will likely outweigh the benefits.

There are no data on whether parenteral nutrition should be continued or not intraoperatively. However, the stress of surgery often causes hyperglycemia, which may be exacerbated by the continuous infusion of glucose. This hyperglycemia may worsen neurologic deficits occurring intraoperatively if there is intraoperative hypotension or decreased cardiac output.

Enteral nutrition
- Supports normal gut flora.
- Decreases infectious complications in surgical patients.
- May preserve the gut mucosal barrier and prevent bacterial or endotoxin translocation.
- Cheaper than parenteral nutrition, with less metabolic and infectious complications.
- Early institution of enteral nutrition does not increase patient morbidity or mortality, and may in fact decrease mortality [50].
- There is no role for routine "nil by mouth" orders following uncomplicated gastrointestinal surgery [50].

Numerous systematic reviews and meta-analyses have demonstrated that, as long as the gastrointestinal tract is functional, enteral feeding is superior to parenteral feeding after gastrointestinal surgery [51]. Enteral feeding offers the following advantages overall compared with parenteral nutrition:

- reduced overall complications,
- reduced infectious complications,
- reduced anastomotic leak,
- reduced intra-abdominal abscess,
- reduced hospital length of stay.

Gastrointestinal cancer patients have a decrease in morbidity and hospital length of stay when fed an "immunonutrition" formula (containing arginine, omega-3 fatty acids, and nucleic acids) pre- and postoperatively [52].

High-risk gastrointestinal surgery patients frequently need postoperative care in an ICU. The use of enteral nutrition in hemodynamically unstable patients is controversial. Patients on moderate to high doses of vasopressor medications may have a decrease in cardiac output and splanchnic blood flow, which could predispose them to bowel ischemia. This ischemia will be exacerbated by a metabolically active gut (i.e. a gut that is being fed). However, it is also risky to *not* feed critically ill patients, as negative energy balances are associated with an increased complication risk, particularly infectious complications [53].

Surgical aspects

Stress response to abdominal surgery

- The intensity of the stress response is related to the degree of tissue trauma, i.e. minor surgery stimulates a minor, transient response whereas major abdominal surgery may stimulate a stress response lasting days to even weeks. Other factors promoting the stress response after major abdominal surgery include gut stimuli via the sympathetic nervous system, local tissue factors and cytokines. Hemorrhage, hypothermia, sepsis, and acidosis will all exacerbate the response.

- The response is multi-factorial, thus neuraxial blockade will not completely prevent it.

  The role of the stress response is to mobilize substrate and acute proteins for wound healing and the inflammatory response. Possible detrimental effects of a profound stress response following major surgery include increased demands on organs which may have reduced reserve, pulmonary complications, thromboembolism, and pain and fatigue. The appropriateness of an unmodified response is, therefore, debatable.

- Intraoperative regional anesthesia may only delay the development of the stress response. The optimum duration of blockade is not known.

- Epidural analgesia has significant modifying effects on the hormonal and catecholamine responses to lower abdominal surgery.

- The effects of epidural anesthesia on the stress response following upper abdominal and thoracic surgery are less impressive. This could be due to failure to adequately block all afferent stimulation.

- Spinal opioids have less effect on the stress response. Their effect on morbidity is unclear but is likely to be less due to lesser effects on stress response.

Hepatic resection

These patients often present with multiple co-morbidities. Respiratory function may be compromised by ascites and volume status should be carefully assessed. Hepatic dysfunction may present with coagulopathy secondary to impaired factor synthesis and potential glycemic derangement. Intraoperatively, there is the potential for significant blood loss and fluid shift. Postoperatively, complications can include hepatic dysfunction, hemorrhage, electrolyte imbalance, hypoglycemia, hypothermia, DIC, and pulmonary insufficiency.

Inflammatory bowel disease

Many of these patients will be very ill, febrile, dehydrated, and septic. Nutritional state and wound healing will likely be poor. They may be young, have undergone abdominal surgery before, and be undergoing complex, prolonged reconstructive surgery. If fistulae are present, fluid, electrolyte, and protein losses can be considerable. The patients have often been managed preoperatively with steroids and/or immunosuppressive agents. Chronic pain is likely to be an issue in addition to acute surgical pain.

Perforated intra-abdominal viscus

These patients are often elderly with co-existing medical conditions. Many perforations will be secondary to diverticular disease or malignancies. As the presentation may be unclear, many of these patients languish for several days on medical wards before presenting to the surgeons with marked sepsis. Large volumes of fluid, pus and/or fecal matter may be present in the abdominal cavity. Operative mortality is high.

Bowel obstruction

Large volumes of fluid may be sequestered in the dilated loops of bowel. With high obstruction the risk of aspiration at the induction of anesthesia is marked. With prolonged obstruction perforation will occur, leading to worse sepsis. Splanchnic blood flow will be reduced and inflammatory mediators released.

Percutaneous drainage of intra-abdominal abscesses

Radiological techniques for drainage of intra-abdominal collections are constantly advancing. Unfortunately there are no prospective randomized trials comparing "open" drainage versus percutaneous drainage. Retrospective comparisons suggest that there are no differences in morbidity and mortality [54]. Thus, it seems appropriate to prefer radiologically guided percutaneous drainage of abscesses and other collections where possible.

Further reading

Kumar C M, Bellamy M, eds. *Gastrointestinal and Colorectal Anaesthesia*. New York, Informa Healthcare, 2006.

References

1. Urbach DR, Bell CM, Austin PC. Differences in operative mortality between high- and low-volume hospitals in Ontario for 5 major surgical procedures: Estimating the number of lives potentially saved through regionalization. *CMAJ* 2003; **168**: 1409–14.

2. Margenthaler JA, Longo WE, Virgo KS, *et al.*
Risk factors for adverse outcomes following
surgery for small bowel obstruction. *Ann
Surg* 2006; **243**: 456–64.

3. Eagle KA, Guyton RA, Davidoff R, *et al.*
ACC/AHA 2004 guideline update for
coronary artery bypass graft surgery –
summary article: A report of the American
College of Cardiology/American Heart
Association Task Force on Practice
Guidelines (Committee to Update the 1999
Guidelines for Coronary Artery Bypass Graft
Surgery). *Circulation* 2004; **110**: 1168–76.

4. Lenhardt R. Monitoring and thermal
management. *Best Pract Res Clin
Anaesthesiol* 2003; **17**: 569–81.

5. Werawatganon T, Charuluxanun S. Patient
controlled intravenous opioid analgesia
versus continuous epidural analgesia for pain
after intra-abdominal surgery. *Cochrane
Database Syst Rev* 2005; CD004088.

6. Karayiannakis AJ, Makri GG, Mantzioka A,
Karousos D, Karatzas G. Postoperative
pulmonary function after laparoscopic and
open cholecystectomy. *Br J Anaesth* 1996; **77**:
448–52.

7. Sellick BA. Cricoid pressure to control
regurgitation of stomach contents during
induction of anaesthesia. *Lancet* 1961; **2**: 404–6.

8. Neelakanta G. Cricoid pressure is effective in
preventing esophageal regurgitation.
Anesthesiology 2003; **99**: 242.

9. Neilipovitz DT, Crosby ET. No evidence for
decreased incidence of aspiration after rapid
sequence induction [Aucune donnee
probante concernant l'incidence reduite
d'inhalation apres l'induction en sequence
rapide]. *Can J Anaesth* 2007; **54**: 748–64.

10. Vanner RG, O'Dwyer JP, Pryle BJ, Reynolds
F. Upper oesophageal sphincter pressure and
the effect of cricoid pressure. *Anaesthesia*
1992; **47**: 95–100.

11. Wraight WJ, Chamney AR, Howells TH. The
determination of an effective cricoid
pressure. *Anaesthesia* 1983; **38**: 461–6.

12. Vanner RG. Tolerance of cricoid pressure by
conscious volunteers. *Int J Obstet Anesth*
1992; **1**: 195–8.

13. Smith KJ, Dobranowski J, Yip G, Dauphin A,
Choi PT. Cricoid pressure displaces the

esophagus: An observational study using
magnetic resonance imaging. *Anesthesiology*
2003; **99**: 60–4.

14. Smith KJ, Ladak S, Choi PT, Dobranowski J.
The cricoid cartilage and the esophagus are
not aligned in close to half of adult patients.
Can J Anaesth 2002; **49**: 503–7.

15. Warner MA, Warner ME, Weber JG. Clinical
significance of pulmonary aspiration during
the perioperative period. *Anesthesiology*
1993; **78**: 56–62.

16. Asai T, Barclay K, Power I, Vaughan RS.
Cricoid pressure impedes placement of the
laryngeal mask airway. *Br J Anaesth* 1995; **74**:
521–5.

17. Li CW, Xue FS, Xu YC, *et al.* Cricoid
pressure impedes insertion of, and
ventilation through, the ProSeal laryngeal
mask airway in anesthetized, paralyzed
patients. *Anesth Analg* 2007; **104**: 1195–8,
tables of contents.

18. Asai T, Goy RW, Liu EH. Cricoid pressure
prevents placement of the laryngeal tube and
laryngeal tube-suction II. *Br J Anaesth* 2007;
99: 282–5.

19. Hartsilver EL, Vanner RG. Airway
obstruction with cricoid pressure.
Anaesthesia 2000; **55**: 208–11.

20. Haslam N, Parker L, Duggan JE. Effect of
cricoid pressure on the view at laryngoscopy.
Anaesthesia 2005; **60**: 41–7.

21. MacG Palmer JH, Ball DR. The effect of
cricoid pressure on the cricoid cartilage and
vocal cords: An endoscopic study in
anaesthetised patients. *Anaesthesia* 2000; **55**:
263–8.

22. Hodgson RE, Gopalan PD, Burrows RC,
Zuma K. Effect of cricoid pressure on
the success of endotracheal intubation
with a lightwand. *Anesthesiology* 2001; **94**:
259–62.

23. Meek T, Gittins N, Duggan JE. Cricoid
pressure: Knowledge and performance
amongst anaesthetic assistants. *Anaesthesia*
1999; **54**: 59–62.

24. Flucker CJ, Hart E, Weisz M, Griffiths R,
Ruth M. The 50-millilitre syringe as an
inexpensive training aid in the application of
cricoid pressure. *Eur J Anaesthesiol* 2000; **17**:
443–7.

25. Kopka A, Robinson D. The 5 ml syringe training aid should be utilized immediately before cricoid pressure application. *Eur J Emerg Med* 2005; **12**: 155–8.

26. Krogh B, Jorn Jensen P, Henneberg SW, Hole P, Kronborg O. Nitrous oxide does not influence operating conditions or postoperative course in colonic surgery. *Br J Anaesth* 1994; **72**: 55–7.

27. Akca O, Lenhardt R, Fleischmann E, *et al.* Nitrous oxide increases the incidence of bowel distension in patients undergoing elective colon resection. *Acta Anaesthesiol Scand* 2004; **48**: 894–8.

28. Badner NH, Beattie WS, Freeman D, Spence JD. Nitrous oxide-induced increased homocysteine concentrations are associated with increased postoperative myocardial ischemia in patients undergoing carotid endarterectomy. *Anesth Analg* 2000; **91**: 1073–9.

29. Myles PS, Leslie K, Chan MT, *et al.* Avoidance of nitrous oxide for patients undergoing major surgery: A randomized controlled trial. *Anesthesiology* 2007; **107**: 221–31.

30. Mauermann WJ, Nemergut EC. The anesthesiologist's role in the prevention of surgical site infections. *Anesthesiology* 2006; **105**: 413–21; quiz 439–40.

31. Greif R, Akca O, Horn EP, Kurz A, Sessler DI. Supplemental perioperative oxygen to reduce the incidence of surgical-wound infection. Outcomes Research Group. *N Engl J Med* 2000; **342**: 161–7.

32. Pryor KO, Fahey T Jr, Lien CA, Goldstein PA. Surgical site infection and the routine use of perioperative hyperoxia in a general surgical population: A randomized controlled trial. *JAMA* 2004; **291**: 79–87.

33. Belda FJ, Aguilera L, Garcia de la Asuncion J, *et al.* Supplemental perioperative oxygen and the risk of surgical wound infection: A randomized controlled trial. *JAMA* 2005; **294**: 2035–42.

34. Holte K, Sharrock NE, Kehlet H. Pathophysiology and clinical implications of perioperative fluid excess. *Br J Anaesth* 2002; **89**: 622–32.

35. Alpert RA, Roizen MF, Hamilton WK, *et al.* Intraoperative urinary output does not predict postoperative renal function in patients undergoing abdominal aortic revascularization. *Surgery* 1984; **95**: 707–11.

36. Brandstrup B, Tonnesen H, Beier-Holgersen R, *et al.* Effects of intravenous fluid restriction on postoperative complications: Comparison of two perioperative fluid regimens. A randomized assessor-blinded multicenter trial. *Ann Surg* 2003; **238**: 641–8.

37. Lobo DN, Bostock KA, Neal KR, Perkins AC, Rowlands BJ, Allison SP. Effect of salt and water balance on recovery of gastrointestinal function after elective colonic resection: a randomised controlled trial. *Lancet* 2002; **359**: 1812–8.

38. Nisanevich V, Felsenstein I, Almogy G, Weissman C, Einav S, Matot I. Effect of intraoperative fluid management on outcome after intraabdominal surgery. *Anesthesiology* 2005; **103**: 25–32.

39. Holte K, Klarskov B, Christensen DS, *et al.* Liberal versus restrictive fluid administration to improve recovery after laparoscopic cholecystectomy: A randomized, double-blind study. *Ann Surg* 2004; **240**: 892–9.

40. Arkilic CF, Taguchi A, Sharma N, *et al.* Supplemental perioperative fluid administration increases tissue oxygen pressure. *Surgery* 2003; **133**: 49–55.

41. Ernest D, Belzberg AS, Dodek PM. Distribution of normal saline and 5% albumin infusions in cardiac surgical patients. *Crit Care Med* 2001; **29**: 2299–302.

42. Prien T, Backhaus N, Pelster F, Pircher W, Bunte H, Lawin P. Effect of intraoperative fluid administration and colloid osmotic pressure on the formation of intestinal edema during gastrointestinal surgery. *J Clin Anesth* 1990; **2**: 317–23.

43. Gan TJ, Soppitt A, Maroof M, *et al.* Goal-directed intraoperative fluid administration reduces length of hospital stay after major surgery. *Anesthesiology* 2002; **97**: 820–6.

44. Conway DH, Mayall R, Abdul-Latif MS, Gilligan S, Tackaberry C. Randomised controlled trial investigating the influence of intravenous fluid titration using oesophageal Doppler monitoring during bowel surgery. *Anaesthesia* 2002; **57**: 845–9.

45. Arbous MS, Meursing AE, van Kleef JW, *et al.* Impact of anesthesia management characteristics on severe morbidity and mortality. *Anesthesiology* 2005; **102**: 257–68; quiz 491–2.

46. Morisot P, Loygue J, Guilmet C. [Effects of postoperative decurarization with neostigmine on digestive anastomoses]. *Can Anaesth Soc J* 1975; **22**: 144–8.

47. Holte K, Kehlet H. Epidural analgesia and risk of anastomotic leakage. *Reg Anesth Pain Med* 2001; **26**: 111–7.

48. Marret E, Remy C, Bonnet F. Meta-analysis of epidural analgesia versus parenteral opioid analgesia after colorectal surgery. *Br J Surg* 2007; **94**: 665–73.

49. Jorgensen H, Wetterslev J, Moiniche S, Dahl JB. Epidural local anaesthetics versus opioid-based analgesic regimens on postoperative gastrointestinal paralysis, PONV and pain after abdominal surgery. *Cochrane Database Syst Rev* 2000; CD001893.

50. Andersen HK, Lewis SJ, Thomas S. Early enteral nutrition within 24h of colorectal surgery versus later commencement of feeding for postoperative complications. *Cochrane Database Syst Rev* 2006; CD004080.

51. Mazaki T, Ebisawa K. Enteral versus parenteral nutrition after gastrointestinal surgery: A systematic review and meta-analysis of randomized controlled trials in the English literature. *J Gastrointest Surg* 2008; **12**: 739–55.

52. Braga M, Gianotti L, Nespoli L, Radaelli G, Di Carlo V. Nutritional approach in malnourished surgical patients: a prospective randomized study. *Arch Surg* 2002; **137**: 174–80.

53. Villet S, Chiolero RL, Bollmann MD, *et al.* Negative impact of hypocaloric feeding and energy balance on clinical outcome in ICU patients. *Clin Nutr* 2005; **24**: 502–9.

54. Bufalari A, Giustozzi G, Moggi L. Postoperative intraabdominal abscesses: Percutaneous versus surgical treatment. *Acta Chir Belg* 1996; **96**: 197–200.

Index